# THE

# EFFECTIVE

# HEALTH CARE

# SUPERVISOR

## Sixth Edition

## Charles R. McConnell, MBA, CM

Human Resource Consultant
Ontario, New York

JONES AND BARTLETT PUBLISHERS
Sudbury, Massachusetts
BOSTON     TORONTO     LONDON     SINGAPORE

*World Headquarters*
Jones and Bartlett Publishers
40 Tall Pine Drive
Sudbury, MA 01776
978-443-5000
info@jbpub.com
www.jbpub.com

Jones and Bartlett Publishers
Canada
6339 Ormindale Way
Mississauga, Ontario
L5V 1J2
CANADA

Jones and Bartlett Publishers
International
Barb House, Barb Mews
London W6 7PA
UK

Jones and Bartlett's books and products are available through most bookstores and online booksellers. To contact Jones and Bartlett Publishers directly, call 800-832-0034, fax 978-443-8000, or visit our website www.jbpub.com.

**Library of Congress Cataloging-in-Publication Data**
McConnell, Charles R.
   The effective health care supervisor / Charles R. McConnell.—6th ed.
      p. ; cm.
   Includes bibliographical references and index.
   ISBN 0-7637-3951-0 (alk. paper)
   1. Health facilities--Personnel management. 2. Supervision of employees.    I. Title.
   [DNLM: 1. Personnel Administration, Hospital. 2. Health Facility
Administrators. 3. Personnel Management--methods.    WX 159
M478e 2007]
   RA971.M43 2007                            362.11068'3—dc22    20060080866048

6048

**Production Credits**
Publisher: Michael Brown
Production Director: Amy Rose
Associate Production Editor: Rachel Rossi
Associate Editor: Kylah Goodfellow McNeill
Marketing Manager: Sophie Fleck
Manufacturing Buyer: Therese Connell
Composition: Pageworks
Cover Design: Kristin E. Ohlin
Printing and Binding: Malloy, Inc.
Cover Printing: Malloy, Inc.

Printed in the United States of America
10 09 08 07 06         10 9 8 7 6 5 4 3 2 1

*Once again, and as always, to Kate,*
*for more than 30 years of support and encouragement.*

# Table of Contents

# Preface

In preparing each previous edition of this book it has been the practice to seriously consider a number of user comments and suggestions and to solicit editorial direction from the publisher. This sixth edition was approached in like manner; every effort was made to make it more useful to both students who employ it as a text and working individuals who might use it for continuing education purposes or simply as a reference for information about supervisory practice.

A new chapter has been inserted. Chapter 28, "Living With HIPAA," addresses a presently active concern within health care organizations: the effects of the Health Insurance Portability and Accountability Act. This legislation was passed in 1996 but its greater impact, for which the name of the law offers no clue, did not descend on health care providers and related services until April 2003. It is certain that numerous readers of these words have encountered some of the ramifications of the HIPAA Privacy Rule, which has in many ways altered and restricted the handling of personal health information. Some of the requirements and provisions of HIPAA have yet to be fully implemented, so this topic is likely to loom larger still in the working lives of some health care supervisors.

Some choices had to be made based on user feedback. In this book's use as a text, for example, it is likely that no single course uses all chapters, although each individual chapter is used in some courses. The most difficult choice faced with every chapter has always been depth of topic coverage. Most chapter topics addressed in this volume could be, and in most instances are, the topics of entire books. But if every topic addressed herein were given in-depth treatment, the book would be impractically long and, more to the point, the book's intent—that of a comprehensive introduction and overview—would be defeated.

In addition to the new chapter, other additions and changes have been made throughout the book. Chapter format has been altered slightly. Each chapter still begins with a "Situation"—a case study to consider while reading the chapter, to be addressed at a later point in the chapter after the information relevant to its assessment has been provided. Each chapter also still ends with a single case or exercise. Preceding this final activity in each chapter, several "Review Questions" have been added to encourage consideration of some of the points made in the chapter.

Also, a number of changes have been made to clarify and, in some instances, expand on, or update, information presented in the previous edition. Every effort has been made to make the book more useful by making parts of its message clearer and easier to absorb and apply. Also, an effort has been made to maintain simplicity of language wherever possible, in the firm belief that information presented in a conversational tone is more readily absorbed.

A word about terminology is in order, specifically about the two terms used most frequently throughout this book. The terms in question are *supervisor* and *manager*. These terms have long generated widely varying perceptions among people who use them regularly, and even among people who simply encounter them in written material. The problems arise from the conflict of the essential generic meanings of these terms with their frequent uses as organizational titles.

Taken simply as words in the English language, manager and supervisor have essentially the same meaning. This can be verified in any dictionary, and every available thesaurus lists each as a synonym for the other. Both refer to overseeing the activities of others. Management may be simply but accurately described as getting things done through people. Likewise, supervision may be described as overseeing the activities of people in the performance of work. In both instances the process is the same: providing the people who are doing the work at the next lowest organizational level with the guidance, instruction, support, and assistance they need to get the job done. And in both instances, the higher-up—whether called manager or supervisor—bears responsibility for the output of the subordinates.

The greatest conflict in the varying perceptions of manager and supervisor is in the tendency of many people, perhaps the majority, to believe that somehow manager is a "higher," and thus better, title than supervisor. This perception is most likely owing to the manner in which the terms are used as titles within work organizations, creating the basic conflict with generic meanings. Much of the time this perception is accurate; manager, as an organizational title, is superior to supervisor in some hierarchies. On occasion, however, the situation is reversed. In some places, supervisor is used as superior to manager and various other position titles.

Since manager and supervisor have different meanings for different people and are subject to varying uses in different organizations, this volume attempts to establish consistency through the use of generic meanings. Therefore, throughout this book the terms supervisor and manager are used interchangeably, as are supervision and management. At times some qualifying term may be used, as in denoting "top management" or perhaps "first-line management," "first-line supervision," or "middle management," but whether one says manager or supervisor, in all instances the reference is to the person who is responsible for the output of those at the next lowest organizational level.

Much of what appears in this book is applicable to all kinds of business organizations, but much of the material reflects the unique character of the health care organization. The book is intended to be read and used by first- and second-line supervisors and middle managers, those with or without formal training in management, and potential supervisors. It also can serve as a refresher text for managers at all levels of the health care organization. It is pertinent as well to many upper-level managers—the people who supervise the supervisors of the supervisors—in terms of lending perspective to the top-down view of what happens at lower levels.

Use this book for general enlightenment about health care supervision. Use it as a reference, seeking out specific topics through either the index or the table of contents. Use it as a textbook for management development classes.

There is no absolutely correct topic order for the material in this book. Although it is divided into a significant number of chapters by topic, it is really not possible to deal with any single topic separate from all others. Each is implicitly or explicitly part of perhaps several other topics. Communication is a case in point; it is the primary topic of several chapters, yet the principles of effective communication make their presence felt in a dozen or more additional chapters.

Chapters can be read selectively, but it may be most helpful to begin with the first four chapters for the sake of obtaining an overall perspective. Then read those chapters on the topics that interest you, that appeal to you, or that touch on a problem you are experiencing. For instance, if the last meeting you attended was a disaster and you would like to learn about effective meetings, go straight to Chapter 20. Do not worry about skipping chapters that simply do not apply to your situation—just as long as you are certain they do not apply. For example, if you do not have budget responsibility at present, save Chapter 21 until later. Use your valuable reading time for the topics that will do you the most good on the job.

Supervision is often a tough task, and one of the conditions making it so is the appalling lack of solutions to problems. If we were presenting technical task instructions, we could simply say, "Here's how to do it, period." However, the problems of supervision more often than not are problems of people, most of whom are unpredictably, but quite naturally, different from each other. When presented with a specific problem, your "correct" answer may be this, that, the other, or none of the above, depending on the people involved. The technical task worker may spend much time in a world of black and white, but the supervisor spends every day among varying shades of gray. Parts of this book are concerned with what are necessarily gray areas. The book can guide you in making many decisions; it cannot, however, prescribe solutions to "standard" problems, since few such problems exist in supervision.

Whatever value this book possesses lies largely in its potential as a working guide. Use it as your particular questions and needs suggest. If it helps you on the job in any substantial way, even only now and then, it will have served its intended purpose.

Charles R. McConnell

# PART I

# The Setting

## CHAPTER 1

# An Evolving Role in a Changing Environment

*Nothing in progression can rest on its original plan. We might as well think of rocking a grown man in the cradle of an infant.*
—Edmund Burke

## CHAPTER OBJECTIVES

☛ Identify the dimensions in which the health care manager's work environment is changing most significantly, and develop an awareness of the major factors contributing to the evolution of the manager's role.

☛ Review the principal paradigm shifts that are contributing to major change in the management and delivery of health care.

☛ Develop an awareness of the major changes wrought by the advent of managed care and the significant impact of the Balanced Budget Act of 1997.

☛ Review the changes in the managerial role that have occurred in recent years, and offer some projections about future changes in how health care managers will approach their work.

☛ Highlight the importance of flexibility and adaptability as significant determinants of managerial success.

## SITUATION: REINVENTING THE HEALTH CARE ORGANIZATION

You work for a health care organization or are at least somewhat familiar with how some health care providers work. Furthermore, assume that your organization is a community hospital and that you have been asked to participate in an activity intended to produce suggestions for redesigning the ways in which your hospital delivers care. For your purposes consider the desired outcome of the hospital's processes to be the preservation of life and the restoration of health through medical and surgical interventions in both inpatient and outpatient settings.

*Instructions*

In either words or diagrams, or perhaps both, develop an organizational structure for accomplishing the foregoing objective, designating the functions you believe will have to be performed. You can do this individually, but this activity may be more fruitful when undertaken by small groups (perhaps three or four people). Spend 10 minutes or so identifying functions for your redesigned hospital, and then consider the following three questions as you proceed through this chapter:

1. Did you find yourself using the names of so-called "traditional" hospital activities (emergency, medical records, admitting, etc.) to describe the functions of your redesigned hospital? Why might you have done so?

2. Why do you suppose you can experience considerable difficulty trying to envision new ways of achieving a hospital's desired outcomes?

3. Previously here we described desired outcomes as including "preservation of life and restoration of health." In what ways might we hear this phrase challenged in describing the apparent purposes of the health care system of the early twenty-first century?

## THE (WHIRL)WINDS OF CHANGE

It seems as though you have more work facing you than ever before. Your hospital's occupancy has been falling steadily, but outpatient volume has been increasing on all fronts. You have lost some of your more effective employees and have attempted to replace them. However, because of periodic "hiring freezes" and other delays that remain frustratingly beyond your control, your department has been chronically understaffed for months. On your last attempt to obtain approval for replacement hiring, you were told that the open positions would probably be eliminated. As if that were not enough, you just learned that the middle manager you have reported to for several years is leaving under circumstances unknown to you and that the position is to be eliminated.

Does the foregoing scenario describe your present working circumstances in some respects? Or does it reflect any of what you might have gone through in recent years or that you have reason to believe might await you and your organization just around the corner? If so, you are far from alone. First-line managers, those who supervise the people who do the hands-on work, are caught up in a period of bewildering change that some, whether by choice or involuntarily, will not survive. It is a period that will see the role transformed in ways that most of today's working managers could never have anticipated when they entered the health care work force.

## THE BROADEST SHIFTING PARADIGMS: A WHOLE NEW ENVIRONMENT

As far as the world of work is concerned, the paradigms of the generations of workers who entered the American work force during the 1930s, 1940s, 1950s, and part of the 1960s have come under severe attack. To these generations, specialized higher education or employment in certain kinds of settings were principal requisites of job—and thus income—security.

One message that young people were bombarded with for decades concerned higher education: for a secure job with a good income, get a college education. There is, of course, still considerable truth in that advice; in the long run the well educated still fare better than those who are not as well educated. However, in recent years it has become apparent that a college education is not nearly as effective as it once was in ensuring employment that is both well paid and stable.

Another widely held belief was that securing a job with a large corporation would usually lead to employment security. For years it was assumed that getting a job with one of the major manufacturing firms could secure one's income for 20 or 30 or more years and lead to a comfortable pension. This was true for many who entered the manufacturing work force as early as the middle to late 1930s or during World War II. A significant number of these people put in their 30 years and retired comfortably during a time when all were being encouraged to aspire to retirement at younger and younger ages. Why wait until 65 ? Many retired by 60, and those who followed were primed to expect the retirement age to drop to 55 in time for them to take advantage of it.

Take a close look at the overall status of college graduates in today's job market, and look as well at the numbers of people presently employed in manufacturing. With the exception of a few occupations, college graduates have been out beating the bushes for employment rather than being recruited on campuses as they were in earlier decades. A great many of the people presently seeking jobs in manufacturing count themselves lucky to find steady work—"steady" meaning that it might last a few years—and are overjoyed should they also be able to obtain benefits such as health insurance.

In brief, to a generation or two of Americans the control was in the hands of the individual: Get into a good company, follow the rules, and be loyal, and you were set for life. However, the paradigms of these past generations are crumbling. Products and even entire technologies come and go, companies come and go, and when economics and the need for survival prevail, the rules mean less than they once meant; loyalty, both personal and organizational, comes in a far second after the bottom line.

## ORGANIZATIONAL PRIORITY ONE: THE BOTTOM LINE

It is a common contention of many health care workers today that top management cares only about the bottom line. The critics point accusingly at even the most prestigious of the not-for-profit, supposedly humanely motivated, health care organizations and charge that patient care has taken a back seat to financial viability. They also can and do point at the government and the other major third-party payers and accuse them of compromising health care quality by cutting back on reimbursements and by applying other pressures to reduce costs. Changes in many organizations have prompted some to claim that the concern for money has grown out of proportion to the concern for the public's health.

There is really no question that health care costs, however, the growth of which has at times been double or triple so-called "normal" inflation, need to be brought under control. So as a solution, outright resistance to all cost-control pressure is neither practical nor sustainable. For long-run viability a health care organization—or for that matter, any business organization—requires a balance of bottom-line concerns with human concerns. An organization that pays no heed to fiscal concerns will not survive long. An organization that focuses mostly on the bottom line may last longer, but a constant, all-fiscal approach leads to morale problems, increased turnover, and decreasing productivity, all of which can take the organization toward failure as business goes to others. Failure via this route is more gradual but fully as certain. Without balance between financial and human concerns, any organization is headed for problems. Recently the swing of the pendulum has favored the bottom-liners, making itself felt first in businesses other than health care but later in health care as well. Mergers, acquisitions, affiliations, and other combinations have frequently created an organizational distance in which layers of structure separate profitability issues from people concerns. This condition, when combined with the occasional oversupply of some kinds of labor, guarantees that some more exploitative employers will exercise the upper hand in work relationships. The management attitude frequently suggests that if you are unhappy with the way the place is being run, there are plenty of others out there willing to do your job. This exclusive bottom-line focus uses up people.

## THEN CAME REENGINEERING

Today most organizations call it "reengineering." A few might call it "repositioning." Some might still call it "downsizing," "rightsizing," or simply "reorganizing." Regardless of the label applied to the process, however, the intended result is the same: the systematic redesign of a business's core processes, starting with desired outcomes and establishing the most efficient possible processes to achieve those outcomes.

There has been much talk of reengineering, and there have been a considerable number of exercises that have borne that label. Many of these, however, have been little more than cursory exercises in reorganizing, as a few functions are combined, some functions are eliminated here and there, and a number of positions are done away with. In some instances, there are actual layoffs; in others, sufficient planning and thought have gone into the process to allow the decision makers to manage normal attrition over a period of time and thereby reduce the work force without involuntary separations. In either case, however, it sometimes appears as though the only constant in all of these reengineering efforts is the inevitable reduction in the work force.

True reengineering, beginning with a clear focus on desired output and working backward to determine how best to achieve that output, consumes large amounts of time and energy. It also frequently requires considerable amounts of money in the form of consultant costs and other expenses. But more often than not it is embarked upon when financial circumstances are poor and there is an anxiously perceived need to do something quickly to stave off disaster.

As numerous management consultants have discovered, rarely has there come a need that makes outside consultants' services as valuable as does reengineering. It is not, however, any special wisdom or experience that makes the outsider important in reengineering. Rather, it is perspective; the outsider can see what the insider cannot see. The person inside of the organization is hampered by the internal perspective, and is frequently unable to see much beyond the processes of which he or she is an integral part and in which he or she has a significant personal stake that can be as basic as continued employment.

There is also a lurking dread in the supervisor's knowledge that "reengineering is coming." This is the fear that one's own position is going to be eliminated, a fear often borne out as reengineering proceeds. Can one expect a supervisor to plunge willingly into a reengineering effort when it might mean the loss of his or her job? How many people will honestly and enthusiastically work themselves out of their jobs?

Faced with the reality of reengineering, today's health care managers are hampered in three significant dimensions: (1) they are at risk in the process, and this manifests itself as fear and uncertainty; (2) they are internal to the organization and cannot step back and objectively view what so intimately involves them; and (3) they are affected far more than they might ever be able to acknowledge by some long-held paradigms that are presently under concentrated—and largely successful—attack.

Further implications of reengineering are discussed in Chapter 25.

## CAN WE "REINVENT" THE HOSPITAL?

What you have been encouraged to recognize and to think about in "Situation: Reinventing the Health Care Organization" is the difficulty involved in true reengineering. Most who ponder this exercise will discover that they cannot avoid using names of a number of so-called traditional activities to describe the redesigned organization. Although true reengineering calls on us to begin with the desired outcome and find the apparently most efficient path to that outcome, we are swayed by our familiarity with the path that already exists. It is as though our present knowledge and understanding form walls around us—walls we cannot readily see beyond. We are in a box, as it were, giving rise to the often-heard admonition of the need to "think outside of the box," which is a phrase that has reached cliché status in recent years. Yet thinking outside the box is extremely difficult because we so often fall victim to the implicit assumption that "the box" represents the limits of our world. We do not readily see a new path to our desired outcome because of the existence of the path already utilized.

Certainly the "preservation of life and restoration of health" may presently be challenged in a number of ways. Although it must remain a primary outcome of the system as a whole and of most individual organizations, it is seen by some as secondary to, or at best equivalent to, a financial purpose that may be as basic as organizational survival. Like it or not, finances are a major driving force in health care. There are those who will say, not completely without justification, that patient care concerns are secondary to financial considerations, and this feeling will prevail as long as limits exist on resources available for health care. For-profit health care providers cannot be expected to provide care if there is no profit in doing so, and even not-for-profit providers, comprising the majority of hospitals and a significant percentage of long-term-care facilities, need to stay financially solvent to continue serving their purpose in achieving their desired outcomes.

## THE MANAGED CARE "SOLUTION"

### A Brand New Look: Restricted Access

Aside from technological advances, most of what has occurred in recent years in the organization of health care delivery and payment has been driven by concern for costs. Changes have been inspired by the desire to stem alarming cost increases and, in some instances, to reduce costs overall. These efforts have been variously focused. Government and insurers have acted on health care's money supply, essentially forcing providers to find ways of operating on less money than they feel they require. Provider organizations have taken steps to adjust expenditures to fall within the financial limitations that they face. These steps have included closures, downsizing, forming systems to take advantage of economies of scale, and otherwise seeking ways of delivering care more economically and efficiently. It was in this cost-conscious environment that managed care evolved. Managed care, at least in concept, seemed to offer workable solutions to the problem of providing reasonable access to quality care at an affordable cost.

The introduction of managed care placed, for the first time in the history of American health care, significant restrictions on the use of services. The public was introduced to the concept of the primary care physician as the "gatekeeper" to control access to specialists and various other services. Formerly an insured individual could go to a specialist at will and insurance would usually pay for the service. But with the gatekeeper in place, a subscriber's visits to a specialist were covered only if the patient was referred by the primary care physician. Subscribers who went to specialists without such a referral suddenly found themselves billed for the entire costs of specialists.

By placing restrictions on what services would be paid for and under what circumstances they could be accessed, managed care plans better controlled some health insurance premium costs for employers and subscribers. In return for controlled costs, users had to accept limitations on their choice of physicians, having to choose from among those who agreed to participate in a given plan and accept that plan's payments, accept limitations on what services would be available to them, and, in most instances, agree to pay specified deductibles and co-payments.

Managed care organizations and governmental payers brought pressure to bear on hospitals as well. Hospitals and physicians were encouraged to reduce the length of hospital stays, to reduce the use of most ancillary services, and to meet more medical needs on an outpatient basis. Review processes were established, and hospitals were penalized financially if their costs were determined to be "too high" or if their inpatient stays "too long." Eventually payment became linked to a standard or target length of stay so that a given diagnosis was compensated at a predetermined amount regardless of how long the patient was hospitalized.

As managed care organizations grew larger and stronger they began to negotiate with hospitals concerning the use of their services. Various plans negotiated contracts with hospitals that would provide the best price breaks for the plan's patients, and price competition between and among providers became a reality.

Cost concerns moved even the federal Medicare program along more controlled directions. As managed care grew and placed limits on providers for their subscribers, these same providers began to feel the financial pinch from Medicare as well. When Medicare began in the mid-1960s, its projected 1990 cost was about $10 billion. Actual cost, however, had attained a level of $100 billion per year by the early 1990s; by 1998 they had reached $230 billion, making Medicare the largest single third-party payer for health care services. Medicare represents the first time in American history that a government benefit was separated from any form of financial control, and steps had to be taken to bring expenditures under control.[1]

During late 1998 and early 1999 approximately 160 million Americans were enrolled in managed care plans, encompassing what may well be the overwhelming majority of people who were suitable for managed care. In-and-out participation of some groups, such as the younger aging and Medicaid patients, was anticipated. However, the bulk of people on whom managed care plans could best make their money—the 160 million cited above—were already enrolled.[1]

### Approaching the Managed Care Limit?

Much of the movement into managed care was driven by corporate employers attempting to contain health care benefit costs. The movement was rapid. In 1994, half of the covered work force came under managed care plans, but by 1998 this proportion had grown to 85 percent.[2] However, during the same period, the number of managed care plans experiencing financial problems grew steadily.

It appears that managed care was able to slow the rate of health insurance premium increases throughout most of the 1990s. As the decade ended, however, the cost of insurance coverage was again climbing at an alarming rate. The climb has continued; it was reported in 2005 that health insurance premiums could increase in some areas by more than 12 percent for 2006, making 2006 the fifth straight year of double-digit premium increases for many.[3]

By the end of the 1990s it appeared that the majority of average middle-class subscribers had reached a negative consensus about managed care. This caused some damage to the political viability of for-profit managed care and hurt managed care overall. Indeed, it seemed increasingly likely that managed care might not be financially affordable in the long run. Experts have expressed the opinion that this first decade of the new century will not see a stable health care system that provides adequate care to an overwhelming percentage of citizens.[1]

The year 2000 was a grim 12 months for the relationship between managed care plans and Medicare. As a result of decisions made during the year, on January 1, 2001, nearly a million beneficiaries in 464 counties of 34 states lost their coverage when 118 health maintenance organizations (HMOs) withdrew from Medicare. In addition, many of the plans that remained in Medicare increased premiums and reduced benefits, in response to what plan managements described as "ever-rising costs and the effects of cuts in reimbursement rates made by Congress in 1997."[4(p.11)]

Perhaps reacting to the severity of the 1997 reductions, in December 2000 Congress voted for billions of additional dollars for Medicare HMOs, supposedly to reduce premiums or increase benefits to subscribers. However, wording of the legislation also allowed HMOs to pay more to their networks of hospitals and doctors, thus consuming the majority of the additional funds. As a result, very few HMOs—just 4 of the 118 that withdrew—returned to Medicare.[4]

Managed care has undoubtedly had its benefits and has had the effect of moderating health care cost increases—at least for a time. However, it is becoming increasingly likely that managed care plans will not be able to sustain their promises of delivering efficient and cost-effective care. An aging population, newer and more expensive technology, newer and higher priced prescription drugs, new federal and state mandates, and pressure from health care providers for higher fees will significantly limit the savings from managed care enjoyed by employers and subscribers alike.[5]

## THE BALANCED BUDGET ACT OF 1997

### Major Cuts Affect Medicare Providers

The Balanced Budget Act (BBA) of 1997 was adopted in part because of the following: the increased fiscal pressure caused by the growth of Medicare payments, concern over Medicare over-payments, the desire for more rational payment methods, and a stated wish to offer beneficiaries greater choice. By mandating that federal revenues and federal expenditures be balanced each fiscal year, the BBA fundamentally altered the rules of fiscal policy making in the United States.[6] There is, of course, a certain amount of wisdom in wishing to balance income and expenses; surely most individuals would not long prevail if they were spending more than they were earning. However, it is the manner in which budget balancing was implemented that forced disproportionate reductions in health care reimbursement. In terms of its overall effects, the BBA became the most significant piece of health care legislation since Medicare and Medicaid were established in 1965.[7]

The reductions required to balance the budget were not taken uniformly from all elements of the budget. More than half of the federal budget—specifically including Department of Defense spending, Social Security, and interest on the federal debt—was insulated from cuts, meaning that the entire balancing reduction would have to come from the remaining less-than-half of the budget. Recall from the previous section of this chapter the information that Medicare had some time ago attained the position of the nation's largest third-party payer for health care services. As a direct result of the BBA, drastic cuts occurred in Medicare reimbursement, therefore affecting the income of health care providers. The BBA required $122 billion in spending cuts over a 5-year period beginning with 1998, with the overwhelming majority of reductions—95 percent or $116 billion—coming from one single source: Medicare. And most of the reductions were attained by eliminating or reducing payment to actual providers of health care.[8]

### Widespread Hardship

The elements of the health care system that have been most affected by the BBA seem to be a matter of opinion, specifically the opinion rendered according to where one may be situated in the provider population. According to some sources, the reductions of the BBA clearly targeted post–acute care services, especially skilled nursing facilities and home health agencies.[9] Certainly a number of health care professionals have been affected by the BBA, including physical therapists, occupational therapists, and speech pathologists who have had reimbursement for their services severely capped. The BBA cap on combined rehabilitation services, effective January 1, 1999, had the effect of dramatically reducing the number of rehabilitation professionals employed in long-term care facilities and also resulted in the closing of some facilities.[10]

Those in post–acute care who felt specifically targeted were not alone; persons responsible for operating a great many hospitals likewise felt singled out for significant reductions in reimbursement. For most hospitals, Medicare had long ago become a significant source of income; for a great many, it had become their largest third-party payer. Depending on various reimbursement systems in place, in some states, for years Medicare had been the single significant payer that essentially contributed the full cost of care and helped these institutions remain financially viable. However, the BBA's arbitrary reimbursement reductions forced many acute care institutions into the red, increased pressures for cost reductions, brought about closures, and inspired an increased number of mergers and other affiliations.

Some degree of relief from the BBA arrived in the form of the Balanced Budget Refinement Act (BBRA) of 1999, arising perhaps out of recognition that the act itself went too far in reducing reimbursements. The BBRA became law in November 1999, and it suspended the cap that had been placed on outpatient rehabilitation services and paved the way for the design of a new payment mechanism.[11] Also contributing some relief for providers was Congress's December 2000 infusion of cash in recognition of many managed care plans' abandonment of Medicare participation (as cited in the previous section). Regardless of these positive steps, however, the effects of the BBA remain widespread among health care providers.

## HEALTH CARE PARADIGMS AND THEIR EFFECTS

In terms of how we handle incoming information, as a set of rules or beliefs or expectations, a paradigm can be both a clarifier and an obstacle. Incoming information that fits within our paradigms is seen clearly because it confirms our expectations. Information that is inconsistent with our paradigms, however, cannot be seen nearly as readily and, in some instances, can hardly be seen at all. The inconsistencies disturb our equilibrium with our environment, and our reactions include fear, uncertainty, frustration, resistance, and the inability to imagine any good resulting from the pressures we are experiencing.

Today's health care managers are caught up in some dramatic paradigm shifts. Consider just a few of the long-held beliefs that are crumbling under present-day pressures:

- The acute care hospital will always be the heart of the health care system (clearly no longer true as the "system" takes over).
- The way we presently deliver care is the best, most cost-effective way available (only to those who cannot see another way).

- We work in an essential industry; times might get tough, but we will never be allowed to disappear (tell that to the former employees of all the hospitals that have merged, downsized, or just plain closed).
- All people have a right to the latest and best that medicine has to offer (contradicted by the steady increase in rationing forced by economics).
- Free choice must always prevail, so managed care—HMOs and such—can go only so far (contradicted by the growth of managed care options).
- Physicians will (and should) always control the use of the health care system (but they too are being swept along by the same changes affecting everyone else).
- "But we can't reduce cost without adversely affecting quality," is a reflection of perhaps the strongest paradigm of all, and certainly it is the one causing the most frustration on the part of persons subject to the pressures of change.

In true reengineering it is necessary to begin with the determination of necessary outcomes and work backward to determine what should be put in place to achieve those outcomes. In any organization—in this respect health care is no different from any other business—the people within its systems are limited in their ability to see the possibilities because their paradigms are products of their individual experiences and beliefs.

In working backward from desired outcomes to appropriate processes, at times it is necessary to force our thinking along different paths, to deliberately turn away from what we know and follow a line of thought that feels wrong and that causes discomfort. Assistance from outside the organization, whether from professional consultants or others, can be helpful in forcing us to get out into the uncomfortable territory where the creative solutions are to be found.

Managers working in health care can best ensure their futures by becoming paradigm breakers and by refusing to remain satisfied with the status quo for very long. We have heard repeatedly that necessity is the mother of invention. Perhaps so, although if this were strictly true we would be seeing the world's greatest advances coming out of the areas of most dire need, and this certainly is not happening. Perhaps instead, the parent of invention, or at least of innovation, is dissatisfaction. Dissatisfaction with the status quo appears to be the strongest force available for breaking out of our paradigms.

## MARKETING HEALTH CARE

Marketing within the health care industry is seen by many as a relatively recent phenomenon, and opinions concerning the place of marketing in health care run the gamut from complete acceptance to total rejection. The range of attitudes perhaps exists in part because to many people "marketing" is simply "advertising," and traditionally professions, especially the health professions, did not advertise. True marketing, of course, consists of more than just advertising, but to a significant portion of the population these terms are likely to remain synonymous.

The marketing process essentially guides potential customers in differentiating the organization's products and services from those of competing organizations. Accepting this as a thumbnail definition of marketing, we might then proceed to ask: Is this sort of differentiation necessary in health care? At one time in the recent past many would have said that such differentiation was not particularly necessary. Today, however, marketing is a fact of business life in many health care organizations. As health care becomes more volatile, as medical practice changes and some providers strive to fill unused capacity, as payment mechanisms and forms of provider organizations proliferate, competition will continue to intensify between and among elements of the health care system.

Competition in health care essentially involves access, cost, and service quality. What becomes complex is the consideration of who is being courted for their favor at any given time. Patients are the ultimate consumers of health care; it is for them that the system exists. But since most patients neither select their own health care nor directly pay for their care, a number of different relationships enter the marketing equation, including the following:

- Physicians admit patients to hospitals, so hospitals have a stake in getting a certain number and kind of physicians on their admitting staffs.
- The diminishing use of inpatient hospitalization has brought some hospitals into direct competition with each other as unused capacity grows.
- Hospitals supply patients to rehabilitation and long-term care facilities, which thus have an interest in cultivating relationships with the hospitals.
- Managed care plans (HMOs, etc.) and traditional insurance plans, both for-profit and not-for-profit, attempt to sell themselves to employers, individuals, and care providers.
- Providers, in turn, endeavor to sell themselves to the plans they feel will best serve their needs.
- An increasing number of medical group practices, free-standing surgical centers, clinics, and the like, most being products of the recent quarter century, vie with each other for patients either directly or through physicians' referrals.
- Pharmaceutical companies vigorously promote their products with the physicians who prescribe medications for patients. Since the late 1990s pharmaceutical companies have engaged in widespread advertising aimed at encouraging patients—those ultimate consumers—to ask their physicians for specific medications.

All of the foregoing suggest that marketing is becoming increasingly important to the health care organization and that the rapidity of change occurring within health care is subjecting providers to the same uncertainties that most other industries face in the normal course of business. Today's health care organization cannot afford to go forward without the benefit of a well-thought-out and regularly updated marketing plan.

## THE EVOLVING ROLE OF THE HEALTH CARE MANAGER

### Changes in Health Care Management Lead the Way

One could argue at great length whether management skills in and of themselves are most important in managing in health care or whether one should have a solid grounding in one of the various health care disciplines. It is the age-old and generally irresolvable controversy: Who makes the better manager, the functional specialist or the management generalist?

The specialist-versus-generalist argument has probably been more prevalent in health care than in other arenas, although for many years the external view of health care did not especially recognize that conflict. Rather, much of the external view of health care held that almost anyone could manage there and that the "real" managers managed in "industry," primarily in manufacturing but certainly in the for-profit sector (see Chapter 2).

Of course there is nothing new about this tendency to look down on other fields as somehow lesser than one's own. Thus, for-profit looks down on not-for-profit; within for-profit, manufacturing looks down on banking while banking looks down on insurance and real estate; within for-profit and not-for-profit, everyone looks down on the public sector (government); and so on. What is significant, however, is how past general perceptions of health care as a "lesser" field have led some people to assume an expertise they have never possessed. Perhaps because they remember the days of health care of 35 to 40 years ago, or at least health care pre-1970 when people of greatly varying backgrounds and qualifications managed health care organizations, countless displaced managers with no health care expertise whatsoever have offered themselves to health care with the attitude that anyone can do it. ("I managed in XYZ Corporation for years, so I'm obviously qualified to manage a hospital or one of its departments.")

The perception external to health care severely lags the internal reality. The years when "industry dropouts" could gravitate to health care's management ranks are decades past. In fact, in recent decades a cycle of sorts has been experienced. Specialized graduate-level training in health administration grew and expanded, which furnished many master's-degree–trained managers to health organizations. Such programs proliferated to a point where colleges were turning out many more master's-prepared, would-be managers than the system could absorb. Yet hospitals continue to receive applications from new master's-degree holders who are attempting to enter at general administrative levels but are finding that opportunities are dwindling while the competition is intensifying; they find themselves competing with an increasing number of experienced—and unemployed—health care managers.

For the foreseeable future, the best preparation and background for the new manager within health care will be training and experience in one of the various health care specialties, or at least in one of the few non–health specialties regularly applied within health organizations (finance, for example) plus graduate-level education in health administration. The days when a newly graduated master of hospital administration (MHA) could count on entering directly into an administrative position are largely gone. Rather, one should expect to spend some time in the ranks and in management at the department level. Because of the current health care climate and the dramatically increased competition for administrative positions, a pure health administration education (without benefit of prior, specialized education and experience) is no longer as valuable as once it was.

## The Flattened Organization

Health care managers are in a period when one of the most prominent indicators of change is the elimination of layers of management in their organizations. This reduction can be difficult for many to deal with because it is a change that occurs abruptly when compared with the condition it is correcting.

The management hierarchy usually develops gradually over a period of time. This growth always happens for what are apparently good reasons; in times of success or at least financial stability, top managers react to what seem to be valid needs, and positions are created to serve certain purposes. Each position created becomes interrelated and, to some extent, interdependent with others in the hierarchy. Some tasks accrue to the new position from other positions in the hierarchy; some develop solely as a function of the new position.

There is always some useful purpose served by a newly created management position. However, the process of establishing multiple layers of management has some negative and sometimes extremely damaging effects. The multiple layers breed duplication of effort as the same problems and issues are addressed at successive levels. Responsibility is diluted and diffused as these levels become involved. Communication needs—not to mention the potential for communication breakdowns—expand and intensify as levels proliferate.

The presence of multiple levels of management tends to push decision making up the chain of command. This is in direct contradiction with one of the tenets of Total Quality Management and with today's prevailing management belief in general that decisions are most effectively made at the lowest possible organizational level. The manager who makes few real decisions because of the presence of two or three higher levels of management can hardly be described as capable of feeling ownership of the job.

For years many health care managers had the benefit of job titles and position perks without having to worry a great deal about accountability. They simply "played supervisor" to the extent that they were visible members of management who could count on their supervisors to relieve them of the responsibility of making difficult decisions or dealing with troublesome issues. Now, this condition is rapidly changing. First-line managers are assuming—and will continue to assume—increased responsibility as layers of management are removed and the organization is flattened (a term that is best appreciated when one views organization charts of the same structure in "before" and "after" circumstances).

A frequent victim of reorganizing that involves flattening is the middle manager, the occupant of that intervening layer of management between the supervisor and the top. In reengineering or reorganizing, middle managers sometimes disappear from the organization as their positions are eliminated.

Sometimes they remain within the structure but at a lower level, becoming first-line managers.

Middle management might have multiple layers (for instance, consider the nursing department run by a vice president, four directors, two dozen nurse managers [head nurses], and a number of assistant nurse managers, not to mention staff who, on occasion, are assigned as charge nurses). Or middle management might be a single layer (as in the case of the billing supervisor [first line] reporting to the business office manager [middle] who in turn reports to the director of finance).

Middle management is frequently shown to be the last level created in the hierarchy, evolving from apparent necessity as the spans of supervisory control broaden to seemingly intolerable dimensions. As middle-management positions are cut, a few duties flow upward, but the bulk of what remains—that is, the essential part of what remains—flows downward to the first-line manager. At first, it would seem that the span of first-line control is again increasing as middle management thins out, but what is primarily happening today—or at least should be happening, in organizations that have reengineered sensibly—is that the properly empowered supervisors (always considering the term supervisor as synonymous with first-line manager) are empowering their employees and spreading authority and responsibility across the work group.

In any case, a flatter organization means a broader scope of responsibility for the individual supervisor and often also means more employees to manage.

### Some Constants to Hang Onto

Although this discussion deals primarily with ways in which the supervisory role is changing, it is necessary to point out some fundamentals that should never change in the relationship between manager and employees.

It will always be important for the manager to be visible and available to the staff. The employees need to know that their primary source of job guidance and organizational communication is readily accessible when needed.

Closely related to visibility and availability is the matter of the manager's organizational orientation: Does this person face upward or face downward? The temptations to face upward, that is, to orient oneself in the direction from which recognition and rewards are perceived as coming, are numerous. However, the upward-facing supervisor is usually perceived as aloof and unapproachable. It is the downward-facing supervisor, the one who identifies with the work team and behaves as part of the team, who will be most successful in moving the group in productive directions.

The individual must be a practitioner of a true open-door policy. We are all aware that there hardly exists a manager at any level who has not said, "My door is always open." This is, however, more readily said than accomplished. The open door is largely an attitude, once again related to visibility and availability. Too often the door may be physically open but the manager's attitude suggests that one had better make an appointment through proper chan-nels before approaching. The manager who is not readily reachable by direct-reporting staff for a few minutes now and then is sending a message of self-importance, saying through actions that he or she is more important than the staff.

The manager should accept a role as a key team member and resist the temptation to behave as though he or she is the most important team member. Terms that accurately describe the present first-line supervisor include the likes of "coach" and "counselor." In fact, the term coach suggests a strong similarity between the coach-and-team relationship and the supervisor-and-group relationship. A team can indeed play without a coach; it may play raggedly and without unified purpose or direction, but it can nevertheless play. But a coach cannot coach without a team. Thus a team without a coach is still a team, but a coach without a team is without a job. Similarly, a counselor with no one to counsel is unneeded.

If the manager is no more important than the team members, then why is this person paid more than the team members? The answer to this lies in the amount of responsibility borne. Regardless of how far staff empowerment progresses and how much decision-making is done in the ranks, the person who directly supervises the staff remains responsible for what is done and for instructing, coaching, and leading the staff in getting it done.

A leader should never set himself or herself above the employees except in one critical dimension—the bearing of responsibility.

## Self-Motivation and the First-Line Manager

Because of the ways in which the supervisory role is changing and because of the dramatic changes in health care that are causing the alteration of that role, the individual is caught in a classic motivational crunch. Hospitals are cutting back their staffs and thinning out the ranks of management. Attendant to this, employee morale is worsening. This contributes to declining productivity; employees can hardly be expected to give their undivided attention to high-quality output at a time when they fear for their employment. All of this—declining morale and decreasing productivity—tends to occur at precisely the time when productivity should be expected to increase for the sake of organizational survival.

The supervisor occupies a difficult place in today's health care organization because he or she is susceptible to the same negative pressures on morale as the nonsupervisory staff. Yet he or she is expected to be sufficiently self-motivated to help lift the employees' level of motivation. As a key team member and the one most responsible for the output of the group, the supervisor can have a significant effect on the group's outlook and effort. It is important that the supervisor do everything possible to be "up" when the group members are "down." This leader must be a cheerleader at a time when the employees might feel there is nothing to cheer about.

Surely this seems like one is expected to put up a false front for the employees. Why, one might ask, should the supervisor not feel the same frustration and lack of confidence in the future that the employees feel? Simply stated, trying to be optimistic is necessary for all concerned. If the supervisor's behavior reflects only the doom and gloom the staff members feel, you can be guaranteed that this will dramatically affect employees' behavior—and not in positive directions.

Improving morale is presently an uphill struggle in many health care organizations. Poor morale has been cited as the worst human resources problem in the hospital industry, with the main cause of the problem being layoffs.[12]

Morale and motivation are, of course, complex considerations that at any time can depend on a variety of factors. It is fairly safe to say, however, that the attitude and approach of the leader can have significant effects on the attitude and approach of the group. It is part of the leader's responsibility for the entire group to recognize that the group can be influenced in either positive or negative directions by the attitude brought to the job every day.

This is easily said, but not so easily accomplished. We can readily say, "Cheer up!" but if you are gloomy it is not so easy to force a reversal of mood. So much of what is related to the supervisor's ability to self-motivate will depend on that individual's personal relationship with the elements of the job. If you genuinely like the work, and if you can find satisfaction and fulfillment in the tasks you must perform, then you have a running start on successfully motivating yourself and serving as a positive example for the group members. If, however, one has been lured into the role primarily by title, status, pay, and perks, in all probability this person will not rise to the challenges of the shrinking organization and the flattening management structure.

### Some Honest Empowerment

In management circles and in the literature there is always a great deal of attention paid to the "flavor of the month." Since the TQM movement arose, one of the principal "in" terms has been "empowerment." In all that we do concerning reengineering and total quality management—somewhat curiously, because these are concepts that frequently work against each other—we speak of appropriately empowering employees.

In terms of a supervisor empowering employees, empowerment is no more than that old standby delegation—but delegation performed properly (see Chapter 5). The problem has been that most of what we have called delegation was not delegation performed properly, so delegation as both a term and an observed management practice has acquired a tarnish that no amount of polishing can remove. However, it is pointless to engage in controversy over what such a term might mean. What is important is that any group's leader must truly be empowering in relationships with employees by delegating properly and fully to the fullest extent of his or her capacities.

In these days when management structures are becoming leaner and leaner, empowerment is essential. Empowerment stands as the only practical way to expand and extend the leader's effectiveness and to pursue the constant improvement that is expected in the present environment. When it comes to seriously improving the ways the group's work is accomplished, empowerment acknowledges the fact that no one knows the details of the work better than the person who performs it every day.

The leader needs all the help that can be gotten from the group because chances are the group will be larger than in the past. Leaner management structures will mean more employees within a supervisor's responsibility, thereby automatically increasing the potential for employee problems and expanding the supervisor's involvement in personnel management issues. More time on such matters means less time to devote to other concerns.

New concerns and involvements are arising. In the emerging environment, the supervisor may be called on to undertake tasks that were never before part of the role, such as actively participating in a reduction-in-force and actually designating individuals for layoff.

For the most part, first-line supervisors have traditionally been seen as doers, the working leaders of groups of people whose concentration is on getting today's tasks accomplished. In the leaner, flatter organization, especially the organization that has eliminated its middle-manager positions, the first-line supervisor will take on much more of a planning role than previously experienced. This provides even more reason for the supervisor truly to be empowering staff; while the employees look after today, the leader will spend more time preparing for tomorrow.

## JOB SECURITY IN THE NEW ENVIRONMENT

As pointed out earlier in this chapter, the old paradigms of job security involved education, loyalty, and stability. These paradigms have shifted; education does not guarantee employment, loyalty has lost its meaning in terms of organizational attachment, and it is impossible to pursue a stable career and employment relationship when entire technologies and occupations can come and go within a few years, and organizations can vanish almost overnight.

The only things that will give you job security in a changing environment are skills.[13] Job security—at best a relative commodity, if it exists at all in any absolute sense—no longer lies in constancy and predictability. Rather, job security today lies in one's flexibility and adaptability. The manager who can continually learn and grow and change is most likely to survive to work in the new environment.

It has been said repeatedly that the primary thrust of TQM involves the determination always to do the right things and always do them right the first time. This is a highly appropriate belief for both the individual and corporate entity. After all, whether for an individual or an organization, the best security for continuing success lies in performance.

---

### REVIEW QUESTIONS

1. How does true "reengineering" differ from "reorganizing," "downsizing," and other concepts of organizational restructuring?
2. What is the significance of a supervisor's visibility and availability?

3. What is meant by the claim that job security now resides in flexibility, adaptability, and performance?
4. What are the forces encouraging a supervisor to "face upward?"
5. Define "paradigm."

## EXERCISE: RESPONDING TO EXTERNAL PRESSURE

"Due to concerns over quality and access to care, the move to shorter (inpatient) stays is being monitored by patient-advocacy groups and legislators. It is imperative that facilities turn their attention to tighter control over the cost of ancillary services to meet the expectations for controlling the costs of health care."[14(p.4)]

### Exercise Questions

1. Why do you believe ancillary services might be specifically targeted for cost reduction?
2. In your view, what impact will the significant reduction in the use of ancillary services have on the quality of care? Why?

**NOTES**

1. E. Ginzberg et al., "Healthy Debate," *Human Resource Executive* (May 5, 1998): 57–59.
2. "Public Anger at HMOs Is Hot Political Issue," *Rochester (New York) Democrat & Chronicle*, 17 May 1998.
3. "Premiums for Health Insurance Up 12.7%," *Rochester (New York) Democrat & Chronicle*, 31 August 2005.
4. P. Barry, "HMOs Return 'Little' to Enrollees," *AARP Bulletin* 42, no. 3 (2001): 11.
5. M. W. Toran, "Paradigm Lost," *Human Resource Executive* (July 1998): 52.
6. K. M. Paget, "The Balanced Budget Trap," *The American Prospect* (November/December 1996): 1–2.
7. W. H. Ettinger Jr., "The Balanced Budget Act of 1997: Implications for the Practice of Geriatric Medicine," *The Business of Medicine* 46 (1998): 530–533.
8. L. McGinley, "Usual Enemies Trade Roles in Medicare Funds Battle," *The Wall Street Journal*, 11 May 1999, A24.
9. M. Rovinsky, "How IDSs Can Turn BBA Postacute Care Provisions to Their Advantage," *Healthcare Financial Management* 9 (1999): 31–33.
10. L. McGinley, "Medicare Caps for Therapies Spark Protests," *The Wall Street Journal*, 26 April 1999, B1.
11. K. B. Enchelmayer et al., "The Impact of the Balanced Budget Act of 1997 on the Physical Therapy Profession," *The Health Care Manager* 19, no. 3 (2001): 68.
12. J. Duncan Moore Jr., "Morale Hits New Low," *Modern Healthcare* 25, no. 50 (1995): 52.
13. K. Lumsden, "Will Nursing Ever Be the Same?" *Hospitals and Health Networks* 69, no. 23 (1995): 31.
14. "Hospitals Must Move to the Cutting Edge," *Trustee* 50, no. 2 (1997): 4.

## CHAPTER 2

# Health Care: How is it Different from "Industry"?

*The end product of all business is people.*
*—Rensis Likert*

## CHAPTER OBJECTIVES

☞ Examine management in health care and in "industry" for similarities and differences.

☞ Provide criteria for describing or "typing" organizations according to genuine differences rather than by product or service.

☞ Identify the various settings in which present-day health care is delivered.

☞ Establish an appropriate overall perspective of the organization of the health care institution.

☞ Identify several key departmental characteristics that serve as determinants of individual "management style."

## SITUATION: THE CASE OF THE STUBBORN EMPLOYEE, OR, "IT ISN'T IN THE JOB DESCRIPTION"

George Morton, manager of the maintenance department, was experiencing increasing frustration with mechanic Jeff Thompson. Morton considered Thompson a good mechanic, and this opinion was usually reinforced by the consistently high quality of Thompson's preventive maintenance work and by his success in accomplishing difficult repair jobs. Morton's frustration centered about Thompson's apparent lack of motivation. Thompson always had to be told what to do next after completing each job. If he were not so instructed, he would take a prolonged break until Morton sought him out and gave him a specific assignment.

Morton's frustration peaked one day when a small plumbing problem got out of hand and suddenly became a large problem. He knew that Thompson had to have seen the leaking valve because it was right beside the pump that Thompson had been servicing. However, when Morton asked Thompson why he had done nothing about the valve, Thompson said, "Plumbing isn't part of my job."

"You could at least have reported the problem," Morton said.

Thompson shrugged and said, "There's nothing in my job description about reporting anything. I do what I'm paid to do, and I stick to my job description."

"You certainly do," said Morton. "Jeff, you're one of the better mechanics I've seen. But you never extend yourself in any way, never reach out and take care of something without being told."

"I'm not paid to reach out or extend myself. You're the boss, and I do what you tell me to do. And I do it right."

"I know you do it right," Morton agreed. "But I also know that you sometimes stretch out the work. I know you're capable of giving a lot more to the job, but for some reason you seem unwilling to work up to your capabilities."

Again Thompson shrugged. "I stick to my job description and do what I'm told."

*Instructions*

Initially, imagine yourself in George Morton's position and think about how you might wish to address employee Thompson's attitude. Then consider the following questions as elements of appropriate responses are developed throughout this chapter:

1. What are the characteristics of a position like Jeff Thompson's that should influence the group manager's style and approach?

2. Should Morton's management approach focus primarily on the task to be done (production centered) or the person assigned to the task (people centered)?

3. Do you basically agree or disagree with Thompson's literal adherence to his job description? Why?

4. Again imagining yourself in Morton's position, describe one or two ways in which you might go about getting this employee to perform more in line with his capabilities.

## PROCESS VERSUS ENVIRONMENT

### The Controversy

To begin consideration of the health care environment, we briefly examine the opposing sides of an age-old argument:

> It doesn't matter how well it worked in a factory, it won't work here—this is a hospital [or nursing home, urgent care center, or whatever].

> versus

> Good management is good management no matter where it's practiced. What worked elsewhere will work in a health care organization as well.

Since we plan to discuss management in the health care organization in some detail, it would seem sensible to decide first which side of this frequently encountered argument, if either, is the determining consideration and should thus govern our approach to supervising people in the health care environment. Should we focus on management and thus agree that "good management is good management no matter where it's practiced," or should we give the most weight to the environment, agreeing that health care is sufficiently different to warrant a completely different approach to management?

Health care managers are clearly divided on the fundamental issue of process versus environment. Listen carefully to the comments you are likely to hear regarding the introduction of certain techniques into the health care organization by people in fields other than health care. Often all organizational considerations are split into two distinct categories, which are then assumed to be inconsistent with each other. These considerations can be condensed to health care versus "industry," with the latter category including manufacturing, commercial, financial, retail, and all other organizations not specifically devoted to the delivery of health care. Further, in this simplistic comparison, "industry" frequently becomes something of a dirty word. ("After all, we deal in human life.")

## The Nature of the Health Care Organization

It is not at all surprising that the process versus environment argument exists when we consider the evolution and character of the health care organization. The function of the hospital as we know it today is largely a product of the past 100 years. Many of the health care institutions of the past century provided only custodial care. They were places where the sick, usually the poor and the disadvantaged, were housed and cared for until they died. Physicians practiced very little in hospitals, and most persons fortunate enough to be able to afford proper care were tended at home or in private clinics.

In the hospital of the past there was only one medical profession: nursing. The mission of the organization was nursing care, and essentially the only management was the management of nursing care. Also, most health care institutions were charitable organizations operated by churches or social welfare groups, and little thought was given to operating a health care institution "like a business."

The modern health care organization is vastly different from its counterpart of a century or more ago. What used to be the major purpose of a hospital—maintaining sick people in some degree of comfort until they died—is now the primary mission of only a relatively few health care organizations created for the care of the terminally ill (for example, hospices and certain other specialized institutions). The role of the hospital evolved into that of an organization dedicated to restoring health and preserving life with an increasing emphasis on the prevention of illness.

The hospital of the past had a unique mission, which it fulfilled in a simple, one-dimensional manner that had no parallel in other kinds of organizations. The only similarity with the activities of other organizations was the direct supervision of the nurses who delivered care: the basic process of getting work done through people. However, the modern health care organization is far from one dimensional. There is a large variety of functions to be performed, and numerous complex and sophisticated specialized skills are involved. Also, a great many "business" functions, which are not specifically part of health care but which are critical to the delivery of health care, are present in the health care organization. We find that in many respects the health care organization of today very much resembles a business. In fact, in recent years the proliferation and growth of for-profit hospital corporations, health maintenance organizations, and other health care chains demonstrate that health care is indeed a business—and one of significant proportions.

## The Dividing Lines

It should initially be conceded that many health care organizations are coming to more closely resemble business organizations of other kinds. This is evident in two dimensions: marketing and competition. In the not-too-distant past, marketing and even modest advertising were virtually unheard of in health care—at least in the not-for-profit arena (the largest health care provider component). Now, however, health care, up to and including the services of high-level professionals, is advertised and marketed like any other product or service. This activity, of course, relates to the intensifying levels of competition which are evident in health care as provider organizations vie with each other for a share of the market.

However, even the growth of competition and marketing does not essentially make management in health care appreciably different from what it has long been. The traditional views—from inside health care looking out, or outside health care looking in—have not changed. Those inside of health care are more likely to claim uniqueness of management; those outside of health care are more likely to cite universality of management.

The argument of health care versus industry is frequently organized along functional lines, with the health care professional leaning toward the uniqueness of the field and the so-called outsider inclining toward generic management. Indeed, it may seem natural that polarization of outlook might take place along medical and nonmedical lines.

Many employees in nonmedical activities in health care were originally trained in other kinds of organizations or educated in schools where they were concerned with some general field. These people, essential to the operation of the health care institution, include accountants, personnel specialists, building engineers, food service specialists, computer specialists, and others. While acquiring their skills in school and perhaps later practicing them in other settings, these individuals may have no idea of applying these skills in health care until they have an opportunity to do so. They see their functions as cutting horizontally across organizational lines and applying to health care, manufacturing, or any other field.

Health care professionals, however, come into their fields by somewhat different routes and with different goals in mind. A health care discipline will ordinarily be pursued with the intention of applying that discipline in the health care environment; for instance, a student of nursing will become a working nurse. However, a student who pursues accounting may do so with no idea that he or she eventually may be applying this skill in a health care organization.

Part of the process versus environment argument seems to stem from the background and experience of medical and nonmedical personnel as well as the vertical versus horizontal view of organizations. Nonmedical employees may have applied their education and training in other lines of work before entering health care; this reinforces the horizontal view of organizations and encourages the belief that basic skills are transportable across industry lines. However, the health care professional's education and training lie in the health care environment only, and most health care professionals who work in other kinds of organizations do so in entirely different capacities. Consider, for instance, the person who leaves a job as a bank teller to go to nursing school and eventually takes a position in a hospital. The path followed into nursing and eventually to the hospital strongly reinforces a vertical view of organizations because the skills involved are specific to that kind of organization and are not readily transportable across industry lines.

Certainly there are some fundamental differences between management in health care organizations and management in other organizations. However, in claiming the existence of such differences we may perhaps oversimplify the problem and make the mistake of attempting to classify organizations according to product, output, or basic activity. There are some important differences found in health care, but these differences are not based simply on the contrast of "health care" with "industry," with health care being set apart because of its uniquely humane mission.

## IDENTIFYING THE REAL DIFFERENCES

### A Matter of Need

Organizations are created to fill certain needs. Business organizations of all kinds—including health care organizations—continue to exist because they provide something that people want or need. Hospitals exist because people need acute care, and nursing homes exist because of the need for long-term health care. In the same manner, food wholesalers and grocery stores exist because people need food.

It should follow that if a set of human needs can be fulfilled in a number of different ways, the organizations that do the best job of responding to those needs will be the ones most likely to continue to exist. It has long been true in manufacturing and in retailing, where competition is ordinarily keen, that the organization that can meet customers' needs with the best products at the best prices will stand the best chance of success. Now that competition in health care is largely a fact of business life, health care providers are vying with each other to serve the same customers. This suggests that in one critical respect all business organizations are alike: to continue to exist, they must meet people's needs.

### "Typing" Organizations

The basic error in considering health care organizations as different is the classification of organizations by type, that is, by mentally assigning organizations to categories such as health care, manufacturing, retail, commercial, financial, and so on. Such classification is simply not sufficient to allow us to judge the applicability of supervisory practices across organizational lines. Rather, we need to examine organizations for the degree to which certain kinds of activities are present.

Disregard organizational labels and look at the processes applied within organizations and the kinds of activities required to manage these processes. Look not at what business we do, but rather look at how we do business.

### Two Theoretical Extremes

In one of the timeless classics of management literature, *New Patterns of Management*, Rensis Likert developed a view of organizations based on how they do the things they do.[1] He expressed much of his work in the form of a "scale of organizations" running from one extreme type to another.

At one end of Likert's scale is a type he called the job organization system. This system evolved in and applies to industries in which repetitive work is dominant, such as the many manufacturing industries complete with conveyor belts, assembly lines, and automatic and semiautomatic processes. This system is characterized by an advanced and detailed approach to management. Jobs lend themselves to a high degree of organization, and the entire system can be controlled fairly closely. If you are involved in assembly line manufacturing, it is possible for you to break down most activity into specifically described jobs and define these jobs in great detail. You can schedule output, deciding to make so many units per day and gearing the input speed of all your resources accordingly. A great amount of structure and control is possible. All this calls for a certain style of management, a style suited to the circumstances.

At the other end of Likert's scale is the cooperative motivation system. This system evolved in work environments where variable work dominates most organizational activity. Management itself is considerably less refined in this system. Jobs are not readily definable in detail, and specific controls over organizational activity are not possible to any great extent. For instance, in a hospital, although we can make reasonable estimates based on experience, it remains difficult to schedule output. (Picture, if you will, a predetermined number of patients, cured of their ills, dropping off the end of a conveyor belt each day.) Within the cooperative motivation system there is much less opportunity for close control than there is in the job organization system.

What makes these differing organizational systems work? Likert contends that the job organization system depends largely on economic motives to keep the wheels turning. That is, everything is so controlled that the only remaining requirement is for people to perform the prescribed steps. Therefore, what keeps the wheels turning are the people who show up for work primarily because they are paid to do so. These people are not expected to exhibit a great deal of judgment; they need only follow instructions.

In the cooperative motivation system, however, there are no rigid controls on activities. Jobs cannot be defined down to the last detail, activities and outputs cannot be accurately predicted or scheduled, and the nature of the work coming into the system cannot be depended upon to conform to a formula. In the cooperative motivation system it is not sufficient that employees simply show up because they are being paid. This system depends to a much larger extent on individual enthusiasm and motivation to keep the wheels turning.

Examined in their extremes, therefore, the job organization system and the cooperative motivation system can be seen to differ in several important ways. The most important difference, however, lies in the role of the human element—the part that people play in each kind of system. Under the conditions of the job organization system, the system controls the people and essentially drags them along; under the cooperative motivation system, however, the people control the system and keep it moving.

Regardless of an organization's unit of output—whether automobiles, toasters, or patients—we need to look at the amount of structure that is both required and possible, and at the variability of the work itself. There are few, if any, pure organizational types. As already suggested, an example of a pure job organization system would be the automated manufacturing plant in which every employee is a servant of a mechanized assembly line. At the other end of the scale, an example of the cooperative motivation system at work would be the jack-of-all-trades, odd-job service in which any type of task may come up at any time. Within health care, the office of a physician in general practice may be very much a cooperative motivation system, with patients of widely varying needs entering the system in unpredictable order.

### The Real World: Parts of Both Systems

Most organizations possess elements of both the job organization system and the cooperative motivation system. For instance, the automated manufacturing plant could have a research and development department describable by the elements of the cooperative motivation system.

The organization of the modern health care institution leans considerably toward the cooperative motivation system. There are, however, internal exceptions and differences related to size and degree of structure. A small hospital, for instance, may be very much the cooperative motivation system. On the other hand, a large hospital will include some departments organized along job organization system lines. For example, the housekeeping function of a hospital is highly procedural—there is a specific method prescribed for cleaning a room, and the same people repeat the same pattern room after room, day after day. Food service in a large health care institution usually includes conveyor belt tray assembly, the principles of which are essentially the same as those for product assembly lines in manufacturing. A large hospital laundry will include repetitive tasks that are highly procedural, and repetitive functions may be found as well in some business offices, clinical laboratories, and other functions directly supporting the delivery of health care.

### HEALTH CARE SETTINGS

Earlier in this chapter it was suggested that at one time there were few health care organizations, except for hospitals, that were little more than places where the terminally ill, mostly poor or disadvantaged, were maintained until they died. At that time there were but two or three other kinds of health care organizations. There were private clinics—mostly small and usually associated with the practices of one or more physicians and available to persons who could afford to pay for their care. There were institutions known primarily as asylums, publicly or religiously operated, that did little more for the mentally ill and seriously impaired than keep them contained—often in fairly grim circumstances. And there were other organizations, again publicly or religiously operated, whose mission was the housing and supervision of older persons and the infirm. These were usually known as homes of various kinds (rest home, county home, church home, etc.).

Many of the examples used throughout this book are drawn from the hospital setting, but other settings are referred to as well. The modern acute care hospital uses the broadest range of health care occupations of any health care setting. Hospitals continue to employ the greatest percentage of health care workers of most occupations, but this percentage has been shrinking steadily as health care workers are able to find employment in a growing number of other settings. In addition to both general and specialty hospitals, largely not-for-profit but some for-profit, privately, governmentally, or religiously operated organizations, we find health care workers today employed in the following:

- Long-term care facilities, including nursing homes, and a range of designations generally indicating the levels of care provided or the kinds of populations served
- Rehabilitation facilities, sometimes free-standing (for example, a physical therapy practice) as well as often part of acute care or long-term care organizations (for example, a hospital's cardiac rehabilitation program)
- Medical and dental practices, ranging from solo practices to large groups that may be either generalized (family practice, internal medicine, etc.) or specialized (obstetrics/gynecology, prosthodontics, etc.)
- Free-standing surgical centers, where an increasing number of surgical procedures are being accomplished without hospitalization
- Walk-in clinics, urgent care centers, and other designations, essentially free-standing medical practices that patients utilize without appointments
- Health centers, collections of medical practices and ancillary services sharing location and clientele
- Home health agencies, both privately and governmentally operated, using an increasing number of nursing and rehabilitation personnel as home-based health care services proliferate
- Free-standing clinical laboratories, including commercial, governmental, and shared not-for-profit entities
- Hospice programs, caring specifically for the terminally ill, both as free-standing and palliative care units of larger entities
- Insurance companies, managed care plans, professional medical review organizations, and government agencies (health departments and other regulatory bodies), all of which employ health professionals to some extent
- Suppliers to health care providers and their patients, including pharmacies, pharmaceutical manufacturers, equipment manufacturers, medical transportation companies, and numerous others that provide the materials and services that keep health care functioning

The style of management one might employ may well differ from one setting to another depending on the nature, size, and how a particular function happens to be organized. However, it should be clear at this point that most of health care tends strongly toward Likert's cooperative motivation system, and that most health care management will necessarily be people centered rather than production centered.

## IMPLICATIONS FOR MANAGEMENT

### Environment and Management Style

A given technique borrowed from the non–health care environment may not apply in health care at all. If this is the case, however, it is not because "this is health care," but rather because of the effects of variability, controllability, and structure.

The concept of Likert's job organization system tends considerably toward production-centered management; the essential interest is in getting the work done, and the people who do the work are more or less swept along with the system. This system is rigid, and the people who keep the system going need only show up for work. On the other hand, the concept of the cooperative motivation system suggests people-centered management. People—the employees—are needed to do the work, and more is required of them than simply showing up. They have to take initiative, perhaps make individual decisions and render judgments, and in general must accept a measure of responsibility for keeping the system moving.

It is perhaps unfortunate that businesses that evolved along the lines of the job organization system sometimes tend to overemphasize production while largely ignoring people. Under the cooperative motivation system, however, it is not so easy to ignore people—even by default—since the organization may function poorly or, in the extreme, not function at all if people are not cooperative.

Decision-making can be vastly different in the job organization system as opposed to the cooperative motivation system. In the former, it is more likely to be procedural, with many decisions being made "by the book." In the latter, specific procedures often do not exist (and cannot exist because of the variability of the work), so it becomes necessary to rely heavily on individual judgment.

### Where Does Your Department Fit?

Decide for yourself what kind of department you work in. Does it look like a job organization system or does it approach the cooperative motivation system? How your department measures up in terms of certain essential characteristics will have a strong influence on the style of supervision necessary to assure proper functioning. Examine the following characteristics:

- Variability of work. The more the work is varied in terms of the different tasks to be encountered, the length of time they take, and the procedures by which they are performed, then the more difficult it is to schedule and control. Tasks that are unvarying and repetitive require supervisory emphasis on scheduling inputs and resources; work that is variable requires supervisory emphasis on controlling the activities of the people who do the work.

- Mobility of employees. If all the employees work in the same limited area and usually remain within the supervisor's sight, the supervisor need not be concerned with certain control activities. However, as employees become more mobile and move about in larger areas, there is a need for the supervisor to pay more attention to people who are out of sight much of the time.

- Degree of professionalism. There can be a vast difference in supervisory style depending on whether the majority of employees supervised are unskilled, semiskilled, or skilled. Many departments in a health care institution are staffed with educated professionals who are able, and expected, to exercise independent judgment. Managing the activities of professionals is considerably different from managing the activities of unskilled workers whose primary responsibility lies in following specific instructions.

- Definability of tasks. The more structure possible in work roles, the more rigid the style of supervision may be. For instance, the job of a sorter in a large laundry may be defined in every last detail in a few specific steps on a job description. Since the job is completely definable, the supervisor need only assure that a well-trained worker is assigned and then follow up to see that the work is accomplished. However, as any nursing supervisor who has attempted to write a job description for a staff nurse is aware, because of task variability, the need for independent judgment, and other factors, the job description for the nurse is not written as easily as that of the laundry sorter. The job of the staff nurse is considerably less definable, so there is likely to be more need for the supervisor to provide case-by-case guidance when necessary and also more need to rely on the individual professional's independent judgment.

In general, the organization of the modern health care facility leans well toward Likert's cooperative motivation system, since the activity of a health care organization is mostly variable and centered around people. However, elements of the job organization system must be recognized as being present. This suggests that within any particular institution there may be the need for different supervisory approaches according to the nature of the functions being supervised.

## RETURNING TO "THE STUBBORN EMPLOYEE"

Concerning the "Situation" described at the beginning of the chapter, the characteristics of Thompson's job that should influence manager Morton's style and approach are as follows:

- Variability, because Thompson's tasks, although all mechanical repairs, can differ greatly from one to the next

- Mobility, because the mechanic's tasks take him everywhere in the facility and he is out of sight most of the time

Thompson's tasks may be only broadly definable because there are so many different kinds of repairs possible that they can never all be detailed in a job description. But most of Morton's frustrations probably concern professionalism, specifically an apparent lack thereof. Morton may believe he has every reason to consider Thompson, an apparently skilled tradesperson, to be capable of the professional behavior desired of someone who must work as independently as Thompson.

Morton's approach to Thompson should, of course, be primarily a people-centered approach. Fortunately, quality of output is not a problem. The problems are amount and timeliness of output, factors that are entirely employee controlled.

George Morton might look into revising the job description, adding a line calling for the reporting of other maintenance needs encountered, and perhaps adding a standing instruction concerning what to do when a job is finished (such as pursue certain preventive maintenance tasks). Most managers will basically disagree with an employee's rigid adherence to the letter of a job description, preferring to see a certain amount of flexibility and initiative. However, job description changes are not always easy; in a union shop, for instance, it often takes a significant change in equipment or procedures to revise a job description.

Beyond consideration of the job description, the manager also might want to check for weaknesses in the department's work order scheduling practices. Conscientious scheduling might cut down on the opportunity for prolonged breaks, and a work order control system that captures elapsed time, material costs, and other information for each job might reveal whether Thompson is taking more time than is reasonably required for a given job.

All of the foregoing add up to the need for Morton to provide closer supervision of the employee, especially since much of the problem can be seen as residing in the employee's attitude. One can only guess at the reasons behind Thompson's attitude, but the manager does have at least one strong positive factor to build on—the employee's confidence in his own ability to do the job.

Overall, manager Morton should consider the following actions:

- Strengthening the job description and improving scheduling and control procedures
- Supervising Thompson more closely
- Stressing the employee's positive efforts and good results
- Getting to know the employee on a one-to-one basis, expressing an interest in the employee as a whole person as well as a producer

The rest is up to the employee. At worst, Thompson's productivity may improve, even if no attitude change occurs, because of closer supervision. At best, his attitude will improve over time as he is drawn into a relationship in which he sees that he and his skills are respected.

## A WORD ABOUT QUALITY

There is always room in a discussion such as this for the consideration of quality. Considering again the contention that all organizations exist to serve people's needs, it follows that quality should always be a primary consideration regardless of the form of the organization's output. Businesses basically organized along the lines of the job organization system tend to have frequent built-in quality checks at points in the process. As many manufacturers have discovered, however, quality must be built into a product—it cannot be inspected into it. Organizations tending toward the cooperative motivation system also have their quality checks, but these are less numerous and less specific. In the kind of organization that relies heavily on individual enthusiasm and motivation, there is considerably more reliance on the individual employee to produce acceptable quality.

## EXTERNAL PRESSURE: AN AREA OF INCREASING CONCERN

The "health-care-is-different, period" argument generally does not succeed in differentiating health care from other lines of endeavor. However, there are some legitimate differences that have made themselves felt in health care more than in other fields. These differences have come in the form of pressure from sources outside of the health care organization.

This is not to claim that health care has a monopoly on external pressure. Every work organization that serves people in any way experiences pressure from outside, even if that pressure is as basic as competition from others in the same business. We will not even claim for health care the burden of maximum external regulation. Although health care, or at least health care's hospital sector, may well be the most strictly regulated business in the country, other businesses such as insurance, banking, and public utilities are highly regulated as well. However, very few businesses overall are as highly regulated as those just mentioned, and factors in addition to regulation conspire to make health care quite different in some ways.

Growing regulatory intrusion, increasing financial constraints, and mounting public attention to health care costs have combined to create a unique, frequently high-pressure work environment for the supervisor. A product of recent decades, this high-pressure environment will prevail for some time to come.

The health care organization understandably has a strong interest in maintaining the level of income necessary to provide its services and remain solvent. However, health care costs have continued to increase at a rate exceeding the overall inflation rate. In recent years, nonhealth businesses' major concern with health care has been with ways of slowing the growth in the amount paid for health care coverage. Thus health care management has been caught in a rather elemental squeeze between external limitations on income and the need to pay open-market prices for the products and labor needed to continue delivering service.

Some undeniable forces have entered the health care system and are reshaping the way that supervisors do their jobs:

- Health care costs are being capped in several ways in a continuing effort to prevent them from growing unchecked.
- Competition, once a negligible factor in health care, has become a way of life.
- Continued high-quality health care will be demanded despite constant pressure to contain or reduce costs.

Again, no particular form of external pressure is the province of health care alone. However, virtually every form of external regulation and intrusion is present in health care, making health care one of the country's most regulated activities. This places pressure on the manager to continually strive to produce more with less, and since the health care organization tends toward Likert's cooperative motivation system with its dependence on individual employees to keep the work progressing, it means that the manager must inspire the employees to willingly work under increasing pressure while conserving scarce resources.

Some have claimed that a preponderance of rules and regulations should make management easier; one has only to follow what is prescribed. To the contrary, burgeoning rules and regulations have made health care management considerably more difficult, because they mean that health care's desired outcomes—quality service with fiscal viability—come only through creatively finding a way through the obstacles.

## YOUR SUPERVISORY APPROACH

We should not be misled by what we see as differences between types of organizations. Health care organizations are indeed unique in terms of the output they produce, but they are not necessarily unique in terms of the management processes employed. Again, examine your own department—how it is put together and especially the variability of the work and the degree of structure required. Your approach will be determined not by the fact that "this is a hospital, not a factory" but rather by the kinds of employees you supervise and the nature of their job responsibilities.

---

## REVIEW QUESTIONS

1. What is the impact of employee mobility on supervisory style?
2. What primarily keeps the organization working toward its goals within Likert's Job Organization System?
3. Why may supervisory style vary with the degree of professionalism present in the work group?
4. Why does the Cooperative Motivation System depend largely on individual enthusiasm and motivation?
5. How is health care different from manufacturing in immediacy of service to customers?

## EXERCISE: WHERE DOES YOUR DEPARTMENT FIT?

Take a few minutes to "rate" your department according to the four characteristics discussed in the chapter: (1) variability of work, (2) mobility of employees, (3) degree of professionalism, and (4) definability of tasks. Although this assessment will necessarily be crude, it may nevertheless suggest which end of the "scale of organizations" your department tends toward.

Rate each characteristic on a continuous scale from 0 to 10. The following guides provide the ends and the approximate middle of the scale for each characteristic:

### Variability of Work

0 = No variability. Work can be scheduled and output predicted with complete accuracy.

5 = Average condition. Workload predictability is reasonable. Advance task schedules remain at least 50 percent valid.

10 = Each task is different from all others. Workload is unpredictable, and task scheduling is not possible.

### Mobility of Employees

0 = No mobility. All employees remain in sight in the same physical area during all hours of work.

5 = Average condition. Most employees work within or near the same general area or can be located within minutes.

10 = Full mobility. All employees continually move about the facility as part of normal job performance.

### Degree of Professionalism

0 = No professionals are employed in the department.

5 = About half of the employees are professionals by virtue of degree, licensure, certification, or some combination of these.

10 = All the employees are professionals.

### Definability of Tasks

0 = All jobs are completely definable in complete job descriptions and written procedures.

5 = Average condition. There is about 50 percent definability of jobs through job descriptions and procedures.

10 = No specific definability. No task procedures can be provided, and job descriptions must be limited to general statements.

Take the average of your "ratings." This may give you a rough idea of whether your department leans toward the job organization system (an average below 5) or the cooperative motivation system (an average above 5).

## Exercise Question

- Assuming that your "ratings" of the four characteristics are reasonable indications of the nature of your department, what can you say about your supervisory approach relative to each characteristic?

## Suggestion for Additional Activity

Try this exercise with a small group of supervisors (perhaps three or four) who are familiar with your department's operations. Try to arrive at a group rating for each characteristic.

---

**NOTE**

1. R. Likert, *New Patterns of Management* (New York: McGraw-Hill, 1961).

## CHAPTER 3

# The Nature of Supervision: Health Care and Everywhere

*As we are born to work, so others are born to*
*watch over us while we are working.*
*—Oliver Goldsmith*

## CHAPTER OBJECTIVES

☛ Define the two-sided role of the supervisor as both "functional specialist" (worker) and "management generalist" (manager).

☛ Explore likely reasons for a supervisor's tendency to emphasize one side of the role at the expense of the other.

☛ Introduce the overall responsibilities of health care management in general.

☛ Establish the nature of health care supervision as a strongly people-oriented process unavoidably concerned with day-to-day problems.

---

## SITUATION: PAID TO MAKE DECISIONS?

Sandra Dolan, a registered nurse with 11 years of management experience, was hired as nursing supervisor of the emergency division of Community Hospital. Her style was to gain insight into how to manage a given operation by putting herself into the action and becoming immersed in the work. However, she quickly discovered that her deep involvement in hands-on work drew reactions from staff that ranged from surprise to resentment. She soon learned that her predecessor, who had been in the position for several years, had been referred to as "The Friendly Ghost"—friendly because she usually seemed to be just that, and ghost because she was seen rarely and then only fleetingly.

Despite the legacy of "The Ghost," Sandra provided a constant management presence and seemed determined to remain deeply involved in the work of the department. She also was determined to improve the level of professionalism in the department, a quality that had struck her from the first as decidedly lacking.

In a short time, Sandra had moved to reinstate a long-ignored dress code, eliminate personal telephone calls during working hours except for emergencies, curb chronic tardiness by some staff members, bar food and drink and reading materials from work areas, and halt the practice of changing scheduled days of work after the time limit allowed by the policy.

Sandra found her efforts frustrated at every turn. As she said to her immediate superior, "I can't understand their reaction. All I've done is insist that a few rules be followed, rules that have been there all along, yet the bitterness and lack of support—and even resentment—are so strong I could slice them. I'm getting all-out resistance from a few people I would still have to describe as good, professional nurses at heart."

36

Sandra's boss, the director of nursing, said, "Do you suppose you may be pushing too hard, hitting them with one surprise after another without knowing how they feel and without asking for their cooperation?"

"That's possible," answered Sandra, "but now I'm committed on several fronts and I can't back down on any of them without looking bad."

"Don't think of this as a competition or a test of wills. It may be necessary for you to back down temporarily in some areas, or at least hold a few of your ideas for later. It may not hurt to involve a few of your staff members in looking at the apparent needs of the department."

With a touch of impatience in her voice Sandra said, "Oh, I've heard all this stuff about participative management. That may be the way for some, but that's never been my style. I'm paid to make decisions, so I make them— I don't try to avoid responsibility by encouraging employees to make my decisions."

*Instructions*

As you proceed through this chapter, consider how well you believe Sandra is coping with the demands of being both a professional nurse and a manager of nurses. Comment on how well you believe she is functioning in the essential task of getting things done through people, and describe what she appears to have been doing that might be approached more constructively.

## BORN TO WORK OR WATCH?

We often create problems for ourselves by behaving as though Oliver Goldsmith was, in fact, correct when he made the statement quoted at the start of the chapter. Perhaps we can safely assume a bit of cynicism or resignation in Goldsmith's words, but certainly those of us who work for others (as opposed to working for ourselves) are occasionally inclined to agree. Regardless of some appearances to the contrary, however, no one is "born" either to work or to oversee the work of others.

Also, by separating work and watch, Goldsmith's words convey the impression that overseeing is not to be considered work. Unfortunately, many people nurture the feeling that managing or supervising is not real work. We usually find, however, that people who hold this belief are not and have never been supervisors.

Although we cannot say that someone is born to work or born to supervise, we can, however, suggest that supervision is an activity for which a person can exhibit a talent. Many people are called on to become supervisors because they have exhibited talent for certain kinds of work—usually the same kinds of work they are asked to supervise. However, talent for doing manual, technical, or professional work is no guarantee of the presence of talent for supervision. Although the supervisory and nonsupervisory work both may be closely related to the same human activity, doing one well does not guarantee that the other will be done equally well. If you consider the occupations of cook and kitchen supervisor, for instance, you will find that the two are closely related positions, but that it is not necessarily true that the talented cook will automatically be a talented kitchen supervisor.

## THE SUPERVISOR'S TWO HATS

Most first-line supervisors in health care institutions function in the dual capacities of worker and supervisor. They are constantly required to fill two roles, which we shall identify as the functional specialist and the management generalist.

The functional specialist is the worker who is responsible for doing some of the basic work of the department. The registered nurse, the laboratory or X-ray technician, the telephone switchboard operator, the medical record transcriptionist, the maintenance mechanic, the accountant, and many others are required to perform hands-on tasks involved in delivering patient care or supporting the delivery of care. Almost everyone in the organization is or has been a functional specialist of some kind. In any given department, the specialist is ordinarily concerned with some function that is unique or very nearly unique to that department.

The management generalist, on the other hand, is concerned with activities that are common to many departments and to most situations in which someone must guide and direct the work of others. Regardless of whether the manager began as a nurse, technician, accountant, maintenance mechanic, or whatever, running a department requires that the manager be concerned with staffing, scheduling, personnel management, budgeting, and other activities that apply to many departments.

The nonsupervisory employee is a pure functional specialist. Only in some instances, however, is the manager a pure management generalist. Certainly there are few if any management generalists among first-line supervisors. Generally, the smaller the organization or department, the more likely is the supervisor to be both worker and manager. The supervisor of a four-person maintenance department will probably be a maintenance mechanic and jack-of-several-trades as well. The manager of a three- or four-person medical records department will spend considerable time on nonmanagerial tasks. The head nurse in a 30-bed medical unit may spend more time providing hands-on patient care than performing managerial duties. Only in the upper levels of management are we likely to find a few generalists.

The first-line supervisor, then, is both worker and manager and needs to recognize this fact. However, this recognition alone is not enough, for sometimes wearing these "two hats" is fully as difficult as wearing two real hats at the same time.

A natural leaning toward one of the supervisor's two roles is created by the nature of management itself. Management is not nearly as well defined in its own right as are many of our working specialties. When we consider specialties such as nursing, accounting, and engineering, we are able to categorize these rather neatly according to certain characteristics. We associate each with an expected amount of education and training and perhaps the awarding of a diploma, degree, or license. For instance, a registered nurse may be fairly well defined as someone who has successfully completed a certain number of years of higher education, received a diploma or degree, and passed a licensing examination. Especially among the professions, specialties are well defined in this manner. Even in nonprofessional occupations we can find a considerable degree of definition through simple instruction, on-the-job training, and experience.

Management as a separate field, however, defies the kind of definition just described. Although a few people trained as so-called management generalists may be identified in the middle and upper levels, in management's lower levels there are no sound criteria for defining "manager" without instantly raising the question, "Manager of what?"

Thus, we are not especially well prepared to think of management as a legitimate field in its own right, which requires a certain amount of skill, education, and training. We are not willing to accept management as a profession since it is not readily definable and is not restricted by specific qualifications. Since one requires no particular background to enter the practice of management, many people are inclined to believe that anyone can do it.

We readily recognize that to be a manager one must manage something. This causes us to consider the individual's functional specialty. It also leads to another consideration: Who is best qualified to supervise the work of the department? Should this be the role of the functional specialist or the management generalist? Is it more important for the supervisor to be knowledgeable of all aspects of the department's work, or should the supervisor's strengths lie in the general functions of management?

After brief consideration, we might reasonably conclude that the first-line supervisor should be proficient in both management and the functional specialty. Indeed, it is usually the individual who becomes well rounded in both areas of activity who makes the more effective supervisor.

Concerning the "Situation" described at the beginning of the chapter, one might be tempted to start listing apparent shortcomings of Sandra's management style. First, however, it is only fair to state that Sandra may be demonstrating balance between being "both a professional nurse and a manager of nurses." Sandra appears to wear both of her hats as necessary, attempting to manage and also joining in the performance of the hands-on work (as most first-line nurse managers do). This may be disconcerting at first to some of the staff—Sandra's predecessor apparently did not help out as Sandra is doing—but they will become accustomed to it. It may well be that in the eyes of the staff the most positive facet of Sandra's behavior is her willingness to pitch in and work with them when that extra pair of hands is needed.

## THE PETER PRINCIPLE REVISITED

Almost all first-line supervisors have worked as functional specialists. Although it is true that some people begin their working careers as supervisors, this usually occurs in natural "two-hat" situations in which the person enters a small department as both a supervisor and a worker. Usually, however, a person is offered a supervisory position because of past performance in some specialty. Ordinarily it is the better workers who become supervisors.

However, the fact that one person is a good worker does not guarantee that this same person will be a good supervisor. It is precisely this dilemma that Laurence J. Peters was concerned with in *The Peter Principle*.[1] Peter's tongue-in-cheek, but nevertheless serious commentary contains a great deal of truth.

In brief, his "principle" states that "in a hierarchy, every person tends to rise to his level of incompetence."[1(p.26)] Recognizing that it is the good worker who is singled out for promotion, Peter reasons that the outstanding worker at any level is likely to be promoted to the next level in the hierarchy. This process may continue until the individual reaches a level where performance is mediocre at best. Here all promotions stop and the person is left, perhaps until retirement, a notch above the level of proven capability for good work.

The best workers do not necessarily become the best supervisors. Although promoting outstanding employees will continue to make more sense than promoting mediocre producers, this practice will never guarantee the presence of effective supervisors.

Much of the problem lies in the individual and organizational attitude toward management of "anyone can do it." Confident individuals step into supervisory positions assuming that all they need to do is begin giving instructions and commands. Likewise, higher managers promote workers and then go about their business believing they have created supervisors by simply conferring titles.

The supervisor's hedge against arriving at a level of incompetence is management development. Whether pursued in the institution or outside, through organizational programs or by individual effort, formally or informally, the supervisor must learn much about the second hat before it fits as well as the first hat. Most people enter their functional specialties sufficiently well trained to do the jobs for which they have been hired. However, most workers who become supervisors do so with little or no preparation. Management then becomes a sink-or-swim proposition. A few catch on and perform remarkably well after a short period of time. A few sink rapidly. Many generate enough motion to enable them to stay afloat but then continue spending most of their energy simply keeping their heads above water.

The player-to-coach transition in the world of professional sports offers an appropriate analogy to the worker-to-supervisor transition. Most successful coaches gained experience as players at some level in the sports they coach. However, only a few outstanding coaches were star performers in their playing days; most were infrequently noticed, solid, dependable team players. Knowing how to play the game well is not enough. The differences between working and supervising are as fundamental as the differences between doing and teaching, and are as great as the essential difference between following and leading.

## THE WORKING TRAP

The working trap poses a hazard to every supervisor whose job includes the performance of both managerial and nonmanagerial duties. Much of the reason why any person is titled and paid as a manager is to see that a certain amount of work gets done through the efforts of other people. This requires that the supervisor primarily be a member of management. Any person charged with the responsibility for directing the activities of others is a manager and must firmly believe this is so.

It is all too easy for the supervisor to feel and behave more as a worker than as a manager. This is understandable when half or more of the supervisor's duties may be nonmanagerial to begin with. However, this leads to a state of favoring one hat over the other—spending much of the time thinking and doing as a worker rather than behaving as a manager. Falling into the working trap can leave a supervisor's time and energy stretched too thinly over numerous technical tasks while some of the department's workers remain underutilized for lack of solid supervisory direction.

## NOTHING TO DO?

The following nine points were excerpted from a list of "supervisory activities" that a nursing supervisor was kind enough to share with the instructor and the class in a management development program.

As everyone knows, the supervisor has practically nothing to do except:

1. Decide what is to be done, and assign the task to someone.
2. Listen to all the reasons why it should not be done, why it should be done differently, or why someone else should do it.
3. Follow up to find out whether it has been done, and discover it has not been done.
4. Listen to excuses from the person who should have done it.
5. Follow up again to determine if it has been done, only to discover it has been done incorrectly.
6. Point out how it should have been done, and prepare to try again.
7. Wonder whether it may be time to get rid of a person who cannot do a job correctly; reflect that the employee probably has family responsibilities and that a successor would probably behave the same way anyway.
8. Consider how much simpler it would have been to do the job one's self in the first place.
9. Sadly reflect that it could have been done correctly in 20 minutes, but as things turned out it was necessary to spend 2 days to find out why it took 3 weeks for someone else to do it wrong.

The foregoing is more than just a tongue-in-cheek recounting of some of the frustrations of supervision. Implicit in the nine points are a number of considerations important in the overall supervisory task. For instance, point two suggests that the assignment of work to an employee is more than simply assigning a person a task and giving the orders. Proper delegation, which is discussed in Chapter 5, includes thoughtful matching of person and task, thorough instruction, and assurance that the employee understands why the job must be done.

Although follow-up is an extremely important part of all supervisory activity, point three might make us wonder how timely the follow-up was in the situation described, since late follow-up can be as bad as none at all. Point five, again dealing with follow-up, might prompt us to ask whether corrective action has been taken and thorough instructions have been provided, or if once again the employee was simply told to do it.

Point six states to "point out how it should have been done." If this is the first time instructions were offered or efforts were made to find out if the job was understood, then the supervisor has far more trouble than even these few frustrations suggest.

The musings of point seven are likely to be uncalled for at this stage. The supervisor must do considerable self-assessment before writing off any employee as incapable. Furthermore, if honest evaluation does lead to consideration of firing, the rationalization that a successor would probably behave the same way is completely without foundation.

Point eight simply illustrates the thought processes that allow the supervisor to fall into the working trap, and the "sad reflection" of point nine does not carry far enough—it should perhaps go on to include: "Why, then, can't I get an employee to do a simple job like this within a reasonable timeframe?" Otherwise, it suggests that the supervisor has compounded some personal errors and attempted to rationalize them away by tagging the employee with the failure.

## THE RESPONSIBILITIES OF HEALTH CARE MANAGEMENT

At this point we will broaden our view of management to take in the entire body of people who are responsible for directing all activities that move employees toward the institution's goals. Consider "management" as a single composite "person" responsible for running the institution. This "person" has several major responsibilities.

First, management is responsible to the patients of the institution to assure that these all-important people receive the best possible care at the lowest possible cost. At the same time, management is responsible to the institution's employees and must recognize their reasonable needs for security, approval, a sense of accomplishment, assurance of their reasons for being there, and fair treatment and fair compensation for their efforts.

Management is also responsible to the board of trustees in their legal capacity as guardians of the organization's resources. Beyond the trustees, management is responsible to the community for determining how best to meet current health care needs. To follow the thread of responsibility completely through to the end, we can also say that management has an important responsibility to itself to strive continually to upgrade its capabilities and adapt as necessary to the constantly changing health care environment.

Although fulfillment of the foregoing responsibilities may be directed toward a common objective—the preservation or restoration of health—there is likely to be conflict in their fulfillment. To appreciate the implications of such conflict, felt most severely at management's highest levels, put yourself in the position of our composite "person" and furthermore imagine that you must do your job while answering to four or five different bosses. To some extent, health care managers at all levels find themselves caught in conflict situations, many of which involve the needs of the patients, employees, or community, as opposed to the reality of what can or cannot be accomplished within the limits of available resources.

## THE NATURE OF SUPERVISION

In Chapter 2 it was established that supervision may differ from one organization to another according to various characteristics, and that such differences may occur among departments in the same organization. Generally, the style of supervision in health care will be more dependent on people-centered attitudes than on production-centered attitudes. The tasks involved in delivering health care are more variable than repetitive; units of input and output to and from the institution's systems are not specifically definable, and health care includes a relatively high proportion of partially self-directed professional and paraprofessional workers. Although a manufacturing supervisor has every need to focus strongly on people, the repetitive-task environment may force concentration on processes and techniques. The necessary orientation for the health care supervisor is more toward strength in interpersonal skills.

It was mentioned earlier that the end product of all business is people. In health care and everywhere else, it is necessary to consider the ultimate customer for a product or service. For a mass-production manufacturing enterprise, the customer is likely to be remote, unseen, and unknown, even though there may be health and safety implications of the product or service. In health care, however, the customer is the patient, and the patient is here. The service is hands-on and personal; as such, it is of immediate importance to the patient. In health care, then, much more so than in most other endeavors, there is an immediate focus on the customer and an immediate impact of quality considerations.

Patients are people, and employees are people. To the health care supervisor, patients and employees exist in the here and now, in a face-to-face relationship with the supervisor. Since the vast majority of the problems of health care supervision are people problems, the nature of health care supervision can truly be described as getting things done through people.

That phrase—getting things done through people—is not only descriptive of the role of the first-line supervisor, but also it is the simplest, most all-encompassing definition of management. Also, it holds an important clue to the source of the frustrations Sandra Dolan is experiencing in "Paid to Make Decisions?" Rather than getting things done through people, Sandra is attempting to get people to do things. Sandra knows where she wants the staff to go, and in all likelihood the directions she has chosen are best in the long run. However, Sandra is trying to send them there rather than take them there. The difference between getting things done through people and getting people to do things is as fundamental as the difference between leading and pushing.

Regardless of the organizational environment within which supervision is practiced, successful supervision comes only through conscientious effort. A considerable degree of dedication to the job is necessary, but no one should feel it necessary to become a workaholic. The person who gives everything to the job to the exclusion of all else is most likely using the job as an excuse to fill other needs. Rather, the effective health care supervisor is a person who has a reasonable liking for the work, who has a sincere interest in delivering quality patient care, and who can bring to the job the perspective of a private citizen and sometimes a consumer of health care.

At the end of a management development class in which numerous techniques were discussed, a supervisor said, "I could really get a lot of good work done around here if it weren't for all the problems that pop up every day." When you find yourself feeling that kind of frustration, consider this: the problems—those nagging, unanticipated, annoying difficulties that seem to spring up day after day—are a large part of the reason for your job's existence. If there were fewer problems, we would require fewer supervisors. To a considerable extent, the supervisor is a frustration fighter; if the frustrations did not exist, necessary tasks might well be accomplished without supervisory intervention. The day-to-day problems do exist, and hour-to-hour and moment-to-moment operating decisions have to be made. And the person who must make most of these decisions is the first-line supervisor—the final link between the best intentions of the organization and the actual performance of patient care.

## TRULY PAID TO MAKE DECISIONS?

Concerning the frustrations encountered by Sandra Dolan in the opening "Situation," a few observations can be offered in addition to what has already been said about the way she handles the dual role of manager and worker (the "two hats") and about how she is trying to get staff to respond to her. Issues embodied in these few observations (for example, change and resistance thereto) are treated at length in subsequent chapters.

In her efforts to professionalize the department, Sandra has insisted on adherence to a number of rules and policies that apparently have not been observed for quite some time. Her approach seems to be simply: "You should have been observing these all along, so start doing so now." Official policies or not, however, staff have every reason to question why these rules had not been enforced in years (probably never enforced in the tenure of some of the staff) and why suddenly they must be observed. Sandra could, of course, order compliance and begin disciplining those who do not respond, but this would buy her little more than resentment and intensified resistance. Sandra is attempting to implement change by edict and implement it rapidly, when what she really ought to be doing is taking time to win people over and helping them to understand why certain changes will be to their advantage in the long run.

By saying, "Don't think of this as a competition or a test of wills," Sandra's manager zeroed in on part of the immediate problem. By saying that she could not back down on any of her changes without looking bad, Sandra had made it just that, a test of wills. The effective manager must learn that sometimes the wisest course of action is to back down, and that compromise is not necessarily a dirty word.

By claiming, "I'm paid to make decisions, so I make them," Sandra might just as well have said, "The buck stops here." The "buck" usually does stop with the manager whether this person makes a decision in a vacuum or factors in the input of the entire staff, but what the "buck" really refers to is the responsibility. One of the most important lessons Sandra has to learn is that true participative management is not abrogation of responsibility; it is not weakness, it is strength. Sandra is, of course, paid to make the decisions, but she apparently has yet to learn that the best decisions often result from the knowledgeable input of the people who do the work day in and day out.

## REVIEW QUESTIONS

1. Define "functional specialist" and "management generalist."
2. Why is it frequently difficult for the supervisor to balance the "two hats" of the supervisory role?
3. Describe the hazards to the supervisor of falling into the "working trap."
4. Comment on the claim that "the end product of all business is people." Why is this claim relevant?
5. What is meant by an individual's "level of incompetence?"

## EXERCISE: YOUR TWO HATS

Divide a sheet of paper into two full-length columns. Label one column "Technical," and label the other column "Managerial."

In the Technical column list the tasks you perform either regularly or occasionally in your capacity as a functional specialist. These should be the things you do not primarily because you are a supervisor but because you are a specialist in performing certain kinds of tasks. For instance, you may be a head nurse responsible for the activities of other nurses, but you still obtain a patient's vital signs, or you may be the supervisor of a maintenance crew, but you still replace a malfunctioning light switch.

In the Managerial column list the tasks you perform as a management generalist. In these tasks you are applying techniques that cut across functional lines (although you are doing them specific to the function you supervise). Such tasks might include departmental budgeting, doing performance appraisals, interviewing prospective employees, and untangling people problems.

You may find it helpful to develop your lists over a period of several days, as you are confronted with a variety of problems and tasks, rather than generating them at a single sitting.

### Exercise Questions

- What do your lists tell you about the "two-hat" nature of your job?
- Can you make reasonable estimates as to how much of your time is spent as a working specialist? As a manager?

## Suggestion for Additional Activity

Compare your lists with those of several other supervisors in a group discussion setting, and develop a composite list that is generally descriptive of the roles of the supervisor. Note that the two sides of the supervisor's job represent two distinctly different roles, either of which must be consciously assumed when the occasion demands.

---

**NOTE**

1. L.J. Peters, *The Peter Principle* (New York: William Morrow & Company, 1969).

## CHAPTER 4

# Management and Its Basic Functions

*Good leadership is the act of management, and when it is applied to a corporation or any group adventure, whether military, social, or religious, it calls for more risk than prudence, more understanding than tact, more principle than expediency.*
—A. M. Sullivan

*Wishing consumes as much energy as planning.*
—Anonymous

## CHAPTER OBJECTIVES

☞ Provide a working definition of management.
☞ Relate supervisor and manager to each other and clearly identify the supervisor as a manager.
☞ Introduce and define the basic essential management functions: planning, organizing, directing, coordinating, and controlling.
☞ Establish the importance of each of the basic functions in supervisory practice.
☞ Describe the relative influence of each of the basic management functions on the roles of managers at all organizational levels.

## SITUATION: A TOUGH DAY FOR THE NEW MANAGER

Lydia Michaels was appointed to the newly created position of assistant director of nursing service at James Memorial Hospital, a general hospital serving a suburban community. As a result of a merger with an old and under-utilized hospital not far away, James Memorial is in the midst of an expansion program that will add 70 beds (replacing the other facility's 150 beds) to its present 92 beds. Mrs. Michaels, a registered nurse with 9 years of experience, most recently served as day supervisor. She became assistant director when the first 25 of the additional 70 beds were within 60 days of opening, and it became her task to determine the staffing requirements for these first new beds and ultimately the remainder of the new beds.

Mrs. Michaels developed a master staffing plan based on providing each unit with a core staff set at 90 percent of the staff required at average expected census. To compensate for instances of understaffing, she created a float pool to augment staff as needed.

One Tuesday morning the hospital received word that local flash flooding was a possibility and preparations should be made for flood-related activity. About the same time Mrs. Michaels received word that one of her key people, the head nurse of the largest medical-surgical unit, had fallen seriously ill during the night.

From the float pool, already depleted by vacations and illness, she was able to pull one licensed practical nurse with emergency department (ED) experience. She then located two staff nurses with ED experience and told them they might be called to emergency; if this happened, they could expect to stay after their regular shift. She then made arrangements to cover their normal positions with float personnel should the move be necessary.

As for the unit without its regular head nurse, Mrs. Michaels was tempted to step into the breach herself since she had run the unit for two years and knew it well. However, she had no idea how long this coverage would be necessary, and she did not want to spread herself too thin by assuming an additional burden when she may be needed elsewhere.

After brief consideration she decided to place the unit under the temporary direction of an energetic young staff nurse, Miss Carson. She had been aware of Miss Carson's work for a number of weeks and had in fact considered using her in a charge capacity in the near future.

Local floodwaters rose, driven by heavy rain that also triggered a rash of traffic accidents. Emergency department activity stepped up considerably, and it became necessary to make Mrs. Michaels's planned changes.

That day, in a 7-hour period, the ED handled as many visits as it normally would in a peak 24-hour day, and it did so with patient waiting time no longer than usual. When she was later asked whether the hospital's disaster plan (a number of elements of which had been put into effect) appeared adequate, Mrs. Michaels was able to suggest that some procedures be strengthened in specific ways.

*Situation Instructions*

Keep "A Tough Day for the New Manager" in mind while proceeding through the chapter. Be prepared to associate Mrs. Michaels's actions throughout the day with the basic management functions as they are introduced.

## DEFINITIONS, TITLES, AND OTHER INTANGIBLES

### Management, Manage, Manager

In attempting to define a concept, especially one that is often expressed in a single word, the dictionary is as good a place as any to begin. In Webster's New 20th Century Dictionary (unabridged), management is defined as follows:

- the act, art, or manner of managing, or handling, controlling, directing, etc.
- skill in managing; executive ability
- the person or persons managing a business, institution, etc.

Synonyms for management include treatment, conduct, administration, government, superintendence, and control.

Note that management is defined repeatedly in terms of its root word, manage. The word manage comes from the Latin *manus*, meaning hand. We might feel we are on the right track, since this origin suggests the use of this part of the body in working or doing. However, we then discover that the original English definition of manage is to train a horse in its paces; to cause to do the exercises of the manège (defined as the paces and exercises of a trained horse).

It seems, then, that the word "manage" developed from the description of a specific kind of work. However, among the many definitions of manage are the following: to control or guide; to have charge of; to direct; to administer; to succeed in accomplishing; to bring about by contriving; and to get a person to do what one wishes, especially by skill, tact, or flattery. Synonyms for manage include administer, conduct, control, direct, regulate, and wield. Some of the words we might use to describe manage have appeared throughout the dictionary definitions, and except for an oddity or two we have gained little new information about manage or management—neither the words nor the concept. Unfortunately, it does little good to look up manager, since we learn only that a manager is one who conducts, directs, or manages something. However, the list of synonyms for manager is of interest because it includes the following: director, leader, overseer, boss, and supervisor.

### Supervisor versus Manager

The preceding, somewhat roundabout path was taken to illustrate that at least in some uses the term supervisor is the same as manager. The same dictionary defines supervisor as a person who supervises, a superintendent; a manager; a director. Based on proper use of the English language, then, we can say that supervisor and manager are equal in definition: a manager is a supervisor and a supervisor is a manager.

However, the idea of supervisor and manager being equal may not be agreeable to everyone. All of us have ideas of what a supervisor is and what a manager is, and all of our conceptions are not necessarily the same. Our understanding of what these terms mean—the positioning in the organization of persons who may be called managers, supervisors, directors, administrators, or whatever—is largely determined by the use of these words as titles. It is important to realize that the differences in what these terms mean to us are not absolute. Rather, we and our organizations have artificially created these differences in meaning.

Differences in how we see supervisors in relation to people who run other organizational units interfere with our complete understanding of what is and is not "management." For instance, a maintenance crew chief, when asked to consider enrolling in a management training program, said, "No. I'm not a manager—I'm just a supervisor."

### A Practical Definition

Throughout this book we will be using management to mean the effective use of resources to accomplish the goals of the organization. In simpler terms, management can be described as getting things done through people. Regardless of your title, as long as you are responsible for getting work done at least in part by directing the activities of others, you are a manager. This applies to the working chief of a three-member maintenance crew or the working supervisor of a four-person medical records department as well as to the administrator of a nursing home or the chief executive officer of a hospital. These bottom and top levels both constitute management, just as the people directing the efforts of others at numerous intervening levels also belong to management.

Throughout this book we will speak of management in the broadest generic sense, referring to the processes applied and not to particular job titles. In this context, everyone who directs the activities of others is a manager.

## Organizational Labels

### Label and Level

It is easy to guess how so many different organizational labels for manager developed. It was most likely a matter of organizational convenience, initially adopted to differentiate between managers at different levels or in different roles. It could be quite confusing if all three levels in a particular hospital's business office carried the title of manager. Rather, it makes considerably more sense to identify them as, for instance, controller, business office manager, and accounts receivable supervisor.

The use of manager and its synonyms as position titles did not develop uniformly in all organizations. We are likely to find, for instance, that the health information (medical records) departments of four different hospitals are run by a manager, supervisor, director, and coordinator, respectively. There is little overall comparability of titles from one organization to another. In one institution, a "supervisor" may be the low person on the managerial totem pole and in another may be in the middle or upper part of the hierarchy. Certainly the term manager is most sensitive to this effect in its use as a title, and it may apply anywhere in the organizational pyramid in almost any institution.

### The Supervisor

It is probably fair to say that when we hear supervisor used to describe a working position we usually imagine a position in the lower part of the management structure. For this reason we will regularly use the term first-line supervisor or first-line manager to describe the lowest level of management in the organization—the lowest level at which persons manage the work of other persons. We may also refer occasionally to the second-line supervisor, meaning the second level up—the "supervisor of the supervisor."

### Upper and Middle Management

As the label "top management" suggests, this is the person or persons at or near the top of the organization who are responsible for the entire organization or a major operating unit. Between top management and supervision we may find, depending on the size of the organization, a number of positions generally referred to as "middle management." Middle management may or may not include many people, depending on the size of the organization.

Organization size may render a large part of the "middle management" discussion irrelevant. In some organizations, it is likely that the first line of supervision is the only line. For instance, in a small hospital, the medical records supervisor may report directly to the administrator, so there is no middle management between the top and bottom levels. In this instance, the person who runs the department is a supervisor, department head, or both, depending on the direction from which the position is viewed.

## Line and Staff

It may be beneficial to differentiate among managers as to whether the functions they run are line or staff. A line function is one that advances the accomplishment of the work of the organization; a staff function supports the organization such that it is able to function as intended. For instance, in a hospital the departments of nursing service, radiology, laboratory, dietary, and several others are line activities. The human resources department and the payroll department are two examples of staff activities. The essential difference between line and staff activities is the difference between doing and supporting.

Relating line and staff to managerial titles, a person can be described as a manager of a line activity or a manager of a staff activity. However, whether the overall function of the department is line or staff, the manager, within the individual department, possesses line authority in the management of the department's employees. Within each function there is a line of authority that extends from the department head down to and including the first-line supervisor. For instance, in the nursing service department of a hospital, the line of authority, viewed from the top down, may be: director of nursing service, assistant director, shift supervisor, head nurse, and charge nurse. Each person at each level directs the activities of those at the next lowest level in a manner that may be felt through the entire line of authority; instructions from the director of nursing ultimately result in actions by staff nurses.

Every health care organization necessarily consists of persons working in both line and staff capacities. Often there is confusion about the degree of authority staff persons are to exercise, and problems sometimes arise from the three-way relationship among a line employee, a staff employee, and the staff employee's line manager.

The staff employee, whether professional, technical, advisory, or another type, may appear to be making decisions and following up on them, allocating certain kinds of resources, and even conveying instructions and direction to others. The staff employee occupied in a pure staff function often appears to be the holder and exerciser of all management prerogatives except the critical one that essentially defines a manager—the authority to direct other people. We might even say that an effective staff person often looks, sounds, and acts like a manager. This frequently causes problems for some line personnel because it creates the impression that a person lacking proper authority is intruding into another's territory.

Often line managers do not know how to make fully effective use of the staff assistance available to them. Some line managers tend to view staff people as regulators or intruders rather than use them as the advisers and helpers they really are. Also, some managers behave as though they believe a request for staff assistance—or even an agreement to accept staff assistance when offered—constitutes a weakness or an admission of inadequacy. In short, the line manager who does not completely understand the role and function of staff personnel often tries to go it alone, attempting to be all things in all situations, operating without the available staff assistance.

As far as functions are concerned, the difference between line and staff, as suggested earlier, is the essential difference between doing and supporting. As far as nonmanagerial staff are concerned, line personnel do and staff personnel support. But as far as managers are concerned, managers are all line managers in the operation of their own departments and in the direction of their own employees. Their functions may be clearly definable as staff functions— like accounting, public relations, and human resources—but as managers they are by definition line personnel when operating as managers within their own departmental chains of command.

Many health care institutions are organized along functional lines, giving rise to another way of grouping activities for organizational purposes. We often see health care organizations structured along a three-way division of functions: (1) medical (nursing, radiology, laboratory, and others); (2) nonmedical (food service, housekeeping maintenance, and others); and (3) financial (business office, payroll, general accounting).

### A Title as More Than a Label

We have been talking about titles of managerial positions and the various uses of such titles to differentiate levels of responsibility, but we should also consider the use of titles as "status points" or as a form of "psychic income." Not long ago most hospitals and nursing homes were run by top managers known as administrators. Now, however, we see many chief executive officers, executive directors, presidents, and similar titles in addition to administrators. The functions and responsibilities of a position may have changed little if at all between the days of administrator and executive director, but the latter title may be more impressive to a larger number of people than the former title. It may sound marginally ridiculous, but differences in title do matter in terms of how some people see themselves and how other people view the positions of the title holders.

Title differences are significant only to the extent that they may affect your view of your position. Avoid falling victim to the attitude of the person who said, "I'm no manager—I'm just a supervisor." As a supervisor you are, in fact, a manager, and it is important that you see yourself as a manager and clearly consider yourself to be a member of the collective body known as management.

### INTRODUCING THE MANAGEMENT FUNCTIONS

There are several kinds of activities that all managers pursue in fulfilling their responsibilities. For our purposes, we will break these into five groups, which we will refer to as the basic management functions: (1) planning, (2) organizing, (3) directing, (4) coordinating, and (5) controlling. This five-way breakdown is not original within this work; rather, it has served for years as a reasonable, if somewhat general, description of what managers do.

In the management literature you may encounter other lists of functions that contain four, five, or even more entries and use labels different from those applied here. One different, widely utilized breakdown is found in the work of Theo Haimann, who refers to the basic management functions of planning, organizing, staffing, directing, and controlling.[1] The same five-function breakdown appears in a number of other sources, including Charles Housley and Nancy Nichols writing in *The Health Care Supervisor.*[2] Still another more recent source, *Principles of Health Care Management* by Seth B. Goldsmith, describes a seven-function breakdown: planning, organizing, staffing, directing, controlling, coordinating, and representing.[3] The seventh, representing, described as being a spokesperson for the department, organization, or industry on the outside, is not often encountered as a separately enumerated function.

An interesting four-function breakdown appears in a study guide published in 1985.[4] This division of the management functions at first seems to be only a partial listing of the functions already presented: planning, organizing, directing, and controlling. In this approach, however, directing is subdivided into two categories identified as directing: goals and directing, and motivation.

Other delineations of the management functions to be found in the management literature include planning, organizing, leading, and controlling; planning, organizing, staffing, motivating, and controlling; and other variations. Even as early as 1916 Henri Fayol, the French industrialist and early management theorist, was basing much of his management approach on the simple four-function breakdown of planning, organizing, leading, and controlling.[5]

It is important to appreciate that none of these lists of functions represents someone's belief that a particular listing is the correct delineation of management functions while the others are lacking. Certainly the various lists of management functions are more similar than dissimilar. As evident in the examples cited above, nearly all such lists specifically cite planning, organizing, and controlling, and all such lists begin with planning.

The differences among the lists are simply matters of semantics and matters of how one views some of the elements of management. What is directing in one approach may be leading in another; what is organizing and staffing in one approach may simply be organizing in another; what belongs under both coordinating and controlling in one approach (the one used in this chapter) may all be encompassed by controlling in another.

Why all of these differences? Are there not clearly definable management functions that we can keep separate? The truth is that we cannot clearly differentiate among a number of separately defined management functions in a manner that covers all circumstances. In speaking of management we are speaking of a broad pursuit made up of many overlapping and interwoven activities. The management process is a continuum; the management process is a cycle. All of the business of "defining" management functions is simply a convenience that allows us to examine portions of the management cycle in a way that emphasizes certain kinds of activities.

Regardless of the labels applied, however, it is the concepts that are important. It will be helpful to your understanding of management responsibilities to develop an appreciation of the kinds of activity managers pursue for certain purposes. Later in this chapter we will consider how the emphasis on certain of these basic functions differs according to your position or level in the management structure. Specifically, we will suggest that a manager's organizational position has much to do in determining which management functions are likely to, and perhaps should, consume most of the manager's time and effort.

## MANAGEMENT FUNCTIONS IN BRIEF

Planning is the process of determining what should be done, why it should be done, where it should best be done, by whom it should be done, when it should be done, and how it should be done.

Organizing is the process of structuring the framework within which things get done and determining how best to commit available resources to serve the organization's purposes and carry out its plans. Our consideration of organizing essentially includes what is often referred to as staffing in certain other discussions of the management functions.

Directing is assigning specific resources or focusing certain efforts to accomplish specific tasks as required. Simply stated, directing is running an organizational unit on a day-to-day basis. Directing may be considered to include a great deal of leading, yet leading is woven throughout most of the other functions as well. Directing may also be considered to include motivating and all it implies in getting things done through the unit's employees, yet motivating is certainly a consideration throughout the other functions as well.

Coordinating consists of integrating activities and balancing tasks so that appropriate actions take place within the proper physical and temporal relationships. Coordinating does not appear by name in a number of other delineations of the management functions, yet in all cases it is directly implied in descriptions of the tasks managers perform.

Controlling is follow-up and correction, looking at what actually happened and making adjustments to encourage outcomes to conform to expected or required results. It is controlling that best illustrates the cyclic nature of management and the inseparability of the basic management functions. By its very nature controlling requires directing, coordinating, organizing, and (re)planning, which is itself simply planning, since that activity is also a cyclic process.

## PLANNING

We are planning any time we look ahead at what we might be doing sometime in the future. The "future" may be months or years ahead or it may be only minutes away. Whenever we try to look ahead and predetermine a possible action for a time that has not yet arrived, we are planning. Planning often involves policy-making, objective setting, and developing strategies for reaching the organization's objectives.

Planning can be high level and far reaching, as when the administration and the board of trustees of an institution develop a long-range plan calling for growth and expansion or other major changes. Much planning, however, as it concerns most working managers, is short term and oriented toward near-future applications.

As the development of a 5-year plan for a hospital is an example of planning, so the development of a department's 1-year budget is a representative planning task. Likewise, if you spend half a day developing the work schedule for your department's employees for the coming month, you are actively involved in planning. Even if you simply pause at the end of the day to order your thoughts, sort out the notes on your desk, and jot down a list of items you need to take care of in the morning, you are engaged in planning.

We should recognize, of course, that the future, even when second-guessed minutes before the fact, does not always come to pass as envisioned. Generally, the further into the future we are projecting, the less accurate our planning is likely to be. It stands to reason that we never attain full knowledge of the future until the future becomes the present, so we are always looking ahead with less than perfect information.

## An Imperfect Process

The imperfect nature of planning suggests that plans should be flexible, intended to be changed and updated as the time to which they apply comes closer. If you have done any personnel scheduling, for instance, perhaps you will appreciate the necessity to revise your schedule as you move into and through the period to which it applies.

Although more will be said later about how much planning a supervisor's job might involve, at this point we can suggest that you should keep your planning reasonable in terms of how much you do and how long it takes. Planning is essential to effective managerial performance, but it is possible to fall into the habit of "overplanning." Indeed, some people spend so much time planning that they rarely have time to do anything.

Although much supervisory planning need not be formal or time consuming, it nevertheless pays to be sufficiently thorough and organized to commit your plans to writing. Often the simple act of putting your thoughts on paper will serve to crystallize your ideas and help you decide on the essentials.

## The Plan Is Not the Objective

We are all aware of what happens to "the best laid plans of mice and men." Since our plans, especially those that look more than a few days into the future, seem rarely to generate results exactly as planned, we might reasonably ask, "Why plan at all?"

In defense of planning, we cannot overstress the importance of having well-defined targets at which to aim. Granted we are often going to miss targets because conditions change between the time the plans are generated and the future arrives and because of weaknesses in the planning process itself. When we have a target, however, even when we miss it we have learned something. We at least know by how much we missed the mark and perhaps in what direction we were off, and with that information we can assess both our planning processes and our work practices.

Consider a simple analogy in shooting an arrow toward a target. If the target is simply a blank circle, this whole target is our mark, and as long as we strike anywhere in the circle we really do not know much about where we hit relative to where we wanted to hit. However, when we add a bull's-eye and several target rings, we then have a clearer idea of how much we need to adjust our shots to come closer to where we would like to be.

Keep in mind, however, that when our plans are not realized it could be for any of several reasons. It is possible that surrounding conditions have changed and what was once a good plan is no longer valid in the light of new conditions. It is also possible that the plan was inadequate to begin with. Also, there is always the possibility that the plan was well conceived and fully adequate but failed to work because the implementation effort fell short of what was needed. In any case, whether or not our plans work out well we have always learned something from the experience. It has often been said that plans themselves are not particularly worthwhile, but that the planning process is invaluable. Indeed, what is truly valuable is the cyclic process of examining needs, setting objectives, making plans to reach those objectives, implementing the plans, and following up on the total effort.

Plans should never be regarded as cast in concrete. We sometimes tend to try bending reality to fit the plan so as to arrive at the results we projected. It is true that a certain amount of this kind of effort is called for with some kinds of plans. Departmental budgets, for instance, should be considered as relatively important targets to be met. However, a plan is first and foremost a guide to action—it is not in itself a predestined action.

As a first-line supervisor you may not feel there is a great deal of planning required of you. This may be generally true, but you will find that every management position, even one in the lowest levels of management, requires some planning. A certain amount of planning is necessary to help you run your job properly, and if you do not run your job to at least some extent there is a good chance that your job will run you.

## ORGANIZING

Sometimes it may seem that organizing, much like planning, is not a particular concern of the first-line supervisor. It is true that much organizing has to do with departmentalization, the process of grouping various activities into separate units to carry out the work of the organization. Much of this takes place at high levels in the organization and may not occur very often. However, as a first-line supervisor you engage in acts of organizing similar to departmentalization whenever you make decisions concerning which people within your department are going to handle certain tasks. Whenever you become involved in making decisions concerning division of labor or separation of skills, you are organizing.

### Unity of Command

One basic principle of organizing with which you should be familiar is unity of command. Unity of command requires you to provide assurance, for all the activities within your responsibility, that in all instances specific employees are responsible for certain specific results on a one-to-one basis. That is, it is inappropriate to assign task responsibilities in such a way that your employees have room for doubt concerning who is ultimately responsible for any given task. Likewise, unity of command suggests that no function within your responsibility should be allowed to "drift" without belonging to some specific person.

### Span of Control

Another important concept within organizing—and one over which the individual supervisor has little influence—is span of control. An individual manager can effectively supervise only a certain number of workers, with this number hazily determined by the manager's knowledge and experience, the amount and nature of the manager's nonsupervisory work, the amount of supervision required by the employees, the variability of the employees' tasks, the overall complexity of the activity, and the physical area over which the employees are distributed. For instance, the working supervisor of a five-member medical records department (where all five employees work within the same room) has every opportunity for complete control. The supervisor probably knows all the jobs fairly well, and visual and auditory control of the entire department is relatively easy. On the other hand, a working supervisor in a five-member maintenance department has a limited span of control. This department's employees do many different things and usually do most of their work well beyond the supervisor's visual and auditory control. One supervisor can readily control five employees; the other may have great difficulty controlling five employees. A supervisor can oversee and control more people who do similar work in the same physical area than people who perform variable work scattered over a considerable area.

### Delegation

The most important aspect of organizing to the first-line supervisor is the function known as delegation. Delegation, the process of assuring that the proper people have the responsibility and authority for performing specific tasks, is of sufficient importance to the supervisor to warrant a chapter of its own (see Chapter 5).

### DIRECTING

Directing consists largely of assigning responsibilities on a day-to-day basis, letting your employees know what has to be done, how, and by when. It is the making of all the little but all-important decisions so necessary in the operation of the department; it is, in fact, the process of steering the department. Although we may occasionally get tired of "team" analogies in management, the example of the football quarterback is nevertheless appropriate to directing. The quarterback knows the plays and the strategy as a result of prolonged planning sessions; yet when the quarterback goes onto the field, the exact conditions that will be encountered are unknown. It is only when the quarterback sees what happens on the field that the quarterback can call on what has been learned and respond to the conditions of the moment. It is in this way that the supervisor must behave, making the day-to-day and sometimes hour-to-hour decisions necessary in running the departmental team.

Since much of directing consists of giving advice or conveying instructions, directing is, in a mechanical sense, present along with most of the other management functions. That is, since giving an order is a directing activity, it is really not possible to convey any kind of decision without directing.

Under directing you might logically place an entire management library of discussions about management activities. The foregoing quarterback example should make clear, for instance, that people who are most successful at directing are successful at leading. We can direct without leading by simply giving orders; we can fill leadership positions (although perhaps not very well) without being true leaders. However, direction is more successful when we can truly lead.

Motivation is also related to leading in our consideration of directing. Related in turn to motivation and leadership is all of the advice pertinent to anyone in a position of authority over other persons in an organizational unit. Directing in some way touches on essentially every function, process, or technique ever brought into play in getting things done through people.

## COORDINATING

It has been suggested that coordinating—the blending of activities and timing of events—might legitimately be considered a part of the directing function. We are considering it separately, if only briefly, out of recognition of its importance to the supervisor.

A dinner of five magnificent courses will not be particularly successful if the courses are scattered over two or three hours, the dessert comes second, and the entree arrives last. Likewise, an essential part of many work activities is not the simple fact of their performance but rather when they are performed relative to other activities. Thus we approach a potentially large number of tasks that involve coordination with other tasks.

In health care activities it is always essential that employees, facilities, supplies, and services all be combined in the right relationship to each other for the benefit of the patient. Throughout the department, and certainly between and among the departments of a health institution, it is necessary for activities to be coordinated. It makes little sense to place a full breakfast before a patient who is soon to be given tests requiring fasting, just as it makes little sense to place a patient who is scheduled for an X-ray in the corridor four hours before the department is ready to receive the patient. Effective coordination is one of the keys to supervisory effectiveness.

## CONTROLLING

Plans rarely come to realization exactly as intended, so many moment-to-moment changes are required in pursuit of departmental objectives. In the controlling function we evaluate progress against objectives and make adjustments or new decisions as we go along. The terms most descriptive of controlling are follow-up and action. We take note of how things are going as compared with how they should be going and make new decisions and provide new direction to effect corrective action.

Controlling is often the most neglected of the basic management functions, especially in terms of the strength of follow-up on implementation of earlier decisions. The problems of limited or nonexistent follow-up will be examined further during our consideration of delegation and, later, of supervisory decision making.

## THE MANAGEMENT FUNCTIONS IN ACTION

Returning to "A Tough Day for the New Manager," there are a number of observations that can be made about Mrs. Michaels's hectic Tuesday relative to the basic management functions.

In preparing to bring the new beds into service, Lydia Michaels was actively involved in both planning and organizing in determining what needed to be done for the expansion and in establishing projected staff levels and how the additional staff would be phased in as needs grew. Her master staffing plan activity was primarily organizing, but within this role was planning in that she determined how they might compensate for staff shortages with a float pool.

When Mrs. Michaels pulls from her float pool and locates additional nurses with emergency department experience, she is engaged in both controlling—literally, follow-up and correction—and coordinating. It should be immediately evident that neither coordinating nor controlling can be accomplished without directing as well. By not personally stepping into the vacancy created by the absence of the large unit's head nurse, she avoided a working trap of sorts and kept herself available for continued coordinating and controlling, which were highly likely to be necessary given the day's circumstances.

More controlling, as well as directing, occurred in placing young Miss Carson in the acting head nurse role. And directing was in the forefront when Lydia Michaels implemented the emergency staffing alternative she had planned for earlier.

Lydia Michaels also engaged in a form of controlling when she suggested strengthening the hospital's disaster plan. What was learned from one disaster situation could then enhance the hospital's ability to cope with future disasters.

Controlling, described above as follow-up and correction, ordinarily leads to more planning, sometimes more organizing and coordinating, and always more directing. This illustrates the frequently cyclic nature of the management functions; it also suggests that usually two or more basic functions are experienced together. Only sometimes, as in long-range strategic planning, for example, do any of the basic management functions occur in isolation from the others.

## EMPHASIS

The basic management functions of planning, organizing, directing, coordinating, and controlling were presented in a given order for an important reason.

Generally, the first elements of this list occupy, or should occupy, a proportionately larger amount of the time of people in the upper levels of management. We said "should" because top managers and middle managers are frequently prone to continue behaving in the manner of first-line supervisors; that is, they spend significant amounts of time dealing with day-to-day operating problems when they should be leaving most such problems to the lower management levels. Indeed, managers at all levels in all organizations are frequently prone to "crisis management," expending most of their time and effort in reacting to present events and conditions rather than looking ahead.

Because of the nature of departmental supervision, the first-line supervisor will concentrate more on activities toward the bottom of the list of basic management functions. It is the lower echelons of management who are rightly more concerned with the problems of the moment. Those at the top of the organization should be more concerned with where the organization is going relative to its long-range goals and should be considering courses of action required to support those goals.

However, planning, organizing, directing, coordinating, and controlling are all part of every manager's job. In a large health care organization, top management may spend 70 percent or 80 percent of the time involved in broad-based planning and organizing. In the same organization, except for the regular practice of delegation (a part of organizing), the first-line supervisor may spend 80 percent or 90 percent of the time on a combination of directing, coordinating, and controlling (Figure 4–1).

How you may see your approach to the basic management functions will be largely influenced by the approach you have taken to the job since you have been supervisor. Much of what you do has been determined by the concept of management you held before you became a supervisor, and by whether or not you received any solid orientation to supervision.

## PROCESSES VERSUS PEOPLE

In discussing the basic management functions we necessarily focus on a number of practices that are often described as management processes. In doing so we run the risk of creating an impression that management is strongly process oriented. We might be tempted to believe that to be successful in management we need to learn a number of processes and then apply the appropriate processes to circumstances as they arise.

It is indeed true that planning and organizing are processes. Controlling, delegating, and leading (to name some fairly broad functions) are processes, too, as are controlling absenteeism, scheduling, and interviewing (to name some more narrowly delineated functions). And we could name dozens of other so-called functions or techniques that are processes.

With all of this seeming emphasis on functions and processes, it is appropriate to remind ourselves that the central focus of management is people. We might spend a great deal of time learning management processes—most management education is in fact heavily weighted toward process—and never become successful supervisors. In the long run, success at any level of management will depend on one's ability to work with people.

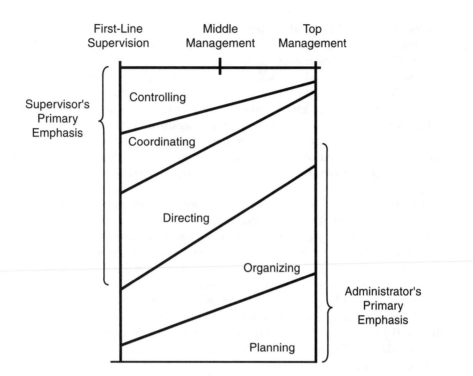

Figure 4-1 Typical Shift in Emphasis on Basic Management Functions from Lowest to Highest Levels of Management

---

## REVIEW QUESTIONS

- Describe the fundamental differences between *line* and *staff*.
- Provide an example of the use of the word *manager* as a generic term and an example of its use as a specific organizational title.
- Considering how the terms *supervisor* and *manager* may be perceived, which would you rather be called and why?
- As simply as you can properly express it, what is the single defining characteristic of *planning*?
- Which of the basic management functions get the most of the supervisor's attention? Why?
- What are the primary characteristics of the management function *controlling*?

---

## CASE: BALANCING THE FUNCTIONS

Betty Wilson was administrative manager of the department of radiology. She was an outstanding example of someone who had come up through the ranks; Betty had been chief technician, a special procedures technician, a technician assigned to routine procedures, and years earlier a student in the hospital's school of radiologic technology.

Because of her broad knowledge gained through experience and additional academic study in matters of radiation safety, as administrative manager she found herself called on more and more to substitute for the hospital's radiation safety officer and to fill in as a special procedures technician when that area was short staffed. More frequently, however, she found herself resisting these technical-work intrusions on her management role, doing so until it became clear that Dr. Arnold, the medical chief of the department, disapproved of her behavior.

One day her manager, the hospital's associate administrator, asked, "What's wrong between you and Dr. Arnold? He claims that you're no longer willing to help out in special procedures, and that the radiation safety committee has just about fallen apart because you wouldn't take the chair and see that things got done. Is your work piling up to where you've got too much to do?"

Betty shook her head. "No, my workload is under control. I know that radiation safety needs help because of Susan's off-and-on health problems, and the turnover in special procedures is killing us because those people are so hard to find in this area just now. What I think the problem really is—I seem to be in a dual role that I'm not comfortable with."

"Meaning what?"

"Meaning that I don't really know if I'm a manager or a technical staff member or neither or both. I know special procedures and radiation safety fairly well, but it doesn't take a manager to serve as radiation safety officer, and if I let it do so, radiation safety alone could take up more than half of my time."

Betty continued, "And I always thought I was a good special procedures tech, but times change and it's been a long time since I did that day in and day out. More than half the equipment there has changed since I worked there full time. One of the last times I was in there at Dr. Arnold's direction, one of the techs—actually the only full-time special procedures tech we have—said he'd rather not have my help because coaching me along would slow him down and he could do it faster without me. Yet Dr. Arnold seems to regard me first and foremost as an extra pair of hands to be put wherever there's staff work to be done."

After a moment Betty concluded, "I've always believed that the basic job of a manager was to get things done through people, and I've tried to practice that ever since I entered management. I guess I really don't know if I'm supposed to be a real manager or just another employee, and I'm afraid that doing all of this technical work is somehow making me less of a manager."

## REVIEW QUESTIONS

1. How is Betty functioning in both line and staff capacities?
2. Do you agree that Betty's performance of technical work as described could be making her "less of a manager," as she fears? Explain your answer.

3. Describe one set of circumstances under which Betty's involvement in the technical tasks described would be fully appropriate.

---

**NOTES**

1. T. Haimann, *Supervisory Management for Hospitals and Related Health Facilities* (St. Louis: The Catholic Hospital Association, 1965, 1973, 1989, 1993, 1997).
2. E. Housley and N. G. Nichols, "The Responsibilities of the Responsible Supervisor," *The Health Care Supervisor* 2, no. 3 (1984): 2.
3. S. B. Goldsmith, *Principles of Health Care Management* (Sudbury, MA: Jones & Bartlett Publishers, Inc., 2005).
4. L. Slagle et al., *Managing (Study Guide)* (Glenview, Ill.: Scott, Foresman & Co., 1985).
5. H. Fayol, *General and Industrial Management* (New York: Pittman, 1949).

# PART II

# The Supervisor and Self

## CHAPTER 5

# Delegation and Empowerment: Forming Some Good Habits

*One of modern management's most important functions—*
*effective delegation of work—is a subject for plenty*
*of preaching but not enough practice.*
*—Earle Brooks*

## CHAPTER OBJECTIVES

☞ Identify delegation and its practice as a major influence on effective supervisory performance.

☞ Place empowerment into perspective with delegation, recognizing empowerment's present-day application as generally totally inclusive of proper delegation.

☞ Convey the importance of empowerment—proper delegation—in terms of its value to supervisors, employees, and organizations alike.

☞ Identify the common reasons behind the failure to delegate, and develop a pattern for proper delegation.

☞ Establish a perspective on delegation that will also help the supervisor when so empowered by higher management.

☞ Encourage the supervisor to form sound delegation habits.

## SITUATION: DELEGATION FOR THE WRONG REASONS, OR "IF YOU WANT SOMETHING DONE RIGHT. . ."

John Miller, manager of laundry and linen for City Medical Center, dreaded the day each month he had to spend doing the statistical report for his department. Miller was responsible for all laundry and linen activities in the 800-bed hospital, two smaller satellite facilities, and several municipal agencies whose linen needs were filled by the hospital. At one time the report had been relatively simple, but as Miller's scope of responsibility grew and administration requested increasingly detailed information each month, the report had become more lengthy and complex. Miller had simply modified his method of preparing the report each time a new requirement was placed on him, so there was no written procedure for the report's preparation.

Faced once again with the time-consuming report—and confronted, as usual, with several problems demanding his immediate attention—John Miller decided it was time to delegate report preparation responsibilities to his assistant, Bill Curtis. He called Curtis to his office, gave him a copy of the previous month's report and a set of forms, and said, "I'm sure you've seen this. I want you to take care of it from now on. I've been doing it for a long time, but it's getting to be a real pain and I've got more important things to do than to allow myself to be tied up with routine clerical work."

Curtis spent perhaps a half minute skimming the report before he said, "I'm sure I can do this if I start out on the right foot. How about walking me through it—doing just this one with me so I can get the hang of it?"

Miller said, "Look, my objective in giving this to you is to save me some time. If I have to hold your hand, I may as well do it myself." He grinned as he added, "Besides, if I can do it, then anyone with half a brain ought to be able to do it."

Without further comment Curtis left the office with the report and the forms. Miller went to work on other matters.

Later that day Curtis stopped Miller in the corridor—they met while going in opposite directions—and he said, "John, I'm glad I caught you. I've got three or four questions about the activity report, mostly concerning how you come up with the counts and percentages for the satellites." He started to pull a folded sheet of paper from his back pocket.

Miller barely slowed, "Sorry, Bill, but I can't take the time. I'm already late for a meeting." As he hurried past Curtis he called back over his shoulder, "You'll just have to puzzle it out for yourself. After all, I had to do the same thing."

The following day when the report was due, Miller found Curtis's work on his desk when he returned from lunch. He flipped through it to assure himself that all the blanks had been filled in, and then he scrawled his signature in the usual place. However, something caught his eye—a number that appeared to be far out of line with anything in previous reports. He took out two earlier reports and began a line-by-line comparison. He quickly discovered that Curtis had made a crucial error near the beginning and carried it through successive calculations.

Miller was angry with Curtis. The day was more than half gone and he would have to drop everything else and spend the rest of the afternoon reworking the figures so the report could be submitted on time. Miller was still working at 4:30 P.M. when Pete Anderson, the engineering manager, appeared in his doorway and said, "I thought we were going to rework your preventive maintenance schedule this afternoon. What are you up to, anyway?"

Miller threw down his pen and snapped, "I'm proving an old saying."

"Meaning what?"

"Meaning, if you want something done right, do it yourself."

*Instructions*

It should be obvious, even at this early point in the chapter, that Miller committed some significant errors in "delegating" the report to his assistant. In proceeding through the chapter, identify Miller's mistakes and decide how he could have approached this task constructively.

## TAKEN FOR GRANTED

Effective delegation has long been a subject of considerable preaching. It is the basis of numerous workshops, seminars, and other educational programs.

One needs only to review a small sample of current management literature to obtain a reasonable idea of how often delegation is discussed in print.

Despite its frequent presentation, however, delegation is often treated lightly, if at all, even by supervisors who are genuinely interested in becoming better managers.

Although subject to much dispensing of good advice, delegation is frequently overlooked when it comes to conscientious practice. All too often our ability to delegate is unconsciously taken for granted, and we tend to assume an expertise that is not present.

Many people who are responsible for the work of others tend to take delegation for granted because:

- They do not fully understand the true nature of delegation.
- They do not recognize, or at least do not fully appreciate, the extent of the power of their own habits in preventing improvement in delegation.
- They have not yet come to view delegation from the perspective of the employee to whom the work is delegated.

## THE NATURE OF DELEGATION

There are some significant problems to be encountered when considering delegation as a management technique. Although most managers believe they should delegate and are convinced they do delegate, these problems exist because much so-called delegation is incomplete and ineffective. Few supervisors believe or will admit that they do not delegate. However, few supervisors delegate significantly beyond simple organizational delegation.

In Chapter 4, delegation was described as part of the basic management function of organizing. Most supervisors are automatically, if passively, involved with organizational delegation. You place a person in a job and give that person a job description or a set of instructions. You have delegated; you have charged an employee with the performance of a number of tasks for which you are ultimately responsible. The job description is, in a real way, the employee's authority to perform certain functions. Any department consisting of more than one person is necessarily subject to organizational delegation because the normal division of activities requires different people to perform various tasks.

In this chapter we are dealing with a major step beyond organizational delegation. Not every task to be accomplished by the department will appear on someone's job description. Indeed, many of the department's activities fall between the lines of the job descriptions or are not listed at all. You will usually find that the job description for a supervisor, as well as the job description for a partially self-directing professional such as a registered nurse, will include a catch-all statement such as "perform all other duties as required." The responsibilities of each department include many tasks not specifically mentioned in the job descriptions. These tasks may be found at various levels within the department, but invariably the supervisor is responsible for ensuring that someone does them.

A supervisor's job description may also contain many tasks that rightly belong there but that need not necessarily be done entirely by the supervisor. There are probably a number of tasks within your responsibility that can be accomplished by you or by someone who works for you. Much of a supervisor's effectiveness is determined by how well the capabilities of employees to accomplish many such tasks properly are utilized by that supervisor.

Delegation is both a process and a condition. It is, in part, the process of assigning work to an employee. The process is generally well understood, but much consideration of delegation stops at this point. The condition of delegation, which must be achieved by going well beyond the process itself, exists when there is thorough, mutual understanding by supervisor and employee of what specific results are expected and how these results may be achieved. Too often delegation is treated as a simple process and no steps are taken to attain the true condition of delegation.

The hows and whys of the delegation process are relatively simple, and it is by understanding and pursuing them that we approach the condition of true delegation. The all-important consideration in effective delegation is practice; like any desirable activity, effective delegation must be pursued conscientiously and intentionally, perhaps for a considerable time, before it becomes a habit. We also must first break some old habits. Unfortunately, most of us are much more accustomed to doing than to having others do.

## WHAT ABOUT "EMPOWERMENT"?

Rising to prominence in the late 1980s and through the 1990s largely in conjunction with the total quality management (TQM) movement, empowerment has become a latter-day buzzword. Business has supposedly been discovering that empowerment is "the thing to do" with employees to enable them to make their best possible contributions to organizational success.

Technically, delegation and empowerment are the same. As may be verified in any comprehensive dictionary or thesaurus, the two words are actually synonyms for each other.[1] Therefore, any differences between them are largely perceived differences, brought about mostly by years of misuse of the term delegation and the recent and present overuse, misuse, and abuse of the term empowerment as one of the "in" terms of modern management and more specifically as part of the language of TQM.

Although empowerment may be described in a variety of ways, its essence, as it is used in work organizations, remains letting employees solve their own problems or letting employees both decide what needs to be done and then go ahead and do it. Therefore, there is no difference between empowerment and delegation; that is, no difference between empowerment and proper delegation.

Too often, however, empowerment is seen—usually by the not-yet-empowered—as the freedom to do one's own thing in one's own way, to redefine one's role in a largely self-satisfying manner, or to emphasize whatever one may see as the more desirable parts of the job while ignoring the undesirable parts. But the truly empowered employee knows the limits within which he or she may operate and does not stray beyond without management direction. And the honest, empowering manager clearly defines the employee's limits and then keeps hands off as long as the employee operates within those limits and delivers the expected results. The essence of empowerment is reflected in defining and communicating the limits.

Although as words both delegation and empowerment have essentially the same meaning, in practice they have been regarded quite differently. With empowerment's force as a buzzword, many people are behaving as though this concept called empowerment is a vast improvement on mere "delegation." But if the concepts are really one and the same, what happened to delegation?

What actually happened to delegation is decades of misuse of the term, decades of regarding delegation as no more than giving someone a task to complete or as no more than giving someone an order. Proper delegation, however, has always consisted of giving someone the responsibility for task completion and also giving that person the authority required to complete the task. True empowerment is identical to proper delegation: One gives an employee a problem to solve or a condition to correct, specifies the desired outcome or acceptable range of results, and provides the employee with the authority or whatever other resources are necessary to accomplish this.

The problem at the heart of most difficulties with delegation is already emerging as a fundamental problem with empowerment. It is a problem of management style and approach by the delegating manager and is a control issue with many higher managers. These managers cannot let go sufficiently to allow delegation or empowerment to work. Their still-authoritarian management styles send one clear message to the employees: You are free to make whatever decisions you want, as long as they are the same decisions we would make ourselves.

Whether referred to as proper delegation or empowerment, this process will work as intended only if the manager—the person who does the delegating or empowering—is committed in advance to accepting the decisions of the employees.

## WHY DELEGATE?

### For Yourself

The old adage, "If you want a thing done well, do it yourself," is largely a fallacy as far as management is concerned. One person, no matter how competent, can do only so much and still continue to do things well. We frequently see supervisors who try to handle so many activities that they are able to hold things together only loosely at best.

You may believe that because you work long hours, take extra work home, and generally try to fill every request that comes along and solve every problem that arises you are a dedicated, effective, hard-working manager. You may be dedicated and hard working, but if this is the way you approach your job, chances are you are not effective.

Failure to delegate effectively is one of the principal causes of managerial failure and is a leading reason why many people in management do not get promoted to more responsible positions. We do not claim that failure to delegate effectively will necessarily halt a management career at the first level, because many persons, by dedication and "workaholism," manage to rise several levels through sheer energy and activity. However, even the workaholic, the manager who continues to do as much as possible alone will eventually reach a level where the job is too big to handle. Failure to delegate effectively is an even greater hazard for higher-level managers than for first- and second-line supervisors. In fact, delegation failure at all levels of management is damaging.

You owe it to yourself to delegate, to ensure that some of your employees are capable of taking care of some of the tasks, problems, and requests that you usually have to handle. You can achieve a measure of peace of mind by knowing that one or more persons can capably act on your behalf when you are ill, on vacation, or busy elsewhere. Delegation can build your image as a leader with your employees and will likely improve your standing with higher management, since as a supervisor you are properly judged not by what you do but rather by what your department does.

Delegating certain tasks can give you more time to concentrate on true supervisory activities. Rarely is there enough time in the supervisor's day for all the thinking, planning, and communicating needed to maintain and improve a department's effectiveness. Generally, the effectively delegating supervisor gains a greater degree of freedom from technical tasks and is able to function as more of a manager more of the time. This could also include sufficient freedom to enable you to assume greater responsibility by taking on functions delegated by your immediate manager.

### For Your Employees

Why delegate? People who are normally weighed down by boredom and frustration during work hours come alive when given a whole job, and their abilities take a quantum jump. It is far better to have champions working for you than zombies.[2]

You owe it to your employees to delegate. As their supervisor you should be seeking to help them learn and grow, rather than acting in a manner that holds them back. You build a department by building individuals.

As much of your fate is determined by your immediate supervisor, so is the fate of your employees largely in your hands. You can guide your employees upward in terms of growth and development, or you can hold them back. You can challenge and interest them by giving them responsibility and opportunity, or you can lock them into routine and boredom.

Most employees would rather be stimulated and interested than unchallenged and bored. Most would rather learn and grow than stagnate. Most would rather be serving useful purposes than doing unimportant or inconsequential work. And most would rather work—because they enjoy work or, at worst, because they wish to pass the time more quickly—than be idle. Proper delegation can be an effective morale builder.

When you delegate, your employees get a taste of greater responsibility and perhaps some decision-making experience. They are likely to take more pride in what they do, reflect higher morale, both individually and as a department, and exercise more individual initiative.

The presence of effective delegation within a department represents opportunity to the employees. All employees will not react the same way to the chance to assume greater responsibility or do different work; some people do not wish to go in those directions. However, the simple presence of the opportunity is a tonic to all employees whether they avail themselves of that opportunity or not. And the absence of such opportunity will affect many employees in a way that eventually affects the outlook of all. Overall, an empowered employee is usually a growing employee.

## FAILURE TO DELEGATE

Managers fail to delegate for a number of reasons, one of which is as simple as a tendency to prefer to do things one's self. But some of the reasons for delegation failure are complex and involve fear of competition from employees or the loss of recognition for task accomplishment, factors of which the supervisor may be only dimly aware. It is often difficult to avoid thinking of yourself as being in competition with your employees, since some employees seem to foster such competition as they attempt to grow in the organization. However, the effective supervisor encourages growth, and a legitimate challenge taken up by an employee can look much like direct competition. The fear of competition from subordinates often goes hand-in-hand with a degree of insecurity, but the presence of two or three eager promotion-oriented employees with their sights set on the supervisor's job can be a stimulus that keeps the supervisor in a heads-up and growing attitude.

Although all employees are legitimately concerned to some extent with how they may be doing in the boss's eyes, as a supervisor your first concern should not be, "Does my boss think I'm doing a good job?" Rather, your concern should be, "Is this department doing a good job?" When your employees perform well, the credit is yours as well as theirs. As the department is recognized, so is the supervisor recognized.

Old habits are a major reason for failure to delegate. Our earliest working years were devoted to the doing of work, and we often fail to deemphasize that habit even though we may have spent more recent years supposedly directing the doing of work.

A great deal of sound advice is available concerning delegation. That is, it is sound advice if it is followed, but most of the time the advice offered in step-by-step approaches to delegation is either not followed or, if followed at all, not conscientiously pursued for a sufficient amount of time to become ingrained in the supervisor's habit pattern.

One of the most significant barriers to effective delegation is habit. If we are to try to adopt a new approach to delegation, we must change our ways of doing things. Such change means altering habit patterns by shedding old habits and replacing them with new ones.

Anyone who has put forth a conscious effort to change a deeply ingrained habit should fully appreciate how difficult it can be. It certainly can be done, depending on how much effort is applied, how long this effort is sustained, and how deeply ingrained the old habit is. Attempts to improve the way we delegate frequently go the same way as attempts to apply what we learn at a time management seminar about improving effectiveness: a flurry of initial activity is followed by stops and starts that diminish and eventually vanish as old ways take over again. This ordinarily occurs because we are only dimly aware of, or perhaps have not thought at all about, the immense barrier presented by habits that may have become so deeply ingrained through years of practice that they are now second nature.

The key to improving your skill at delegation lies in the constant awareness of the need to overcome old habits. It is necessary to start on a small, or at least modest, scale, conscientiously applying the new process to one well-defined task or project at a time and doing so over and over until the new way becomes a habit that is strong enough to keep the old habit from returning.

Another common reason for the failure to delegate, one that many supervisors may readily recognize and admit, is the feeling that available employees simply cannot handle greater responsibility. This is a classic situation: you hesitate to try to give someone more responsibility because you do not know if they can handle it; yet the only way you will find out if they can handle it is to try it. If you find yourself feeling that you do not delegate because you have no one who can handle additional responsibility, ask yourself if you have seriously tried to prepare someone to assume more responsibility.

The most prevalent reason for failure to delegate is also the most obvious reason: lack of time. Here we find ourselves caught in a basic contradiction—we tend to think most seriously about the need to delegate only when the pressure is most intense. The in-baskets are overflowing, problems are coming from all directions, and we realize we need to delegate to improve our effectiveness—or simply to help us get caught up. However, delegation takes time—time to pick people and prepare them, time to prepare the work, time to do several other things—and when the workload is heavy we simply do not have that kind of time. We may promise ourselves to do some serious delegating "as soon as the rush is over." However, when the rush finally goes away so does the feeling of urgency that came with it: "Delegate? The workload is under control, so where's the need?"

The time required to accomplish proper delegation is an investment, an investment that must often be made when there is precious little time available. The returns of delegation are not immediate; it is often necessary to expend an additional amount of time and go even further behind for the sake of improvements that will not appear as real time savings until weeks or perhaps months have passed. However, this hurdle—the "time trap"—must be overcome before improved efficiency through delegation can become a reality.

Consider the case of the administrative supervisor of a large outpatient department who was required to submit a detailed statistical report of activities each month. Each time the supervisor faced the report, which required about 4 uninterrupted hours to complete, this person considered delegating this task to a certain employee who could handle it with proper training. However, the supervisor estimated it would take 8 to 10 hours to go through the report point by point with the employee, so the employee's training was put off until a "convenient time" between reports. However, the convenient time never came, and soon it was time to submit the next report and the pressure was on again.

After rationalizing the way through this time trap several times, the supervisor finally recognized the need to invest extra time and effort. When the time came to do the next report, the supervisor and the designated employee closeted themselves and went through the report number-by-number and line-by-line. It took an entire day. The next month's report took the two of them nearly 6 hours, still longer than it had taken the supervisor alone. The third report was done in the same way in about 4 hours.

The fourth month's report consumed about 6 hours. However, this consisted of 5 hours of the employee's time, working alone, and an hour of the supervisor's time to audit some important statistics. By the sixth month of the new arrangement, the employee was doing the report in 4 hours and the supervisor was spending perhaps 5 to 10 minutes to review and approve the report. Improvement took a long time, but the early investment of time and effort paid off in later returns.

The impact of the failure to delegate can be significant and can be felt well beyond the individual nondelegating supervisor. Consider the case of the business office manager who was not promoted to assistant director of finance primarily because of delegation weaknesses: neither of the two assistants had been tested with responsibility and the department was without a potential successor to the manager. The business office manager had been the only possible in-house candidate, so the organization was forced to search elsewhere for a new assistant director of finance. Because the manager lost out on a promotion, one of the two assistants also lost the chance to become business office manager. In addition, two lower-level jobs that could have been opened up by this promotional chain reaction remained closed. Thus, four people missed out on possible promotions simply because one of them had not practiced effective delegation.

The department of a nondelegating supervisor suffers in a number of ways. Unchallenged people with time on their hands usually do not exhibit high morale. As morale goes down, productivity and quality are likely to suffer. A department so afflicted can acquire a reputation for discontent and unreliability, and once acquired such a reputation is not easily shed. In the extreme case, such a department will begin to lose its better people as they go elsewhere in search of work environments in which there is opportunity for growth and advancement. Employees who do not consider job interest and challenge as particularly important will remain to drift—and complain.

We have repeatedly referred to management as "getting things done through people." This is accomplished through delegation. As a supervisor you obtain your own authority through delegation. It is up to you to learn how to use that authority, including how to redelegate part of it when doing so is in the best interest of the organization.

Finally, it is necessary to remember that there is always some degree of risk involved in proper delegation. If there were no risk at all, the delegated task would be no more than a pointless exercise. In hesitating to delegate, one might fear the risk and balk at the other hazards inherent in the process;

however, regardless of risk and other roadblocks, the supervisor has more to gain than lose by delegating.

## LOOKING UPWARD AS WELL AS DOWNWARD: THE PERSONAL APPROACH TO DELEGATION

The supervisor who sincerely wants to improve at delegation should look both downward and upward: downward toward the employees to whom he or she will delegate and upward toward the higher manager from whom delegated tasks are received. Put yourself in the position of your employees and consider, by looking upward at the same time, how your superior should, or perhaps actually does, delegate to you. It helps to look toward your boss regarding delegation because your employees similarly look toward you.

Although the motivational forces that cause people to work exist in a complex mix that may vary dramatically from person to person, the net effect of these motivating forces is often not all that different between you and most of your employees. For the most part the majority of your employees will want many of the same things that you want; many of them will perhaps aspire to supervision, wishing to rise from the ranks of the work group as perhaps you did.

Not all of your employees are likely to aspire to management, and not all of them will seek challenge in their work as perhaps you do. Generally, however, their motives will parallel yours so that you can deal with them in a manner similar to the way you would like your boss to deal with you.

You are therefore on a reasonable course if you try to pattern some elements of your relationship with each individual employee after an idealized working relationship with your boss. Attempting to do so will put you in a position of being able to work on improving delegation both upward and downward—that is, while you strive to become better at delegating, you can work to achieve a more appropriate delegation relationship with your superior. This is a highly personal approach, because it finds you looking out for your own best interests—as well as the best interests of your employees and the organization—by improving the effectiveness with which you delegate and simultaneously improving your communicating relationship with your superior.

### Ideal Versus Real

In an ideal relationship with your boss, you and that higher manager would both know where you stand with each other at all times and on all matters. In the real world, of course, this relationship may be somewhat less—perhaps even significantly less—than the ideal. However, it is possible to use your knowledge of your needs as a supervisor and your concept of an ideal relationship with your boss to:

- Reshape and generally improve your relationship with your boss, actually guiding your boss along the path toward a more effective delegation relationship with you.
- Establish a new and more effective pattern for how you delegate to your employees.

It is necessary to determine initially how you want to be treated by your immediate superior concerning delegation. This usually means deciding how, as realistically as possible, you need to be treated so that you can fully meet the requirements of your job. What follows after your needs have been defined is the application of the same line of thought to your relationship with each employee in your work group. Constantly envisioning yourself as "in the middle," you can apply a number of considerations to delegation both upward and downward.

## Differing Perspectives

The upward view between adjacent points in the chain of command is not the same as the downward view between those same two points. Looking upward, you are likely to see your superior as a single point of information, advice, and assistance; looking upward, your employees probably see you in the same way. The upward view between adjacent points in the chain of command focuses on a single person, and more often than not that person, an organizational superior, is seen as a source of support. However, the downward view is quite different.

The superior, whether it is you looking downward at your employees or your manager looking downward at you and your peers, sees not one point of contact but several. Furthermore, the superior frequently sees these several points of contact as sources of problems and grief. Every person in the chain of command has one primary upward channel of communication; however, every managerial person in the chain of command has as many primary downward channels as he or she has direct reporting employees.

As the person in the middle of three consecutive points in the chain of command, the supervisor needs to appreciate the differences between the upward perspective and the downward perspective. Therefore, the most constructive view to take when looking up the chain of command is: I am but one of a number of people reporting to this superior, so I need to make it as easy as possible for my superior to communicate with me. Conversely, the downward view suggests: Each of these people who reports to me is looking to me for guidance, so I must show him or her how to relate to me so that I can meet his or her needs as well as possible.

Whether he or she is a rank-and-file employee, a supervisor, or a middle or upper manager, the person looking up the chain of command sees a single point of contact and thus a single and presumably dedicated source of assistance. However, the person looking down the chain of command invariably sees multiple points of contact that, taken together, are capable of making overwhelming demands.

## Not Just Problems, But Solutions

A large part of becoming an effective delegator consists of teaching employees to do their homework before bringing problems and concerns up the chain of command. However, the business of homework, or thorough staff work, as it might be called, can be dealt with both upward and downward by the individual supervisor. The reaction of many employees to the presence of a problem is to take that problem to the boss and ask for advice and assistance. The boss, however, whether it is you or your immediate superior, does not need problems. Rather, the boss needs solutions.

The way not to communicate with one's superior is to say, in effect, "I have a problem and I need your help." Rather, it is necessary to do some homework first: Analyze and isolate the problem, identify causes if possible, develop alternative solutions, and identify specifically what is needed from the boss. Then go to the boss and say, "Here's a problem. This is why I think it's a problem and what probably caused it. Here are two or three possible solutions, and here's the solution I like best and why. This is what I think I need from you in order to proceed. What is your advice?"

To the foregoing the boss often need only answer, "Yes," "No," "Do this," or "Do that." Just as often the problem will be nearly self-solving once you have subjected it to analysis. In any case, you will have made it as easy as possible for the boss to communicate with you, without intruding on the boss's time to analyze the problem and without transferring ownership of the problem to your superior.

In parallel fashion, the supervisor should encourage individual employees to do the same kind of homework to the fullest extent of their abilities. Whether dealing with a specifically delegated task or a problem encountered directly by the employee, the supervisor should instruct the employee in techniques of analyzing and refining everyday problems, offering alternative solutions, and making recommendations. The employee who does the necessary homework does not always relieve the supervisor of sometimes extensive involvement; the supervisor may have input to offer beyond the reach of the employee. However, the employee who does the necessary homework has accepted partial ownership of the problem and has focused the problem so that it can be dealt with more efficiently. At the heart of effective delegation is the need to teach the employees to do as much as possible on their own before calling for help. One highly successful supervisor expressed management's needs well by saying, "Don't bring me more problems, bring me solutions."

### Reasonable Deadlines and Follow-up

Although your superior may be lax with you regarding deadlines and follow-up—no level of management is exempt from such weaknesses—there is no need to be similarly lax with your subordinates. This is another area of supervisory behavior in which you can do much for yourself in improving how you work both upward and downward.

The supervisor who is lax concerning deadlines and follow-up shapes subordinates' expectations accordingly. If the boss says simply, "Take care of this when you can," the subordinate may respond immediately, within days or weeks, or never. And if the superior says, "Let me have this by Friday," but the subordinate knows through past practice that the boss is not likely to mention it again for 2 weeks, it will probably be 2 weeks before the work gets done. Such managers have, through their actions over time, conditioned their employees to expect this kind of behavior. Add to this conditioning the fact that some time-related instructions—"When you get a minute," "Whenever you can," and "Sometime soon"—can mean anything from right this minute to never, depending on the employee's interpretation.

No matter how nonurgent or unimportant it may be, any task that is worth assigning is worth assigning a reasonable deadline. Once a deadline is assigned, regardless of the task's significance, that deadline should never be allowed to pass without some kind of closure taking place. If closure does not occur in the form of delivered results, then the manager who assigned the task and set the deadline should immediately follow up with the employee.

If your manager does not set deadlines for you, set them for yourself. Commit yourself to such deadlines, if possible by promising results to the boss by some given day and time. Do not be too tough on yourself by promising immediate results, but rather allow yourself all reasonable slack. (If your boss is at all fair and effective, he or she will immediately tell you that you are allowing yourself too much or too little time.) If you are unable to deliver when you promised because of circumstances beyond your control, do not wait for the boss to follow up; rather, inform the boss of the delay and its causes.

This notion of applying reasonable deadlines and faithful follow-up is even more important in the supervisor's relationship with the employees in the work group. These are also the steps that ensure the thoroughness and effectiveness of proper delegation. One can assign a thoroughly defined task to a well-instructed employee and still get nothing if there is no specific requirement for completion or follow-up. The supervisor who assigns no deadlines projects a casual attitude toward timely accomplishment of work that can permeate the group. Worse still, if the supervisor usually assigns deadlines but lets them slide by without saying anything, the employees will come to see the supervisor as lax, disorganized, and possibly uncaring. It is this latter condition that is most likely to occur. Apparently, it is easy to assign a deadline when a task is assigned, but it is not quite as easy to remember to follow up on that deadline. Many supervisors fail to follow up on the deadlines they have set, and in doing so, they create credibility problems and other difficulties for themselves.

Assigning reasonable deadlines and following up on them probably represent the areas of performance in which a supervisor can considerably improve his or her managerial effectiveness the most with the least amount of effort. The supervisor can simply set reasonable deadlines for every task that is delegated and faithfully follow up every time a deadline is missed.

## THE PATTERN: THE NUTS AND BOLTS OF DELEGATION

### Select and Organize the Task

As discussed in Chapter 3, your work as a supervisor lends itself to separation into two general categories: technical tasks and managerial tasks. Most of your technical tasks are likely to be subjects for delegation, although there may be a few you should continue to control personally, either because they are of sufficient importance to warrant your personal attention or because they occur so infrequently that any training time you invest would never be paid back. Of your true managerial tasks, however, few if any can be delegated in their entirety.

Most of your pure managerial tasks cannot be delegated; they are among the reasons why you were entrusted with supervisory authority in the first place. For instance, the general personnel management tasks of hiring, firing, promotion, demotion, criticism, discipline, and performance appraisal cannot be delegated. Other managerial activities may lend themselves to partial delegation. For instance, you may obtain staff input and assistance in planning, scheduling, budgeting, purchasing, and other such activities, but the authority to approve, recommend, or implement still calls for the exercise of your supervisory authority.

Take the time to make a list of duties you perform that could reasonably be delegated to an employee. If you consider each workday for a period of weeks, writing down each such task whenever one occurs, you may be surprised at the significant amount of work falling into the category of tasks that can be delegated. Preparing routine reports, answering routine correspondence, preparing service schedules, ordering supplies, serving on certain committees, performing actual patient care or other technical tasks, and many other activities may present themselves as candidates for delegation. List them all, and rank them according to two criteria: the amount of your time they require and their importance to the institution. In short, establish a priority order of tasks for delegation.

Do not, however, attempt to delegate all these nonmanagerial duties at once. Do not even consider working with just two or three of them at the beginning. We are interested in establishing delegation as a habit, and new habits are tough to form.

Pick one task to begin with, preferably that which is either of most importance to the institution or takes the largest part of your time or both. You should plan on delegating a single function, or as much of one as possible, to a single person and thus avoid the situation in which a function is so broken up that no one person is able to develop a sense of the whole job. Also, in considering activities to delegate, concentrate on ongoing functions, on jobs that regularly recur. There is little to be gained by delegating a one-shot activity if you can do it faster and better by yourself.

Determine the specific authority you will have to provide the person to whom you delegate an activity and plan also on defining the limits of that authority. As suggested earlier, operating instructions themselves are often the full "authority" needed to perform a task. However, there are instances in which the person must be able to call on certain resources necessary to do the job. In all cases the authority given should be consistent with the responsibility assigned. For instance, if you make an employee responsible for ordering office supplies you should also give that person authority to sign the necessary purchase requisitions.

Generally, you should consider delegating as much of your technical task authority as possible. Even some of the routine portions of a few of your managerial tasks can be delegated. For example, you can delegate much of the numerical work involved in preparing your departmental budget as long as you maintain final decision-making authority over the complete budget.

**Select the Appropriate Person**

If you happen to be at the second line of management (you supervise one lower level of supervision), keep in mind that when you delegate, it should always be to an immediate subordinate. To bypass that intervening level and delegate directly to an employee two levels below is to undermine the authority of the first-line supervisor. First-line supervisors, however, will not have this problem since all of their employees report directly to them.

Pick the employee you will delegate to by matching the qualifications of available employees with the requirements of the task to be delegated. How well you can do this will depend to a great extent on how well you know your employees' strengths and weaknesses and attitudes and capabilities. For instance, if the task you want to delegate consists of guiding new employees through a department orientation, you should be looking for an employee who knows the rest of the employees well enough to introduce new people to them, knows the department's work well enough to describe it to a newcomer, and is reasonably friendly and adept at conversing with new people. If you wish to delegate a portion of your budget preparation, you should be looking for an employee who appears to have the aptitude for numerical work.

However, it is not enough to simply make a judgmental match between the requirements of the task and what you perceive to be the abilities of the person. Your choice should actually involve additional considerations even more judgmental than the assessment of untested skills. Since the entire process is considerably judgmental, you, personally, need to be as comfortable as possible with your choice. Therefore, you need to consider those of your people whom you believe are probably ready to assume additional responsibility. In short, you need to concentrate on those people you think are sufficiently mature and reliable to give the assignment an honest try.

Beware of either overdelegating or underdelegating. When you overdelegate, the employee to whom you give a task is clearly not ready to handle it. While a modest amount of challenge is certainly desirable, too much challenge can be overwhelming to the employee. Overdelegation frequently leads to an employee's failure in a first attempt at handling increased responsibility, a harsh beginning that is not easily overcome. On the other hand, underdelegation—assigning a task to an employee who is overqualified and can obviously handle it with the greatest of ease—can be fully as damaging. Underdelegation is a waste of an employee's capabilities and often results in that employee's boredom and stagnation. Ideally, delegation should provide a modest amount of challenge, modest but recognizable opportunity for growth, and the opportunity for diversification and expanded usefulness. Also, the employee must be able to see the importance of the delegated task.

You must also be reasonably convinced that the employee you have in mind has the time available to handle the delegated task. Even if person and task are properly matched, you can create a hardship by assigning more work to someone who is already fully occupied.

When selecting an employee to take on a specific task, keep in mind that if delegation is to serve its proper purpose, you, the supervisor, must be willing to accept the employee's decisions as though they were your own.

## Instruct and Motivate the Person

One of the most common errors in delegation is turning an employee loose on a task with inadequate preparation. It is at this point that the pressure of time can set the stage for delegation failure. If the task you are delegating is one you have previously done yourself, and very often this is the case, there may be few instructions, procedures, or guidelines existing in writing. It may be that the only available instructions are those in your mind. In gathering the information you need to turn over a job, it may be necessary for you to put those instructions in writing as well as prepare personally to teach the employee how to do the job.

When you are completely ready to turn a task over to an employee, you should be able to provide satisfactory answers to the following questions:

- Am I prepared to give the reasons for the task, fully explaining why it is important and why it must be done?
- Am I giving the employee sufficient authority to accomplish the results I require?
- Are all the details of the assignment completely clear in my mind?
- If necessary, can I adapt all the instructions and procedural details to the level of the employee's knowledge and understanding?
- Does the assignment include sufficient growth opportunity to motivate the employee appropriately?
- Does the employee have the training, experience, and skills necessary to accomplish the task?
- Are the instructions or procedures sufficiently involved that they should be put in writing?

Assuming that you can answer the foregoing questions satisfactorily, turning a task over to an employee then becomes a critical exercise in two-way communication. When you meet to make the actual assignment, encourage the employee to ask questions. If questions are not readily forthcoming, ask the employee to restate your instructions. Whenever possible, demonstrate those parts of the activity that lend themselves to demonstration and have the employee perform those operations to your satisfaction. Throughout the entire process, emphasize two-way communication.

Last in the process of turning over a task, but extremely important, is the necessity for you and the employee to achieve agreement on the results you expect. The precise methods by which those results are achieved may not be particularly important—several people may do the same task slightly differently—but the anticipated output must be known and agreed upon.

Exhibit 5–1 summarizes the information that should be provided for one person undertaking one delegated task.

## Maintain Reasonable Control

Control of delegation is largely a matter of communication between supervisor and employee. The frequency and intensity of this communication will

**Exhibit 5–1** Information for One Person, One Delegated Task

- Complete definition of the task.
- How long it will last (one-time, some period, forever, etc.).
- When the task starts.
- The results expected.
- How much time it should take.
- How to do it; the procedure.
- What is in it for the employee (motivational aspects).
- The authority assigned.

---

depend significantly on your assessment of the individual. You should know your employees well enough to be able to judge who needs what degree of control and assistance. Your people are bound to be different from each other. Some you may need to check with frequently and monitor their activities with reasonable closeness; with others you may be quite comfortable simply touching base every few days.

Since the degree of control necessary will vary from employee to employee, the hazards of overcontrol or undercontrol are always present. Overcontrol can destroy the effects of delegation. The employee will not develop a sense of responsibility, and you may remain as actively concerned with the task as though you had never delegated it at all. Undercontrol is also hazardous in that the employee may drift significantly in unproductive directions or perhaps make costly or time-consuming errors that you could have helped to avoid.

Having decided the approximate extent of control the individual needs, proceed to set reasonable deadlines for task completion, or for the completion of portions of the task, and prepare to follow up as those deadlines arrive. Two points to be stressed at this stage are: (1) the reasonableness of the deadlines and (2) the timeliness of follow-up. Give the employee plenty of time to do the job, including, if possible, extra time for contingencies. However, when a deadline arrives and you have not been presented with results, take the initiative and go to the employee. You have few, if any, valid reasons for letting a deadline you have set slide quietly past without asking for the results you expected.

Laziness in enforcing deadlines will cause you far more grief than just weakening the effects of delegation. If you let only a few deadlines slide by unmentioned, some employees will automatically adapt to this pattern of behavior and assume that the deadlines you impose are unimportant. On the other hand, if you make it a habit always to follow up on deadlines, your employees will pick up on this pattern and expect you to look for timely results.

Throughout the entire delegation process, try to avoid being a crutch for the employee. Regardless of how much guidance and assistance you are called on to provide, try to avoid solving problems for your employees. Rather, focus on showing your employees how to solve their own problems.

In most instances of delegation failure, the responsibility rests with the supervisor, not with the employee. Some failures are to be expected; delegation is an imperfect, sometimes highly subjective process. However, to keep failures to a minimum you should regularly assess your performance with the following questions:

- Did I assign a task only to take it away before the employee could truly demonstrate any competence at the task?
- Did I maintain too much or too little control?
- Did I split up an activity such that no single person with some authority could develop a sense for the whole?
- Was I overly severe with an employee who made a mistake?
- Am I giving proper credit to the employee for getting the job done?
- Am I keeping the more interesting tasks for myself, delegating only the mundane or unchallenging activities?
- Have I slacked off in my own work as I delegated certain activities, or have I used the time saved to increase my emphasis on managerial activities?

## "IF YOU WANT SOMETHING DONE RIGHT. . ."

Before acknowledging the more obvious errors that John Miller made in turning the report preparation task over to Bill Curtis, first consider Miller's reasons for delegating. Miller would probably say that his primary reason for delegating the report was to save time that he could then spend on other tasks. This is a legitimate reason for delegating, but it should go hand-in-hand with employee development objectives. It is clear that Miller showed no concern for employee development in giving Curtis the report task. Also, a strong and inappropriate reason for handing off the report comes through loud and clear: Miller wants to escape a task that he dislikes. This reason is never a valid one for delegation.

John Miller's significant errors included handing off the task—we can hardly call it delegation at all—without properly preparing the employee. Miller also demeaned the task and clearly indicated that he considered it beneath him. He delegated for his own sole benefit, presented the assignment to Curtis in a negative, demotivating manner, avoided answering Curtis's legitimate questions about the assignment on multiple occasions, and generally set the employee up for failure.

Never having put his procedure for preparing the report in writing, Miller was not in a favorable position for suddenly deciding to assign the job to someone else. What he should have done was complete the current report alone as he usually did, then commit the procedure to writing and prepare to do the next report jointly with Curtis.

Miller presented the assignment to Curtis as though he was dumping an unpleasant chore that required little skill or intelligence. He should actually have presented the task in a positive way as recognition of Curtis's abilities and an expansion of his responsibilities. Based on his knowledge of Curtis's work style and his capacity for learning, Miller might then have effectively presented his newly written procedure along with copies of past reports and then should have gone through the procedure with Curtis or encouraged him to go over it himself and ask questions as necessary.

We can, of course, infer that Miller waited until the report was almost due before assigning it to Curtis. Curtis was deserving of more time to do the job, as well as some knowledgeable assistance in learning how to do it.

Finally, but certainly not least in importance, the report format should have been altered to allow Curtis to sign his work, perhaps with Miller's signature of approval. Task ownership and the opportunity for recognition are crucial in effective delegation.

## AUTHORITY AND RESPONSIBILITY

From time to time you are likely to encounter a difference of opinion as to which is truly delegated: authority or responsibility. In some contexts it is correct to speak of delegation of responsibility, authority, or both. To be strictly correct, however, when you speak of delegation—the assignment of work to an employee—you are talking exclusively about the delegation of authority.

Think of the authority of your position as a physical object that can be cut up and distributed. Your authority is like a pie; you cut out a piece and give it to someone. The chunk of authority necessary to perform that work used to be yours; now it belongs to someone else (although you can take it back at any time). This is delegated authority.

Responsibility, however, is quite another matter. The analogy of the pie does not apply to responsibility. The only workable analogy that comes to mind is in the character of the one-celled creature, the amoeba. When the amoeba subdivides it becomes two one-celled creatures, each equivalent to the other. In delegating the authority to perform a task you make the employee responsible for task completion. However, you remain responsible to your supervisor for the completion of that task. Thus authority is actually delegated, but responsibility is simply duplicated at a lower organizational level.

## FREEDOM TO FAIL

When an employee fails in the performance of a delegated task, the failure is often shared. Sometimes the failure is largely the employee's, for doing something incorrectly or for not following instructions, but many times the fault lies with the supervisor in bringing task and person together and in providing direction and support. Since failures at delegation must be shared, and since we all learn from our failures often far more than we learn from our successes, punishing or overcorrecting an employee who makes a mistake makes little sense. Criticism should, of course, be delivered when deserved, but it should always be constructive and include the means for correcting the errant behavior and avoiding a repetition of the problem. In many patient care situations there is no room for error and thus little, if any, room for the tolerance of mistakes. However, in nonpatient care functions, and in many support and administrative activities, there is indeed room for errors, and they occur frequently.

The employee who is soundly taken to task for making a mistake while exercising reasonable individual initiative will likely shy away from exercising further initiative for fear of punishment. Errors are a natural part of career growth, and we might say that the employee who never makes a mistake is not growing much. This employee—and especially the supervisor who never makes a mistake—is the one who never exercises initiative or tries anything new or different.

A decision to delegate is, at best, a calculated risk. You should be willing to take that risk. After all, you do not know for certain about an employee's capability until you have given that person a chance with an actual assignment.

You should feel a strong incentive to practice delegation. As suggested earlier, you cannot always expect to do everything of importance yourself. However, you should also feel the incentive to exercise reasonable control over the delegation process. Since you cannot shed final responsibility for task performance, you will be held responsible for any serious mistakes the employee may make. Your knowledge of this retained responsibility can be frightening at times, but to function as an effective supervisor you need to recognize the necessity to delegate to get things done through people.

## BUILDING THE HABIT

You begin to build the delegation habit by concentrating on a single activity at a time, working with one employee until that activity has been completely incorporated as a part of the person's job. Proceeding in this fashion, one activity at a time, it may take you a long time to make significant progress with the list of activities you decided you could delegate. However, this methodical approach, conscientiously pursued, is the surest way to learn delegation as a true habit.

Incomplete or improper delegation is an undesirable habit and as such can be difficult to alter. However, the practice of proper delegation, once substituted for your old habits, is itself a strong, useful habit that will serve you well throughout your management career. And you can assure yourself that, having delegated properly, you have empowered.

---

## REVIEW QUESTIONS

1. Differentiate between the *process* and the *condition* of delegation.
2. Why is it essential in delegation to provide both responsibility and authority in equivalent amounts?
3. What is the primary reason for failing to delegate properly, and why is overcoming this barrier difficult for so many people?
4. Cite three reasons why failure to delegate can be harmful to the employees in the group.

5. List the steps in the basic delegation pattern.
6. Why is the supposed *freedom to fail* important?

---

### EXERCISE: TO WHOM SHOULD YOU DELEGATE?

Eight of your staff members are briefly described as follows:

1. Arthur is technically competent, seems to communicate clearly, especially in writing, and pays attention to details.
2. Carol has consistently shown good judgment in matters of finance, particularly in analyzing reports and statements for financial implications.
3. Kate is a dependable employee. Young and fairly new to the institution, she nevertheless appears ready to handle increased responsibility.
4. By both credentials and experience, Harry is your most technically qualified employee.
5. Fred is low key, polite, and a diplomatic "people person." He is clearly your best letter writer.
6. Millie is an empathic individual. People are generally comfortable with her and inclined to speak freely.
7. Ed has displayed both technical and managerial skills. He has successfully run several special projects.
8. Elaine is an organizer. Few if any details of arranging a gathering of people escape her attention.

The functions you can delegate to your employees include the following:

a. Provide technical support on a special hospitalwide study.
b. Manage the special study, including responsibility for technical content.
c. Schedule and organize periodic project review meetings.
d. Review and approve all correspondence relating to the special study.
e. Analyze and approve all expense reports relating to the special study.
f. Write monthly status and progress reports for the special study.
g. Answer all inquiries concerning certain activities of your department and the hospital itself.
h. Locate and screen applicants for potential employment in the department.
i. Requisition standard supplies for the office and assure that the supply room is adequately stocked.

### Instructions

Create a possible pattern of delegation by matching employees and assignments in a manner that appears to make best use of each person's capabilities. Note that there are more assignments than people and that any one person may be capable of taking on more than one of the assignments. (Caution:

Avoid overdelegation—assigning an employee a job for which he or she is probably not qualified.)

|   | | |   | |
|---|---|---|---|---|
| ____ | 1. | Arthur | ____5. | Fred |
| ____ | 2. | Carol | ____6. | Millie |
| ____ | 3. | Kate | ____7. | Ed |
| ____ | 4. | Harry | ____8. | Elaine |

---

**NOTES**

1. M. McCutcheon, *Roget's Super Thesaurus,* 2nd Edition, Writer's Digest Books, F & W Publications, Inc., Cincinnati, Ohio, p. 161, 205.

2. R. Townsend, *Further Up the Organization* (New York: Alfred A. Knopf, Inc., 1984): 53.

## CHAPTER 6

# Time Management: Expanding the Day without Stretching the Clock

*Time is fixed income and, as with any income, the real problem facing most of us is how to live successfully within our daily allotment.*
*—Margaret B. Johnstone*

## CHAPTER OBJECTIVES

☛ Place "time" in perspective as an unrenewable resource that influences all supervisory activity.

☛ Identify the common time-wasting practices encountered in organized work activity.

☛ Identify delegation and planning as key considerations in the supervisor's effective use of time.

☛ Offer practical suggestions to apply in improving one's effective use of available time.

☛ Briefly explore the relationship between time management and stress management.

☛ Isolate the sources of time-wasting pressure inherent in the organizational environment and suggest the supervisor's appropriate response to these pressures.

## SITUATION: THE MANAGER AND THE SALES REPRESENTATIVE

As the door closed behind her departing visitor, Janet Mills, central supply manager, glumly reflected that she had just lost an hour that she could ill afford to lose. She would either have to forego the schedule she was working on or be late for an upcoming meeting.

The hour had been lost because of a surprise visit from a pleasant but marginally aggressive sales representative trying to convince her to try "the greatest little thing ever to come along in this business." Janet, as was her practice, consented to see the representative although she resented the intrusion.

This incident, occurring on a Friday, made Janet realize that she had lost time to four such drop-in visits this week alone. She did not like the idea of simply saying no or otherwise trying to avoid people who wanted to see her, but she was becoming more aware that her work was beginning to suffer because of such demands on her time.

*Instructions*

As you proceed through the chapter, develop some workable guidelines that might help Janet and other managers deal with the problem of drop-in visitors.

## TIME AND TIME AGAIN

Time is, for all of us, a resource of considerable value. Moreover, time is always moving, always going forward regardless of whether we are putting it to some specific use. Dream though we may, we cannot call back a single minute that has gone by.

In addition to being self-consuming, time is a resource that is fixed in amount. There are just so many minutes in an hour and so many hours in a day, but although time is limited, for all practical purposes the demands on our time are open ended.

We have heard all our lives that "time is money." To many people in business, time well spent is the difference between loss and profit. To providers of all kinds of service, time wasted is a waste of cash resources, since salaries and expenses go on even when service is not being rendered. Further, to the health care professional, time is often a critical factor in the fulfillment of the institution's objectives to preserve life and improve health.

In this chapter we will begin with the assumption that few of us, no matter how organized and efficient we may be, could not improve our use of some of the working time available to us.

Supervisors are often ruled by the demands of the job. It may seem as though the work and the hours rarely come out even, there being considerably more of the former than the latter. Supervisors react to this disparity in various ways. At one extreme is the supervisor who continually stays late in an effort to get "caught up," a state that seems never to arrive. This approach is not the answer, and neither is the answer found in the other extreme—walking out the door at quitting time although many problems remain to be solved. Certainly there are days when extra time and effort are the only answer, but when this is relied on as a regular solution it simply turns a full-time job into a full-and-a-half-time job without truly improving the way the department runs.

With exceptions occasionally necessary, the place to begin improving performance is in the use of our regularly scheduled job time. We owe it to ourselves, and certainly to our employers, to get more out of each day by putting more of the proper effort into each day.

Task performance aside, consider where much of the working time goes for many people. Late starts, slow starts, long breaks, long lunches, and especially periods of social conversation are part of many people's working style—supervisors and nonsupervisors alike. Although personal considerations and social relationships are important in a work environment, few people realize the extent to which these things cut into the time for which they are being paid to perform certain duties. Many a supervisor has stretched a coffee break into a half hour while complaining of how much work there was to be done.

Aside from out-and-out nonproductive activity, however, a great deal of time is wasted in the ways we approach supposedly legitimate tasks. After enumerating a few good reasons for becoming more conscious of how we spend our available time, we will briefly highlight the readily identifiable time wasters and offer suggestions for incorporating time savers into our behavior.

## WHY BECOME MORE TIME CONSCIOUS?

The individual reader might logically follow the title question of this section—*Why become more time conscious?*—with a perfectly legitimate personal question: What's in it for me? Everyone who makes a serious effort to become more time conscious and improve his or her use of time stands to gain in a number of dimensions. What's in it for the individual includes:

*A greater level of job satisfaction.* When you successfully manage your time to the extent of getting more done in the time available and increasing the degree of control you hold over the work, you are bound to feel more satisfied with your job.

*Increased productivity.* Multiple benefits result when you manage your time to the extent of getting more useful work done. As noted above, you are likely to feel greater job satisfaction. And your department and organization and their various customers benefit from your increased output.

*Better interpersonal relations.* Improving your use of time increases your output and encourages a more organized and less stressful—less of a firefighting or seat-of-the-pants—approach to the job. The resulting atmosphere of order and control makes for cooler heads and calmer tempers.

*Improved future possibilities.* The individual who has mastered personal time management will exhibit a number of characteristics, including successful delegating and generally running a productive department with a stable, satisfied workforce, that enhance his or her chances for promotion.

*Less job-related stress.* As your use of time becomes more effective, the stress experienced on the job—and off the job, should you be one of the many who cannot help but carry their problems home—diminishes. And as stress diminishes for the supervisor, so is it also likely to diminish for the employees.

*Enhanced health.* We are all aware that the job-related stress wrought by long work hours, endless critical problems, and contentious interpersonal relations can have negative effects on one's health. Improving the use of time can serve to enhance or protect one's health.

The foregoing reasons for becoming more time conscious (summarized in Exhibit 6–1) are, of course, significantly interrelated. For example, increased productivity is likely to be accompanied by greater job satisfaction, and reduced stress and enhanced health ordinarily go hand-in-hand. Overall, however, they add up to a powerful argument for becoming more time conscious.

---

**Exhibit 6–1** The Benefits of Becoming More Time Conscious

- Increased job satisfaction
- Increased productivity
- Improved interpersonal relations
- Better future direction
- Reduced stress
- Enhanced health

## THE TIME WASTERS

### Failure to Delegate

Failure to delegate thoroughly and effectively is one of the greatest time wasters to which a supervisor can fall victim. We will not repeat the cautions of Chapter 5 but will simply remind you of the importance of remaining open to delegation possibilities.

### Failure to Plan and Establish Priorities

You may have heard the term traffic-cop management or perhaps firefighting management. These describe a common approach to supervision: very little looking ahead and not much consideration given to deciding which of a number of tasks is most important. It is usually the problem of the moment that gets the attention or the people making the most noise who get heard. A supervisor can be extremely busy practicing this form of management but can nevertheless be wasting significant amounts of time. Without some rationale for approaching work in a manner consistent with its necessity, tasks of lesser importance consume disproportionate amounts of time while more important tasks are handled too quickly or not at all.

### Overplanning and Overorganizing

Overplanning and overorganizing are two common traps that many people fall into when making what they believe are conscientious efforts to improve their use of time. Because they hear so much about the necessity of planning and the importance of being organized, some supervisors tend to overcompensate for their self-perceived weaknesses by going overboard with plans, task lists, schemes of objectives and subobjectives, and open files, active files, tickler files, dead files, and so on.

We could insert here a psychological treatise exploring the possible reasons behind the tendency to overplan and overorganize. These reasons would probably include avoidance of unpleasant tasks (planning is "good," and while one is busy planning one does not have to be doing), a sense of insecurity, uncertainty concerning how superiors will deal with mistakes, and a fear of failure. Whatever the reasons, a supervisor's personal planning and organizing become time wasters when they occur to excess.

What is excess planning and organizing? Only you know for certain how much is adequate for you and when you are overplanning and overorganizing. But a few examples are clear. Consider the manager who maintained his calendar in duplicate—one a full-size loose-leaf binder and one a version that would fit into a pocket. When asked bluntly by another manager why he maintained duplicate calendars, he could say only that he especially liked the features of the desktop book but that it was too large to carry around conveniently. Thus nudged into thinking about what he had been doing, the manager realized that the effort of maintaining duplicate calendars was not worth the minimal benefit gained.

Many managers engage in many activities that are not worth the benefit or convenience gained. If we update a To Do list daily, fine; but if every day sees the To Do lists—plural, because there are lists A, B, C or 1, 2, 3—revamped, reworked, and reordered, then time is being wasted. And if we are "organized" to the extent, for example, that a task is pulled from the To Do folder, stuck in the Active or Open file, and advanced through three or four other stages, each with its own name and filing system, then organizing has become overorganizing.

Planning and personal organizing are surely important. However, both of these virtues can become excesses. Quite simply, even the noble pursuit of planning should be kept consistent with the expected results. That is, never pour a dollar's worth of effort into assuring a two-bit payback.

### Face-to-Face Contacts

Face-to-face contacts represent the essence of a supervisor's job. However, one-on-one situations readily get out of hand and waste our time.

Aside from social conversation, which you should be able to control within reason, you will experience numerous interruptions during your workday. How you handle these interruptions will influence the degree of effectiveness with which you use your available time. For instance, the last time a salesperson was in the neighborhood and dropped in unannounced, did you drop something else for a meeting? Or the last time you were talking business with one of your employees, did you allow another employee or fellow supervisor who wanted your attention for a moment to interrupt? In short, do you usually give in to the pressures of interruptions and unexpected visits? Other people will readily waste your time if you allow them to do so.

### The Telephone

One of the most useful facilitators of communication ever devised, the telephone, can also be one of the greatest time wasters. The telephone can be of considerable value when effectively controlled, but often the tendency is to allow it to control us.

### The Computer

The personal computer has done more to alter work methods and procedures than any other innovation of the past two to three decades. Computers have replaced typewriters and other office machines almost completely, and they have dramatically changed the way many jobs are performed. Unfortunately, the desktop computer has also opened wide a door to a variety of time-wasting personal uses including games and nonbusiness e-mail (personal correspondence, jokes, inspirational messages, anecdotes, etc.). It is not unreasonable to conclude that much of the efficiency gained through computer use is cancelled out by computer misuse.

## Meetings

Like the telephone and the computer, the meeting is another means of communication that is misused and abused to the extent that its effects are often the reverse of what was intended.

Sometimes it seems as though the modern health care organization runs on meetings, and this appearance might seem to justify the need for more and longer meetings in which to conduct business. However, close analysis of all but a scant few of our meetings will reveal significant wasted time. We will not claim that most of our meetings are unnecessary, although some certainly are, but rather that the majority of meetings are too long relative to the results they produce and too loosely approached to be truly effective.

## Paperwork

Many supervisors must feel as though the in-basket is like the magic pitcher in the children's story of many years ago—no matter how much you took from it, it was always full. We seem never to be caught up on paperwork, and the supervisor who conscientiously tries to keep the in-basket current usually discovers this cuts into time needed for more important tasks.

Like many other activities, paperwork can be essential as well as wasteful. It becomes a time waster when some things get done at the expense of others, items of minor consequence get attention while important items remain in the stack, and items that should be ignored receive attention simply because they are there.

## Personal Habits

Whether you waste significant amounts of time on the activities mentioned above will depend largely on the habits you have formed regarding these activities. You can, for instance, allow your meetings to be loose and rambling simply out of habit—you may have always worked that way, following the path of least resistance.

Beyond your approach to specific activities, however, there is your overall pattern of behavior to consider. Are you perhaps a slow starter, entering the day with an hour's worth of coffee and procrastination until you take hold and begin to produce? Are you in the habit of jumping from task to task, starting many jobs but completing few? When you reach a point in a task when you need information and assistance from others, do you simply stop and wait for them rather than fill your waiting time with productive effort?

For good or for ill, unless you exercise conscious control, your approach to your daily duties will be governed largely by your personal habits.

## THE TIME SAVERS

## Plans and Priorities

To get control of your time, you must first determine what must be done and in what order things should be accomplished. The process of planning and setting priorities, along with the practice of proper delegation, is a major force in the productive use of time. Volumes have been written about planning, but for our purposes some simple suggestions will provide an effective basis for a solid start in supervisory planning.

### Determine How You Really Spend Your Time

Make the decision to analyze critically your use of time to determine if you are really using most of your time wisely. To perform this analysis honestly, a degree of commitment is necessary, and it may also be necessary to accept the likelihood of sacrificing some old habits for the sake of self-improvement.

Check up on yourself. For some period of time (at least 2 weeks but preferably 3 or 4 weeks) keep a record of how you spend your time. This need not be an elaborate scheme in which you write down every 30-second task or record your activities down to the minute. Rather, reasonable entries might look like: weekly staff meeting—90 minutes; interview prospective employee—30 minutes; and prepare monthly statistical report—3 hours.

When you have sufficient information to work with, sort the results and determine the approximate portion of your time spent on routine tasks, unscheduled tasks, and tasks that could be considered emergencies. Routine tasks are those you do on a regular basis, for instance, daily, weekly, or monthly. They are routine in that you know what they are and approximately when they occur. An unscheduled task is one for which you know the what but not the when. For instance, you may know there will be times when you have to write an incident report because of an accident or complaint, but you have no way of knowing when this will occur. An emergency task is one for which you know neither what nor when; you simply know that unplanned events occur and you must respond.

When you have finished analyzing your time record, you should know most of the things you do and the approximate portion of your time spent on routine, unscheduled, and emergency tasks. Further, you should be able to tell which of your tasks are likely candidates for delegation.

One of the first useful pieces of information gained from this process is an appreciation of how much of your time on average goes to emergencies—tasks for which you are aware of neither the "what" nor the "when" in advance. If you are the average supervisor (if there is indeed such a person), you will find a surprisingly high percentage of your time consumed by emergency tasks. Although you cannot ordinarily avoid these tasks, especially those falling clearly within your responsibility, you can learn enough to enable you to allow for them in your planning. For example, if your three-way analysis of several weeks' activity suggests that you spend an average of 35 percent of your time on so-called emergency tasks, then on average you should leave that much of your time flexible to meet emergencies rather than scheduling yourself to the hilt with known work.

Although you cannot do much about emergency tasks—you cannot avoid them, and you certainly cannot plan in advance for their accomplishment—you can maintain flexibility in your scheduling and, whenever possible, allow extra time for the unexpected.

When you have eliminated from consideration those tasks you can delegate, you are left with a number of activities, routine tasks as well as unscheduled tasks, that have recently reached you in the form of demands. The next stage of your planning involves determining how you will approach the tasks you must perform.

### A Personal Planning Gimmick

You may have heard the following suggestion before, but its enduring applicability makes it worth repeating here.

Of the tasks you know you must personally perform within the coming few days, write down in list form the four or five you consider most important. Then spend a few minutes putting these tasks into their order of importance; that is, task number one should be the first task you must accomplish. The result should be a list of the several most important jobs you must do and the order in which they must be done.

The approach is simple: go to work on number one and stay on it until it is done. Granted you may be pulled away for an emergency; however, when the emergency is over, get immediately back to task number one. Turn away all other interruptions, and do not allow your efforts to be diverted. When task number one is completed, move on to task number two and tackle it the same way. You may not get through your entire list as quickly as you would like, but rest assured you will have accomplished more than if you had attacked these several tasks in any other manner. Also, when working this way you are always at work on the most important task of the moment.

Do not forget to allow yourself some planning time. The planning process is essential, urging you to think ahead and establish priorities and determine direction before proceeding. A plan as such need not be elaborate—perhaps a list on your calendar of four or five items to tackle tomorrow. However, the time you devote to planning will ordinarily pay itself back in improved efficiency several times over.

### Set Objectives and Work to Deadlines

It always pays to be working toward a specific objective, whether that objective is the completion of your most important open task or simply the completion of a particular part of a larger task. You need to know where you intend to go; it has often been said that if you plan on going nowhere, that is where you will go.

Any objective, whether organizational, departmental, or personal, should consist of what is to be done, how much is to be accomplished, and when it should be completed. For instance, one of your objectives may be to complete the performance appraisals (what) for all five nursing assistants in the unit (how much) by the end of Wednesday (when).

Related to the when portion of any objective, even if there are no outside time limits, be sure to set a deadline for yourself. As for any deadline for an employee, make your self-imposed deadline reasonable and stick to it.

### Write It Down—and Change It

Even if you are used to doing your day-to-day task planning in your head, commit your plans to paper. Your plan may, and usually should, be extremely simple: a few lines on a desk pad, perhaps a few entries in a pocket notebook. Make sure that your tasks, priorities, objectives, and deadlines exist in writing in a place where you will see them frequently.

However, simply noting 2 or 3 days' planned activity in writing does not guarantee that you will be able to follow the plan as written. Each time some unforeseen event intrudes on your activity and upsets your plan, take the new requirement into account and revise your written plan. Get in the habit of spending a few minutes at the end of each day planning for the following day; at that time you can revise your plan to reflect current needs.

### Face-to-Face Contacts

Face-to-face contacts were described earlier as often being significant time wasters. They need not be such if approached properly.

The biggest waste of time in face-to-face contact is found in the tendency to engage in excessive small talk and social conversation when we should be dealing with business. We are not suggesting that social conversation should be taboo; a certain amount is essential to morale and supportive of good interpersonal relations. However, business can also be conducted on a friendly level, and beyond minor social pleasantries you should make an effort to stay on business in contacts with employees and coworkers.

Much of the supervisor's most important work takes place within the context of the one-to-one relationship with each employee, and developing that relationship with each employee is recognized as one of the supervisor's most important tasks. It is not at all suggested that supervisors minimize contacts with employees or that each contact necessarily advances the business of the department. Listening to a troubled employee may take an hour without apparently advancing the work of the department at all, but the time is well spent if it results in upholding the morale and productivity of the employee. However, talking baseball for an hour with an employee who happens to be an enthusiastic fan and who brings up the topic at every turn is a clear waste of time.

While you should not allow employees to waste your time, neither should you waste their time by delaying them for irrelevancies and nonessentials simply because you happen to be the boss. One of your primary functions is to enhance your employees' ability to accomplish their assigned tasks, and you are not doing this if you are wasting their time.

Another form of face-to-face contact that frequently wastes time consists of the unannounced drop-in visits of salespersons or others from outside the institution. If you get a significant number of such visitors, your productivity will suffer. Visitors from outside, especially salespeople, will adopt the practice of "just dropping by" once they have discovered, after a visit or two, that you will always stop what you are doing to meet with them. However, it takes little effort to refuse politely to see a drop-in visitor, and once you begin to ask for advance warning or scheduled appointments these visits are likely to diminish in frequency or cease entirely.

In the opening Situation, for example, it is stated that Janet Mills "did not like saying no" to people who wanted to see her. In all likelihood the "marginally aggressive sales representative" who cost her an hour she could not afford to lose had learned that Janet would stop what she was doing to meet with unscheduled visitors.

Most health care organizations of any appreciable size try to restrict individual managers' dealings with sales representatives. In many places it is policy to have all outside sales people contact the purchasing department while the department managers deal with purchasing for their needs. If such a policy is in place at Janet's hospital she needs to tell drop-in sales representatives that they must deal with purchasing. If there is no such policy, Janet might suggest that one be put in place.

Therefore, in addressing the problem of drop-in visitors overall Janet should consider the following:

- Refer outside sales representatives to the appropriate point, usually the purchasing department.
- Have potential visitors screened, if her department has a receptionist or other point of control. In fulfilling her job responsibilities Janet has the right to determine whom she needs to see and whom she does not need to see.
- Have the person make an appointment for a more convenient time, if the drop-in visitor is someone with whom she would like to talk.
- Learn to control largely social conversations with other employees who will readily "visit" if allowed without being abrupt or unpleasant.
- Take control of her own job, which means controlling her own time. Her work will continue to suffer unless she learns to say no. She has no cause to feel guilty for not allowing an interruption that threatens to interfere with her priorities and disrupt her day.

## The Telephone

How we make or take telephone calls will determine the extent to which the telephone rules our activities and consumes excessive amounts of time. Granted there are many times when you cannot avoid a telephone interruption. However, many of your calls are controllable with a little effort, although the extent to which you can control calls will vary according to your particular office situation and the features of your organization's telephone system.

When it is possible to do so—that is, when there is a person available to take and screen your calls—and when interruptions would be harmful to what you are trying to accomplish, have incoming telephone calls held. This is especially relevant when you are involved in important personal contacts such as selection interviews, performance appraisal conferences, disciplinary conferences, and employee counseling sessions. Taking nonurgent calls in such circumstances can waste yours and others' time and can lessen the quality of the activity by disrupting a possibly difficult and sensitive interchange. If you are able, at such times have your calls screened and sorted, with whoever is answering for you taking messages and putting through only genuinely urgent calls.

Needless to say, you should never interrupt a meeting with another person to make or return a call simply because you happened to remember the need just then. A surprising number of managers will do just that in the presence of an employee or perhaps a peer (although even the most inconsiderate manager would rarely do so in the presence of a superior). If you happen to remember a call you should have made, make a quick note and follow up after your present meeting.

Simple call forwarding, a feature of most business telephone systems, can be helpful. If nobody will answer your telephone for an extended period—say for a week of vacation or even a day away at a conference—arrange to forward your calls to someone who will be available to take messages.

When you make telephone calls, for all but the simplest messages it is helpful to spend a few seconds organizing your thoughts before you dial. Jot down the points you need to cover, and have these and any necessary references and notetaking materials handy. Otherwise, you are likely to prolong a call unnecessarily only to remember after ending the conversation that there was something else important that you should have mentioned.

As you return to your desk at various times during the day and find calls you have to return, do not always feel it is necessary to return every call then and there. Urgent calls, of course, should be returned at once; however, routine call-backs are most appropriately handled if you pick one particular time of day to do most of your telephoning and go through all possible calls at a single sitting. For someone who works the day shift, the best time is usually from early or mid afternoon until the end of the workday. (This time is a bit more restricted for nursing supervisors, since there is usually a shift report to contend with in the last 30 to 45 minutes before the end of the day shift.) Conversely, the noon hour is probably the worst time to return telephone calls because half of the working world is usually out to lunch.

If your organization happens to be one of the many with a voice mail system, you may find that this technology can be used to your benefit, especially if you do not have the services of someone to answer your telephone. Voice mail provides the capacity for leaving and receiving detailed messages. Properly used, it can save additional calls and reduce the incidence of "telephone tag." You can frequently get a question answered successfully without ever having connected "live" with the other party. Voice mail also catches calls coming in while you are already on your telephone.

If you utilize voice mail, however, utilize it properly. That is, make the greeting you leave on your line pertinent to your present circumstances. Do not, for example, let your usual "I'll return your call soon" greeting remain in place if you happen to be away on vacation. Customize your greeting to the extent that callers will know how and when their needs will be addressed.

Like any other technology, voice mail has its downside. Many people remain resistant to "talking with a computer" and will simply hang up when greeted with a recorded message as they also do with simple answering machines. It is not coincidental that more than a few people who remain resistant to using voice mail on their own telephones are also resistant to using computers in their work. Voice mail can, of course, be used to simply dodge telephone calls when one does not wish to answer. Properly used, however, voice mail can help you use time more effectively.

Use the telephone wisely and it can be one of the best time savers available to you. However, let the telephone use you and you will suffer through lost efficiency and reduced effectiveness.

## Meetings

The subject of meetings is of sufficient importance to warrant a chapter of its own (see Chapter 20). At this point, suffice it to say that meetings should be held only when necessary, planned and organized with specific purposes in mind, started on time whenever possible, kept to the subject, and allowed to consume only the amount of time required to accomplish their specific objectives.

## Paperwork

We suggested earlier that it was all too easy to allow the in-basket to control much of our time. Although we all receive much material deserving attention and action, not everything that comes in is of equal importance.

When you are faced with 1 or 2 days' accumulation of incoming material—and for some health care supervisors this can be a significant amount of paper—rather than simply working on the basket from the top down (or bottom up, for that matter), first sort all the paper into three categories.

Your first category should consist of those few items that genuinely deserve your immediate attention and those that, although not urgent, you can dispose of by noting a quick word or sentence in response. Your second category should include those items that will take you some time to resolve because they require research or extended effort and noncritical items that you can afford to resolve at your leisure. Some of the items you put in this category may become part of your workload of routine or unscheduled tasks and should be worked into your priority planning. Also, a few items in this pile may be clear candidates for delegation. As you come across these, you should be making some tentative decision as to who might be able to handle them.

The third category of incoming material, and often the largest stack, consists of items you can safely discard. Resist the temptation to file every seminar announcement or advertising brochure that comes in; this kind of material, especially vendor information, rapidly becomes out of date. When you later wish to investigate a certain line of supplies or equipment, your purchasing department should be able to come up with current information. Simply screen all this material for topics of special interest, pass along things you think may be of interest to someone else, and throw away the rest. Rest assured; it is more than 99.9 percent certain that the fancy brochure in today's mail will never be more than office clutter or file cabinet filler should you keep it.

## TIME MANAGEMENT AND STRESS MANAGEMENT: INSEPARABLE ACTIVITIES

The causes of stress that can potentially affect the health care manager are many and varied, and stress management is itself a broad area of study that commands entire volumes. Stress arises from conflicts among the roles of the manager, for example, being a leader as well as member of group, having responsibility for output as well as responsibility for employees, being a coach and counselor as well as disciplinarian, and so on. Stress also arises from changes in one's personal circumstances as well as in the requirements of the managerial position and the circumstances of the employer (e.g., layoffs, mergers, new leadership, and such). The stress a person experiences often has at least part of its origins in the individual's personality; clearly, some people cope more effectively than others. There are many factors and conditions that can trigger stress reactions.

Stress arises from work activity in a number of ways including the following:

- Emergency tasks arise, forcing rapid changes in priorities.
- Work piles up so there seems to be no way to get caught up; the backlog seems to get larger all the time.
- Demanding superiors exert additional pressure downward with more assignments, changing priorities, and tighter deadlines.
- Problems arise with employees, perhaps necessitating disciplinary action (difficult and thus stressful for many managers).
- One attempts to do everything that needs to be done but falls short of covering all the bases.
- One experiences a growing feeling of working in the midst of disorganization and confusion.
- One is adversely affected (as are some) by working in an environment in which one is regularly exposed to illness, pain, trauma, and even death.

One of the key words to apply in this brief discussion of stress is *control*. The foregoing several examples of management stress inducers carry with them a sense of loss of control of the job. A manager who has essentially lost control of his or her job is simply swept along with the current, feeling helpless to do more than just remain afloat, and is ultimately susceptible to the physical and psychological problems that prolonged stress can cause or aggravate.

What many of the stress inducers constitute is a sense of too much to do and too little time in which to do it, thus the sense of loss of control. Effective time management is one available means of gaining a measure of control over the job. It may not be the sole solution to the stress experienced by some managers, but it can go a long way toward reducing or relieving at least part of the stress. With effective time management, the pressure of too much to do in too little time is reduced and a measure of control is gained; therefore, stress is reduced. We learn control is possible and that we have a fundamental choice concerning control of the job: We can elect to control our jobs, or we can allow our jobs to control us.

Time management, therefore, is an important element of stress management. By no means is it all of stress management, but it is invariably true that the manager who effectively manages time will experience less stress—and get more done—than the manager who does not.

## TIME-WASTING PRESSURES AND THE SUPERVISOR'S RESPONSE

Time-wasting pressures come toward the supervisor from every direction. Your choice is simple: Give with pressures and bend in the direction they take you, or become a positive force, refusing to bend, and influence others in productive directions. Time-wasting pressures are likely to come from a number of sources.

### Your Boss

At times it seems as though higher management is insensitive to the demands on your time. It seems this way especially when you already feel overloaded and the boss comes along with something else for you to do. However, the manager who places more work with an already overburdened supervisor is not necessarily being insensitive—remember, your boss sits at a different organizational level and does not have full knowledge of everything you have to do. You are the only one who can truly say if the new assignment you were just handed is too much. Depending on your relationship with your immediate superior, perhaps you need not simply accept that new assignment when you are short of time to begin with. Speak up. Let the boss know where you stand in terms of workload and that you do not have time to do it properly. Talk it over; your boss needs two-way communication with you as surely as you need it with your employees. Chances are you will be able to work out something—a compromise, perhaps, or a reordering of priorities that will serve both the manager's purposes and yours. There may be many times when the boss will not really know how much you have to do unless you say so.

### The System

In most work environments, inefficient practices prevail to some extent. In many organizations such practices are rampant. If it seems you are surrounded by people who are disorganized, careless, and always late, then you will be under pressure to behave in the same manner. However, no organizational system was ever made better without someone taking the initiative to start improving one small section first. A few supervisors who are determined not to give in to the time-wasting pressure of the system can begin to apply positive pressure that will eventually be felt beyond their own departments.

### Your Employees

Time-wasting pressure will frequently come from your employees, especially those who may be insensitive to the true requirements of your position. It is true that you are there to help your employees and "run interference" for them. However, you may have many employees, but some of them may see you only in terms of their individual needs. Some supervisors have found they could spend most of their time in unnecessary handholding if they gave way to the pressure. (However, in all fairness to the employees who seem to require handholding, if this pressure is widespread in your department then many elements of your approach to supervision need examination.)

### Yourself

This area is, of course, largely what we have been talking about in this chapter. Inefficient planning, poor approaches to delegation, and poor personal work habits can produce the subtlest and yet the most wasteful pressures of all because they originate with you. Only you can eliminate them.

### THE UNRENEWABLE RESOURCE

Time is a resource you cannot replace. Once an amount of time is used, it is gone forever; if it is not used, it is still gone.

As a supervisor, when you do not spend your time effectively you are not simply wasting your own time. In most instances you are also wasting the time of your employees. Conversely, any time you save may be effective in saving time for some or all of the employees in your department.

In the management of your time, you should most certainly be interested in doing a sufficient amount of planning to ensure that you and your employees do things right. However, even more important is your constant awareness of priorities; you must strive for assurance that you and your employees are doing the right things as well as doing things right.

As far as your use of time is concerned, in the final analysis there are but two options: control your time, or it will control you.

---

### REVIEW QUESTIONS

- What do we mean by the statement: *It takes time to save time*?
- Explain why failure to delegate is often a significant—if not the greatest—waste of a manager's time.
- Explain what is meant by *overplanning*.
- Why should you look at yourself for sources of wasted time and potential improvement?
- What is the principal objective in making a daily list to guide your activities for the day?

---

### CASE: TEN MINUTES TO SPARE?

You are a department manager at Community Hospital. This morning you return to work following a 3-day absence to find your in-basket overloaded and your desk littered with telephone message slips. You are greeted by your secretary, Ellen, who informs you that you are expected to substitute for your boss, the associate administrator, at an outside meeting today. You have to leave no later than 9:30 A.M. to make the meeting on time, and you know you can plan on being gone the rest of the day.

You are left with 1 hour in which to begin making order out of the chaos on your desk before leaving for the meeting. True to your usual pattern, you set about reviewing all the items on your desk—telephone messages as well as in-basket items—and sorting them according to their apparent order of importance. You feel that perhaps you can at least get sufficiently organized to be able to begin work the following day with emphasis on your most important unfinished tasks.

About halfway through your hour of organizing Ellen enters to say, "Mr. Wade, the finance director, is here asking to see you. He says he wants 10 minutes of your time to discuss a minor problem with our last month's expense report. Shall I tell him you'll call him about it? Or that maybe he should send you a memo?"

You cannot help feeling that the last thing you need during this hour is an interruption, especially for a nonurgent reason. It occurs to you that Ellen has briefly suggested two alternatives; to these you add a possibility of your own so that you see three choices:

1. Say that you cannot see Wade right now but that you will call him the following day.
2. Ask for a memo detailing the problem so you can look into it at your convenience.
3. Concede to the request for a meeting then and there, and try to limit the discussion to less than 10 minutes.

### Instructions

1. Enumerate the advantages and disadvantages of each of the foregoing three alternatives.
2. Indicate which alternative you would most likely choose and fully explain the reasons for your decision.

## CHAPTER 7

# Self-Management and Personal Supervisory Effectiveness

*Technical training is important but it accounts for less than 20 percent of one's success. More than 80 percent is due to the development of one's personal qualities, such as initiative, thoroughness, concentration, decision, adaptability, organizing ability, observation, industry, and leadership.*
*—G. P. Koch*

## CHAPTER OBJECTIVES

☞ Round out the review of "The Supervisor and Self" by supplementing delegation and time management with important personal considerations.

☞ Highlight the key influence of individual initiative on supervisory effectiveness.

☞ Review the principal barriers to effective performance.

☞ Discuss the relationship of stress to personal supervisory effectiveness.

☞ Provide suggestions and guidance for organizing for effective performance.

☞ Provide guidelines for assessing one's suitability for a supervisory role, with implications for successful self-management.

## SITUATION: THE CASE OF THE VANISHING DAY

Kay Thatcher, director of staff education, decided she had to get organized. Recently her workdays had been running well beyond quitting time, cutting noticeably into the time required by her family responsibilities, but instead of going down, her backlog of work was growing.

Inspired by an article about planning and priorities, Kay decided to try to plan each day's activities at the end of the previous day. This Monday Kay came to the office with her day planned out to the last minute. During the morning she needed to complete a report on a recent learning-needs analysis, write the performance appraisals of two part-time instructors, and assemble the balance of materials for a 2-hour class she was scheduled to conduct that afternoon. After lunch she had to conduct the class, complete the schedule of the next 3 months' training activities (now 10 days overdue), and prepare notices—which should be posted this very day—for two upcoming classes.

Kay got off to a good start; she finished the report before 10:00 A.M. and turned her attention to the performance appraisals. However, at that time the interruptions began. In the following 2 hours she was interrupted six times—three telephone calls and three visitors. Two of the visitors had legitimate problems, one of them taking nearly 30 minutes to resolve. The other visitor was a fellow manager simply passing the time of day. Neither of the performance appraisals was completed, and the training materials were assembled in time only because Kay put them together during lunch while juggling a sandwich at her desk.

Kay's afternoon class ran 20 minutes over because of legitimate questions and discussion. When she returned to the office she discovered she had a visitor, a good-humored, talkative sales representative through whom the hospital bought audiovisual materials. The visitor just happened to be in the area and dropped in. The visit consumed more than an hour.

After the sales representative left, Kay spent several minutes wondering what to do next. The performance appraisals, the 3-month schedule, the class notices—all were overdue. Deciding on the class notices because they were the briefest task before her, she dashed off both notices in longhand and asked the administrative secretary to type and to post them immediately. She then tackled the training schedule.

When Kay again looked up from her work it was nearly an hour past quitting time. She still had a long way to go on the schedule and had not yet gotten started on the performance appraisals. As she swept her work aside for the day she sadly reflected that in spite of her planning she had accomplished less than two thirds of what she intended to do that day. She decided, however, to try again; when she could get a few minutes of quiet time late in the evening she would plan her next day's activities.

On her way out of the hospital she happened to glance at the main bulletin board. The small satisfaction she felt when she saw the posted class notices vanished instantly when she discovered that both were incorrect—the dates of the two classes had been interchanged.

*Instructions*

As you proceed through the chapter, prepare to describe the principal error that Kay committed in her approach to planning and establishing priorities. Also, in spite of how the day had been planned, suggest what Kay could have done to improve her effectiveness on that day.

## IT STARTS WITH YOU

If you would like to gain true control of the practice of management, do not look to sophisticated management theories or techniques and do not rely on gimmicks. Also, do not expect higher management to wind you up and point you in productive directions. Although a certain amount of management direction is essential, it will not always be there when you believe it should be and it will not always take the form you would like it to take.

For a solid foundation on which to base your development as a supervisor, begin with yourself. Do not presume to manage anything else until you have captured and controlled the essentials of managing yourself.

Every employee is a manager of sorts. Even the worker with a few simple tasks and no subordinates is partly a manager of time, methods, and supplies. Since all resources apply together to influence output, the individual worker has at least a limited amount of flexibility in managing output. For supervisory personnel this flexibility is much greater. Performance expected of managers is more results-oriented and less methods-oriented than what is expected of nonsupervisory personnel, so for many managerial tasks any of several approaches can be taken as long as certain results occur.

Conscientious self-improvement in the use of your personal resources will improve the effectiveness with which you manage yourself and enable you to manage the efforts of others more effectively. These personal resources include initiative, organization, and time.

## INITIATIVE

In his self-motivation film titled, *You, Yourself, Inc.*, J. Lewis Powell referred to a junior manager preparing to take a course using a text called *How To Develop Initiative*. The young man was ready; he was waiting for his boss to tell him to begin. In his example, Powell made reference to the "wheelbarrow personality"—useless unless someone else does the loading, pointing, and pushing.

As supervisors, we should recognize that we cannot always be exercising initiative in all directions because of limits on our authority. However, when it comes to self-improvement the only constraints on our initiative are those we place there ourselves. Even in the area of task performance there is a great amount of initiative to be taken. Some first-line supervisors may counter this claim by pointing out that their managers do not seem to encourage initiative but rather seem content to function as "wheelbarrow pushers" rather than as true leaders. This may be a fact of life at times, but the higher manager who is operating as a wheelbarrow pusher is guilty of misguided performance. What do you suppose will happen when administration decides to eliminate a wheelbarrow pusher and you suddenly find yourself reporting to a manager who expects you to be self-propelled?

Your ability to exercise initiative in self-improvement will depend largely on attitude-related factors that often suggest one critical question: How well do you like your job? There are probably not many supervisors who truly enjoy every minute of every day; our jobs are mixtures of things we like and things we do not like, and we can only hope that the former usually outweigh the latter. If you honestly dislike most of your job most of the time, there is little to be done for you. Dislike of one's job is usually reflected in a poor attitude and, in turn, by the absence of initiative.

In short, you will never improve as a supervisor unless you get moving, driven by the determination to do it yourself. The occasional swift kick administered by higher management has only a temporary effect and usually generates resentment and resistance. You have the source of all learning and growth buried within you; no one but you can tap this source.

We are all occasionally haunted by the realization of the need to do more useful things and do a better job with the tasks we now perform; however, we are always waiting for the right opportunity. You have heard a thousand declarations of what will be done "after the rush is over," "as soon as census goes back down," "when I get more staff," or "after the first of the year." However, true initiative says the time is now, not later, and the first places to go to work making initiative count are in personal organization and the use of time.

## BARRIERS TO EFFECTIVENESS

Before further discussion of personal organization, we must examine some of the traditional barriers to effectiveness (other than those presented by the poor use of time) that can have a bearing on how we approach our work. A few of these may be reflections of our personalities. Some, perhaps, are so deeply ingrained that we may never be able to correct them completely; however, the mere awareness of the presence of these barriers can be valuable in helping us understand our behavior. This understanding can, in turn, lead us to ways of compensating for what we may see as shortcomings in ourselves.

The barriers to effectiveness are discussed after the section on initiative for a particular reason. The degree to which we encounter these barriers may be largely a reflection of our personalities—of who and what each of us happens to be. However, the awareness of these barriers is what often opens the door to possible change. And this change cannot come from outside; it must be self-inspired.

### Fear of Failure

One major barrier to effectiveness is the fear of failure. Perhaps we shy away from taking calculated risks or making certain decisions because we are afraid of losing or simply afraid of being wrong. However, fear of failure generally leads to procrastination and inaction, which in turn lead to ineffectiveness. We need to recognize that there is considerable risk and uncertainty involved in management at all levels. Were this not so, far fewer managers would be needed.

### The Search for Perfection

Another occasionally encountered barrier to personal effectiveness is the search for perfection. This can show up as excess time and energy poured into an undertaking or the drive to continue seeking the "ultimate solution" rather than solving one problem and moving on to the next. Although we should always strive to do the best job possible under the circumstances, the person who is lured by the prospect of perfection is bound to discover that perfection is rarely, if ever, attainable.

### Temper

Another common barrier to supervisory effectiveness in day-to-day working situations is temper. Almost without fail, interpersonal communication is impaired by the intrusion of temper. Generally, as temper increases, true communication decreases, and personal effectiveness suffers.

## ORGANIZATION

For many years a popular cartoon has hung on numerous office walls. It pictures two little men facing each other across a table. Both are leaning back in swivel chairs and both have their feet on the table. The area around them is in general disarray. The caption is, "Next week we've got to get organized." The cartoon touches on the biggest problem in the business of personal organization: although it is frequently thought about, it is usually put off until some more convenient time.

Of course you know that organizing is one of the basic management functions, the process of building the framework needed to accommodate the work your department is expected to do; however, thinking for the moment of managing yourself, you should be organizing those things around you that have a bearing on the way you work.

People vary greatly in how they relate to some degree of order—or lack of order—in their surroundings. Some people are meticulously organized, and others seem to function well in the midst of clutter. However, just about everyone can reach an indefinable point beyond which clutter becomes confusion. Not everyone can be like a certain hospital's engineering manager who never used desk drawers or file cabinets. Most flat surfaces in his office were piled high with ragged towers of unsorted documents ranging from one-page letters to inch-thick reports, but he had the uncanny knack of being able to reach into a stack at the right place and pull out what he wanted at any time. This practice served him well for many years. However, the institution grew, the scope of responsibility of the engineering manager grew, the amount of paper in the office expanded accordingly, and the disordered stacks became truly overwhelming. Things began to get lost and stay lost, so the manager, at last, felt compelled to put things in order.

It is not only the material lying about in the open that cuts into your effectiveness. A great many things out of sight in desk drawers and file cabinets also breed confusion and delay. Someone once referred to a refrigerator as a place to keep leftovers until they are old enough to qualify as garbage. Desk and file drawers are used much the same way.

Go through your desk drawers and file cabinets and clean house thoroughly. Keep as few files as necessary, and consider arranging these according to their importance. First and most accessible should be those things you are currently working on, perhaps a number of one- or two-page items in an "open items" file backed up with a few folders for open tasks of greater size. Next keep a few folders devoted to items pending, on hold, or likely to become active in the near future.

A third personal file section would reasonably consist of some limited files of a general nature. Here you would probably want to keep job-related correspondence that may be in your best interest to retain, and frequently used reference material.

Least important in your personal filing system are those things you believe you may find useful or helpful someday. These are the items you refer to seldom if ever, and they are the things that create most office clutter.

Many supervisors suffer from the pack-rat syndrome. They hesitate to discard anything because they feel it may be needed some day. They are likely to keep outdated reports, notes of meetings and incidents long past, old magazines and professional journals, and suppliers' catalogues, brochures, and price lists.

If you are inclined to be a "collector," consider this: most of what you have saved will never again fill a real need as long as you work for the same employer. The problem, of course, is guessing which things are likely to be important so the unimportant ones can be thrown away. Since there is no sure solution to this problem we tend to save everything.

Clean out your office. Go through the clutter and throw out everything you have not referred to in the past two years and are not likely to use in the foreseeable future. Certainly you are going to toss a few things that might have been helpful some day, but what of it? You cannot possibly cover all anticipated information needs with your own resources. Your best bet lies, rather, in knowing where to go for information when a specific need arises.

Go through your office at least twice each year, purging material and condensing files. You will gain two distinct advantages: (1) you will limit the amount of material you keep, and (2) in the process, you will be updating your memory about what you are retaining and where it is kept.

Do not allow material to pile up on your desk, table, or any other surface in your office. At least once a week review the few things that have accumulated and either file them in appropriate places or get rid of them. Keep the reference material you use most often nearest your usual work place, and consider using a desk-top organizer to keep things straight.

Do your best to avoid becoming a generator of the worst kind of clutter—unsorted and undated notes. Some supervisors generate many pages of handwritten notes each week. This practice is itself no problem, and often it is better to err on the side of too much documentation rather than too little. However, this applies only when the problem or activity is current or the nature of the subject suggests that all documentation should be preserved. When the immediate need has passed, your notes should be sorted down to essentials, assembled in order, properly identified, and filed.

As far as note writing is concerned, there is one small rule you can follow to vastly improve the usefulness of your informal documentation: Whenever you put pen or pencil to paper, first put the date on the page.

## INDIVIDUAL PLANNING AND GOAL SETTING

In the Situation opening this chapter, one important element of Kay Thatcher's approach to improving her effectiveness was fully appropriate: spending a brief part of today preparing for tomorrow and the days that follow. Even if it consists of less than five minutes spent at the end of today listing and prioritizing a few tasks to be attempted tomorrow, it is an activity that is potentially helpful to every manager at every level.

As introduced in the previous chapter concerning time management, it is important to list the five or six most critical tasks that have to be done, number them in order of importance, and, upon beginning work the next morning, go immediately to priority number one and stay with it until it is complete. If you are interrupted by circumstances beyond your control—a regular occurrence with first-line managers—when the interruption has passed, get back to priority number one and stay there until it is complete. In brief, make sure you are focusing your time and attention on the most important task at hand.

This sounds so simple as to be self-evident, but apparently it is not so—any number of managers will allow themselves to be diverted and rediverted repeatedly, rarely staying with one task to completion. Also, many managers have a strong tendency to gravitate toward tasks they like or are comfortable with, somehow managing to put off addressing those tasks that they find difficult or distasteful.

In addition to the brief task list updated each day, it also is helpful for a manager to create and maintain a simple planning calendar for known commitments. This can be part of the same calendar or planning book used to keep the daily task lists, but the planning calendar portion looks beyond tomorrow and this week to future weeks and months. Use it to note regularly scheduled meetings, other known commitments, and deadlines for the completion of various tasks. This planning calendar should be reviewed regularly, with tasks that must be done soon moved to the daily task list. This regular review, taking no more than a minute or so a couple of times a week, is extremely important so that commitments or sizable tasks do not creep up on you, leaving insufficient preparation time. A common mistake of some managers, guaranteed to increase the pressure and stress on the manager who makes this mistake, is waiting until the last minute to prepare for a scheduled meeting or begin an important assignment.

Concerning the use of daily task lists and a planning calendar, try to keep it simple. You should of course resort to a level of detail that you find comfortable and sufficient to your needs, but it is all too easy to turn one's personal planning into yet another time-consuming task. A manager's personal planning is best focused on task identification, scheduled meetings, and commitments and deadlines; what is decidedly not needed is excessive detail.

It also is suggested that the individual manager work against deadlines—even self-imposed deadlines. Set goals (or targets or objectives, as you might characterize them) for yourself. Deal with yourself as you might thoughtfully deal with a direct-reporting employee, remembering that any task worth assigning is worth a specific deadline. Do not leave tasks open ended. For every task you must accomplish, set a reasonable, attainable deadline, and do your best to meet that deadline.

Probably most important in the individual manager's personal planning is the recognition that there must be time for contingencies, time to deal with the unexpected. For most managers, a day that is planned out to the last minute, as Kay Thatcher's day was in "The Case of the Vanishing Day," is destined to fall short of expectations. Kay had willingness, enthusiasm, and a task list for Monday, but she left no time for the unexpected, had no means for resisting others' demands, and had no defense against her own nature. Driven by her best intentions to be efficient, Kay became a victim of her own overplanning. We have to recognize that interruptions and disruptions will occur, many of them legitimate and unavoidable. A realistic plan is one that is sufficiently flexible to accommodate the unexpected. A brief written plan or guide for each day is an important tool in addressing personal effectiveness; without it, one's days can be governed by a collection of minor crises, interruptions, and frustrations.

## STRESS AND THE SUPERVISOR

The classic definition of stress, attributed to Dr. Hans Selye, acknowledged as the world's leading authority on the subject, is "the nonspecific response of the body to any demand made on it."[1] In 1914, years before Selye's work, Dr. Walter B. Cannon defined stress as "the body's ability to prepare itself instantaneously to respond to physical threat." The latter definition describes the oft-cited "fight-or-flight" response.[2]

We now know, of course, that the "threat" Cannon referred to can be emotional as well as physical. Indeed, the demand that triggers stress in the body can be purely physical, purely emotional, or a combination of the two. And we should all be more than passingly familiar with the fight-or-flight response— increased heart rate, faster breathing, tensed muscles, flowing adrenaline, and other signs that the body is ready for action.

We cannot avoid experiencing a certain amount of stress. It is inextricably related to change. Stress is largely the way we respond to change, not through our conscious actions but involuntarily, both physically and emotionally.

Perhaps one of the most useful ways to describe stress is as a feeling of loss of control. When some outside influence—some change—disturbs our equilibrium, we react involuntarily in ways that suggest we no longer have the measure of control we need over events and circumstances.

Stress can be both positive and negative. It is positive when you are "up" for something, prepared and alert and determined to regain control. People who seem to perform at their best when under pressure usually do so out of response to positive stress. Consider, for example, a key presentation you are required to make to top management. The future of your department, as well as your own future in the organization, may depend on how well you do. You feel "up" for the occasion—tense, perhaps anxious, maybe experiencing butterflies in the stomach. In your knowledge of how much is riding on your presentation, you are thoroughly prepared (or one would hope you are) and determined to do a good job. You are taking control, reacting positively to positive stress.

Too much stress, however, can be negative. And no one can identify the events that constitute positive stress and those that constitute negative stress. People vary greatly in their ability to cope with stress in general and to perform well under pressure in a job situation. Whether stress is positive or negative depends largely on how you react after the stressful event has passed. Positive stress, or "good" stress, is invariably followed by relaxation. Negative, or harmful, stress is not followed by relaxation, and you continue to experience tension, anxiety, and the like.

### Sources of Stress

Stress emanates from three general sources: your personal life (life outside work), the total job environment, and yourself—your personality, inherent capabilities, and approach to daily living whether at work or away from work.

Stress arising in our personal lives is highly likely to influence our job performance in some way. We have all known people who seem incapable of leaving the problems of the job at work, instead carrying their frustrations home and allowing them to affect their personal lives. And we have certainly known employees who regularly bring their personal problems to work and allow them to affect their performance. Some of the most frequently encountered employee problems a supervisor faces arise with employees whose performance and interpersonal relations are adversely affected by personal difficulties.

We need to recognize that it is not possible to separate the person on the job completely from the person off the job. People vary greatly in their ability to keep the work side of life from influencing the nonwork side and vice versa. To some people, home is a welcome respite from the problems of the job; they can literally leave their worries on the doorstep. To others, work is a refuge, an escape from a chaotic personal life. To a great many people, however, trouble at work usually means trouble at home, and trouble at home usually spills over into their employment in some way.

The total job environment can induce stress in a number of ways. Factors that seem as simple as physical working conditions—heating, lighting, furnishings, space, noise, and the like—can create stress. Organizational policies and practices that are inconsistent or unpredictable can create stress, as well. These are common sources of stress in supervisors.

A supervisor's feeling of having less than total control over the work situation can induce stress, especially when the supervisor has total responsibility for a given situation without having full authority over all the elements that must be brought to bear to address the situation. It is common among supervisors to find that they have responsibility—at least implied responsibility—but that they have not been given authority consistent with that responsibility.

Much supervisory stress comes from negative practices of higher management. "Bossism," management that pushes rather than leads, and management that is authoritarian, unreasonably demanding, or fault finding all create supervisory stress. And although not necessarily negative itself, a change in management that leaves a supervisor reporting to a new superior can be a stress producer. Frequent change in the chain of command or organizational structure that leaves the supervisor reporting to a new manager every few months is virtually guaranteed to produce considerable supervisory stress.

Finally, a major potential stress producer for supervisors is work overload—the fact, or at least the perception, of having too much to do, not enough time to do it, and not enough resources for its accomplishment. Many supervisors have learned the hard way that they cannot be all things to all people in a finite amount of time.

As functions of personality, capabilities, and approach, the stress producers that can be at work within ourselves include:

- self-doubts; a lack of confidence in our own abilities
- lack of personal organization
- inability to plan out our work and to establish priorities and address them appropriately
- perfectionism; placing excessive and unrealistic demands on ourselves

- the inability to say no to any request or demand
- the tendency to take all problems as indications of our own shortcomings; the tendency to take all criticism personally

If you are never stressed on the job, you may have too little to do and little or no true responsibility. Also, if you are never stressed by the demands of the job, you are probably falling short of doing your best work. Positive stress, in urging you to perform under pressure, produces learning and growth.

To a considerable extent, stress goes with the supervisory territory. But if you are always stressed, if you are chronically on the verge of anxiety, depression, or panic, this stress can lead to personal ineffectiveness and ultimately to physical or emotional illness.

## Coping with Supervisory Stress

To succeed on the job over the long run supervisors must gain as much control over both themselves and the work environment as is possible. Approaches suggested for the supervisor to apply in combating stress include:

- Learn to say no, or at least to speak up, when that last request or demand finally adds up to too much. Your boss is only human and is likely to be as stressed as you are, if not more so. Most bosses will understand, especially if you can suggest alternatives or offer to reorder priorities to serve a pressing need.

- Do not let your pile of accumulated work grow until it becomes totally uncontrollable. Take time to plan. Establish priorities. As suggested earlier, tackle one important task at a time and do it completely. Avoid jumping between tasks, intermittently doing a little on each of several items because you think they're all important.

- Delegate. Take Chapter 5 seriously. Delegate tasks in anticipation of stressful times. Do not wait until the pile is so high that you can no longer see over it to think about the need to train others to do some of the work.

- Vary your pace. Intersperse short, quiet tasks among the more hectic, tension-producing contacts required of you. If you have been discussing and negotiating all morning, allow yourself an hour or two of solitary work in the afternoon. Once in a while reward yourself by working on something that you especially like to do.

- When the going gets rough, take a few minutes to relax. Stretch. Breathe deeply. Find an errand to run and turn it into a short walk. A few minutes spent clearing your head will pay themselves back in efficiency many times over.

As for managing stress outside of work, there is still no advice better than what we have heard time and again: proper nutrition, proper rest, and regular exercise.

Just as problems are a part of work that must be managed, so too is stress. Accept the likelihood of stress as part of the supervisory job. Recognize stress when it strikes. By taking control of your situation and consciously managing the stresses that otherwise threaten to overtake you, you will accomplish more in terms of both quantity and quality, take more enjoyment from your work, and reduce your potential for stress-related illness.

## EFFECTIVE USE OF TIME

A consultant once dropped into the office of a friend who was dean of the health sciences division of a college. The dean was talking on the telephone; he motioned his visitor to a chair at a conference table. The table held about 20 square feet of scholarly clutter among which the consultant spied a book entitled *How To Manage Your Time Effectively.*

When the dean hung up the phone, the visitor held up the book and said, "I was thinking of buying this myself. Is it any good?"

The dean's response was, "I really don't know. I got it 3 or 4 months ago, but I haven't had time to read it yet."

The dean said something we have probably all said to ourselves about learning how to make better use of time: we want to do it, but we do not have the time to learn how. We might just as readily admit that we are too busy doing things inefficiently to learn how to do them more efficiently, or simply that we are too busy wasting time to learn how to save it.

One of the greatest difficulties in learning to manage our time is recognizing that we are usually the biggest culprits when it comes to wasting our time. It is much easier to blame drop-in visitors, meetings, inadequate equipment, paperwork, telephone interruptions, or crises. The real problem lies in our allowing these interruptions. We allow others to waste our time. To make real progress in managing time, we need to be prepared to change habits and willing to make changes in the way we work each day.

In "The Case of the Vanishing Day," in addition to allowing no time for contingencies, Kay Thatcher allowed other people to waste her time. She was visited by three employees; apparently two of these visits were legitimate, though even these caused her some stress because she had left no time for contingencies. But concerning the fellow manager who was simply "passing the time of day," Kay should have been prepared to tell this person, after perhaps a moment or two of pleasantries, that she was really busy and had some overdue commitments hanging over her head. Likewise, there was no reason why Kay had to see the drop-in sales representative at all, let alone allow this person to consume a precious hour. Even though the unexpected would have caused her to fall short of her planned accomplishments, Kay could have gotten much more done this day by simply controlling interruptions and politely and diplomatically refusing to allow others to waste her time.

## HOW WELL ARE YOU SUITED TO THE SUPERVISORY ROLE?

Not all persons who work in supervision are equally effective at all parts of the job, and not all supervisors enjoy all parts of the supervisory job equally. The relative effectiveness of many supervisors in the work force can be directly related to how well, personally and temperamentally, they may be suited to the role of supervisor.

How well does any active supervisor fit into the supervisory role? It is possible to examine a few facts and conclusions about yourself and look at the way you relate to the job so you can decide: (1) How well do I fit the supervisory role? And (2) What can I work on to improve the way I fit this role? This can be accomplished through a thoughtful examination of both your personal orientation and your performance orientation.

**Personal Orientation**

To a considerable extent you will unconsciously approach your everyday job activities in the same manner you approach tasks and activities in your personal life. You are the same person whether on or off the job, and unless you make a conscious effort to behave differently in one or another area of your life you are likely to be governed by the same tendencies in all that you do.

Personal orientation can be illustrated in simplified form as a graph with axes representing ranges of capabilities or tendencies (see Figure 7–1).

The vertical axis of personal orientation is focus, ranging from totally internal at the bottom of the graph to totally external at the top. Focus represents the extent to which one is affected by or actively, emotionally involved in activities or events to which one is exposed or is a party. External focus is typified by detachment; internal focus is represented by involvement.

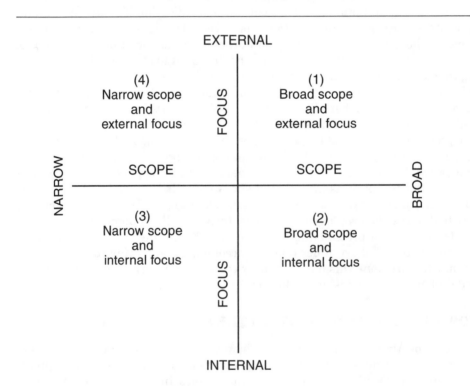

**Figure 7–1** Personal Orientation

As with any rendering of human tendencies or characteristics, this focus axis, as well as other supposed scales discussed here, represents a range with an infinite number of gradations possible between extremes. Rarely do the extremes apply in full. Rather, we can say only that any of us might show a tendency toward one end of the scale or the other.

The individual with an external focus is not personally affected by matters in which he or she is involved, is witness to, or is otherwise party to. An external focus suggests the presence of the ability to keep from taking things personally, and it also suggests the ability to better cope with events and demands that are stressful in some way.

Internal focus is of course the opposite. The person who is internally focused is personally affected by most of what goes on. All events that the individual is party to are internalized, and the individual finds it difficult if not impossible to remain unaffected or unchanged by events.

We may appear to be assessing sensitivity, sympathy, or empathy, but this is not the case. It is possible to be extremely sensitive to another's problem, for example, and to engage in sympathetic involvement, without taking on the full measure of the other's pain. For the externally focused person, that which happens occurs in the world around the self and is to be dealt with and coped with as necessary while being held at a safe emotional distance. For the internally focused person, the self is inevitably affected by events and cannot deal or cope without experiencing others' distress.

As far as the role of the supervisor is concerned, an individual who is totally externally focused may be able to cope rationally with a great many difficult matters, but the result may be a "supervision machine"—a decision maker operating on logic and fact to the exclusion of intuition and all other human consideration. At the other extreme, a supervisor who is totally internally focused probably will not survive for any appreciable time. Considering all of the difficulties that arise in managing people, and recognizing the health care environment as one in which pain and suffering are commonplace, it is easy to accept the internally focused supervisor as a likely candidate for early burnout.

The most desirable focus orientation for the supervisor lies above the origin of the graph, a tendency toward an external focus and thus toward the ability to deal with the various events that come with the supervisory task and to cope with the many problems and other unpleasant situations that are part of the job.

The horizontal axis of personal orientation is scope. Scope simply refers to the kind or amount or variety of activity that an individual can best handle according to temperament or individual ability. The person with a broad scope can "juggle," coping with a variety of tasks in bits and pieces, moving from task to task and back again, and solving unanticipated problems as they arise. Or, to insert a currently popular term that happens to be fully applicable, the broad-scope supervisor is adept at multi-tasking. The broad-scope individual can function in firefighting style without experiencing undue stress and without becoming overwhelmed by a seemingly unending stream of problems or by the inability to truly finish much of what is started.

At the opposite end of the horizontal axis are persons of scope, those who cannot readily function in the scattergun fashion of the broad-scope person but who are most comfortable with and whose talents are best applied to one specific task at a time.

The chances of long-run success in the supervisory role are enhanced if one is possessed of a broad scope and is generally able to constantly reorder priorities and cope with a continuous series of unanticipated demands. Combining the two axes that have been used to describe personal orientation, we can reasonably suggest that one is best suited to the supervisory role if one's personal orientation lies somewhere in the upper right hand quadrant of Figure 7–1—above the origin as far as focus is concerned, and to the right of the origin as far as scope is concerned. The person who is well suited to the supervisory role will tend toward being externally focused, with the ability to deal with most matters at a reasonable emotional distance, and will be of broad scope, with the ability to take what comes as it comes. The supervisor who may be placed by personal orientation in any of the other three quadrants of Figure 7–1 may experience problems of orientation ranging from mild, such as having to remember to avoid giving in to a narrow-scope tendency and staying too long on a pet project, to severe, such as a stress reaction to the internalized pain of others.

## Performance Orientation

Performance orientation can also be described by a pair of perpendicular axes along each of which there can be an infinite number of gradations (see Figure 7–2).

The vertical axis of Figure 7–2 presents emphasis on a continuum from totally personal at the bottom to totally functional at the top of the graph. The higher the degree of functional emphasis evident in a supervisor's performance, the more visible will be that supervisor's degree of attention to activities of highest priority. The supervisor having a strong functional emphasis will ordinarily be attending to the most important task at any given time. On the other hand, the more personal a supervisor's emphasis becomes, the more likely that supervisor is to be giving attention primarily to those tasks or concerns that he or she prefers or enjoys. This may be all well and good when it happens that what the supervisor likes to do and what most needs to be done coincide. However, most of the time the tasks the supervisor favors and the tasks that most need to be done are not the same.

The horizontal axis of Figure 7–2 represents posture along a continuum ranging from completely reactive to fully assertive. The supervisor who tends toward the assertive end of the scale ordinarily initiates action, advances ideas or solutions, and moves to resolve difficulties in their early stages and head off problems before they occur. The supervisor who tends toward the reactive end of the scale ordinarily waits to be told what to do, procrastinates on important decisions until there is no more room for delay, and waits until a problem can no longer be denied before attempting a solution. The assertive supervisor deals in innovation and prevention; the reactive supervisor simply responds when pushed by circumstances.

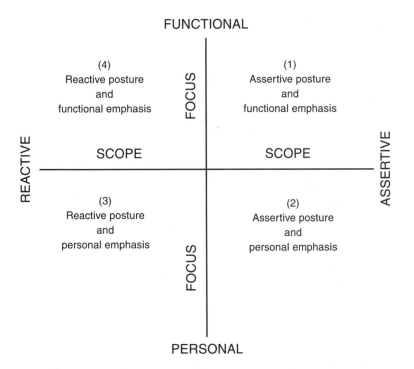

**Figure 7–2** Performance Orientation

The effective supervisor tends more toward functional than personal in emphasis and more toward assertive than reactive in posture. However, emphasis and posture cannot be considered separate from each other; together they exert combined effects that can be described through association with each other in the four quadrants of Figure 7–2.

In the first quadrant (upper right), tendencies toward functional emphasis and assertive posture describe a supervisor who is generally in control of the job and who operates with a noticeable degree of autonomy. In this, describable as the "best" of the four quadrants, the supervisor:

- concentrates on high-priority tasks most of the time
- tackles the important problems in timely fashion even though they may be difficult or unpleasant
- experiences job satisfaction from accomplishment and achievement
- is meeting the needs of the organization in doing what he or she is expected to do as a member of management

A supervisor functioning in the first quadrant is applying the right approach (assertive posture) to the right tasks (functional emphasis), moving in the right direction without being told.

The second quadrant (lower right) suggests the combined effects of a tendency toward an assertive posture and a tendency toward a personal emphasis. A supervisor functioning in this quadrant may frequently be described as pursuing personal preferences or being out of step with reality. In this quadrant the supervisor may:

- be unwilling to delegate, personally monopolizing preferred activities, or unable to delegate out of a sense of insecurity
- take frequent refuge in preferred tasks of low priority as relaxation, self-satisfaction, or escape
- experience goal displacement, being unable to reconcile organizational goals with personal goals
- have little appreciation of job purpose, failing to see how this specific supervisory position is supposed to mesh with others as part of the organizational whole

A supervisor functioning in the second quadrant is generally applying the right approach to the wrong tasks (personal emphasis), moving without being told but going in the wrong direction.

The third quadrant (lower left) is readily describable as the "worst" of the four general situations. The supervisor functioning in the third quadrant may:

- appear to be running fast and working hard while going nowhere and accomplishing little
- exhibit an inability to control interruptions
- be unwilling or unable to say no to any request that comes along, no matter how unreasonable or intrusive it may be
- avoid that which is difficult, complicated, unpleasant, or potentially stressful whenever possible, taking the "easiest" route through most problems
- become disillusioned with the job and the organization

A supervisor functioning in the third quadrant is ordinarily taking the wrong approach (reactive emphasis) to the wrong tasks (personal emphasis), moving only when pushed and then going in the wrong direction.

Because a person falling into the fourth quadrant (upper left) will usually be doing most of the right things, the combination of emphasis and posture evident in this quadrant might present no problems at all if this discussion concerned people employed in any number of nonsupervisory capacities. However, the supervisor falling into the fourth quadrant may:

- experience considerable frustration with a nearly complete lack of autonomy
- feel "out of control," reacting to the seemingly unending and unpredictable stream of demands made by others
- use time ineffectively, moving from task to task and crisis to crisis as directed, having no time left to plan and organize

A supervisor functioning in the fourth quadrant has the proper functional emphasis but is applying an improper reactive approach. As suggested, this may be acceptable in some nonsupervisory employees; although assertiveness is to be desired in many employees, supervisory or otherwise, there are still many jobs in which an employee may best serve by performing as directed. But although a reactive posture may be appropriate—or at least tolerable—in many nonsupervisory employees, such a posture is contrary to what is expected of an effective supervisor.

### How Well Do You Fit?

Many people who did not fit well into a supervisory role have either voluntarily abandoned supervision or failed as supervisors. Many others who also do not fit especially well into a supervisory role have nevertheless remained supervisors, with widely varying degrees of success. It is highly likely that absolutely "perfect fit" supervisors are a minority of the supervisory population of any organization. Therefore it is just as likely that most supervisors have weaknesses that can potentially affect their performance and perhaps ultimately determine whether they succeed or fail in the long run.

Simply identifying one's own weaknesses is a large part of the struggle for improved personal effectiveness. Once these weaknesses are identified, the next essential process is recognizing the difference between those things about one's self that one can actively change and those things about one's self that one cannot readily change but must compensate for or otherwise work around. The final step in the process is acting to remove or guard against one's own weaknesses.

Consider how you believe you must place yourself in regard to personal orientation. You might find, as would most people, that you have more control over your scope than you do over your focus. Although both scope and focus are rooted in personality, focus is much more emotionally based and is therefore much more difficult to alter artificially. Regarding focus, for example, if you are strongly internally focused and truly sensitive to the point of creating intolerable stress within yourself by having to apply firm disciplinary action, you are more prone to minimize this aspect of the supervisory role and thus impair your effectiveness in handling problem employees. Since your focus is emotionally based, unless you are sufficiently near the middle of the graph to allow you to accommodate the occasional emotional stresses of the job, you may be consigning yourself to a working life of strain and unhappiness by remaining in supervision.

Since scope is less emotionally tied than focus, we can all do more to control this dimension of personal orientation. Broad-scope people are team members; narrow-scope people prefer to function as loners. The supervisor needs to be a team member. However, it is acceptable to give in to a tendency to enjoy working as a loner once in a while—as long as one is conscious of the need to be a team member and to willfully function as a team member whenever circumstances demand (which, for the typical supervisor, is most of the time).

Aspects of personality ordinarily have a great deal of influence on both major dimensions of one's performance orientation. Of the two, posture is probably more deeply rooted in personality than is emphasis. Surely there are some whose posture is essentially reactive because they are self-doubting and insecure. Just as surely, however, there are some who are reactive because they lack goal orientation or because they have never been given any clear idea of what is expected of them. Perhaps one's insecurities can be overcome with a great deal of effort and the right kind of assistance and support. However, not nearly as difficult as overcoming insecurity is the deliberate development of goal orientation—which can surely be done if someone wants success strongly enough—and one can pointedly ask for higher management's expectations.

Although unavoidably influenced by aspects of personality, emphasis is more readily altered by the individual than is posture. The key to emphasis is self-discipline, the ability to make oneself give the most attention to the highest priority tasks at hand. The supervisor who can enter each work day by asking, "What is the single most important task I need to accomplish today?" and plan to get that task done and proceed to do it, is on the path of effectiveness. Even the supervisor whose workload may loom as overwhelming is making progress if he or she is always at work on the highest priority task of the moment. To self-discipline one need only add consideration of the need to plan and organize, and to control interruptions while concentrating on priorities, to develop a true functional emphasis.

The self-discipline referred to in the foregoing paragraph is crucial to the improvement of one's personal orientation and performance orientation. To develop an improved personal orientation and to adopt a more appropriate performance orientation is to put oneself in the position of becoming a more effective supervisor. Self-discipline as applied by the effective supervisor is self-management, and self-management comes before the management of others. The person who would aspire to manage others must first become proficient at self-management.

---

## REVIEW QUESTIONS

1. How does the fear of failure prevent someone from being as effective as possible?
2. Why should organization of one's surroundings and materials have an appreciable bearing on individual effectiveness?
3. List at least five forces or factors that can produce stress in the working supervisor.
4. Compare and contrast *personal orientation* and *performance orientation*.
5. Describe the most desirable combination of personal characteristics under *performance orientation*.

## EXERCISE: THE EFFECTIVENESS CHECKLIST

Provide honest, self-searching responses to the statements listed below, using these responses:

U = usually (or always)

S = sometimes

R = rarely (or never)

(Be candid. No one needs to see your answers unless you choose to share them.)

_____ 1.  I put my objectives—and plans for reaching them—on paper.

_____ 2.  My objectives are expressed in specifics: what, how much, and when.

_____ 3.  For sizable tasks, I use checkpoints or subobjectives so I can assess progress along the way.

_____ 4.  I break large jobs into smaller, more manageable pieces.

_____ 5.  I set deadlines for myself and hold myself to them.

_____ 6.  I use written reminders of what must be done today or tomorrow.

_____ 7.  I avoid thoughts or circumstances that might sidetrack my efforts.

_____ 8.  I know my limitations; I do not set objectives I know I cannot achieve or make promises I know I cannot keep.

_____ 9.  I use positive motivation by reminding myself of the benefits I expect from the completion of a task.

_____10.  When facing a disagreeable or difficult task, I am able to distinguish between "I can't" and "I don't want to."

_____11.  I am willing to take risks, to try new ways of doing things.

_____12.  I allow myself the freedom to fail, to make mistakes and learn from them.

_____13.  I keep my personal work area organized and under control.

_____14.  I recognize conflicts for what they are and do not back away from making decisions.

_____15.  I have a sense of priority that allows me to distinguish between what must be done and what I would like to do.

If you gave yourself U on all 15 statements perhaps you had better go through the list again. There are few managers who do not rate S on at least a few items. Each S or R represents a clear opportunity for self-improvement.

**NOTES**

1. S. H. Appelbaum, *Stress Management for Health Professionals* (Rockville MD: Aspen Systems Corporation); 72–74

2. *Stress Management for Health Professionals,* p. 72.

# PART III

# The Supervisor and the Employee

## CHAPTER 8

# Interviewing: Start Strong to Recruit Successfully

*The best man for the job is often a woman.*
—*Anonymous*

## CHAPTER OBJECTIVES

☛ Stress the importance of supervisory involvement in the hiring process.

☛ Offer advice on how to prepare for an employee selection interview.

☛ Present guidelines for interview questioning, specifically identifying kinds of questions that should be avoided and suggesting appropriate lines of questioning.

☛ Describe a recommended general approach to the supervisor's conduct of the actual employee selection interview.

☛ Describe desirable follow-up action to conclude the interview cycle effectively.

## EXERCISE: POTENTIAL INTERVIEW QUESTIONS?

Before proceeding through this chapter, try your hand at rendering a judgment on the legality of each of the following 25 questions. Simply note whether you believe each question is lawful (L) or unlawful (U) to ask an applicant in an interview situation. Answers and comments appear later in the chapter. A number of the answers will seem to be ordinary common sense, but not all will be obvious. See if you can identify a pattern by which all of these questions may be categorized.

1. Have you previously been employed here under a different name?
2. What was your name before you married?
3. Where were you born?
4. Have you any condition that would prevent you from adequately performing in the position for which you are applying?
5. What was your title in your last employment, and who was your supervisor?
6. Do you have any handicaps?
7. Of what country do you hold citizenship?
8. Who is the relative you would designate to be notified in case of emergency?
9. What foreign languages do you read, write, or speak fluently?
10. What other countries have you visited?
11. How did you acquire your foreign language abilities?
12. At what schools did you receive your academic, vocational, or professional education?

13. With what major credit card companies do you have credit?
14. Have you ever filed for bankruptcy?
15. Who would be willing to provide you with a professional reference for the position for which you are applying?
16. Are you a single parent?
17. Have you any commitments or responsibilities that may interfere with meeting work attendance requirements?
18. What relatives of yours, if any, are already employed here?
19. Did you receive an honorable discharge from the military?
20. Why do you want to work here?
21. Where did you live before moving to your present address?
22. Do you own or rent your home?
23. What experiences, skills, or other qualifications do you feel make you appropriate for the position under consideration?
24. Why did you leave your last employer?
25. What organizations, clubs, and societies do you belong to?

## THE MANAGER AND THE INTERVIEW

The personal interview is often not a particularly reliable means of finding good employees. We have no guarantees that the process will always generate positive results. No matter how good we become at interviewing or how much we know about the jobs we are attempting to fill, it frequently remains impossible to separate true ability in a job candidate from the ability simply to "talk a good job." However, in spite of its shortcomings and weaknesses, we must usually rely on the face-to-face employee selection interview for locating new employees simply because there is no other practical means available for approaching the task.

Institutions may vary considerably in the extent to which supervisors become involved in the hiring process. In a few institutions, major departments or divisions will recruit and screen their own job applicants. This practice is a holdover from former days when each department did its own hiring; it survives partially today in some institutions, for example, where the nursing department looks after all aspects of nursing employment while the human resources department sees to the needs of all other departments. In most health care facilities, however, the employment needs of all departments are served to a more or less equal extent by human resources.

Make it a point to know specifically how much of the employment process is yours and how much is done by human resources. Ordinarily you can expect to look to human resources for locating a number of candidates who generally fit the requirements of the open position; that is, the employment staff in human resources find people who have the appropriate academic credentials and minimum required experience and who otherwise fit the hiring criteria you established. In most cases human resources will screen applicants to locate generally qualified candidates and will arrange personal interviews for you.

A very few institutions may still follow the age-old and highly undesirable practice of having a very few people, perhaps only one or two, doing all of the actual employee selection for the entire organization. This outmoded practice is contrary to the fundamentals of supervisory responsibility; we cannot simply "give" an already-chosen employee to a supervisor and expect to facilitate the establishment of the proper employee-supervisor relationship. If the supervisor is to be responsible for an employee's output, then the supervisor must be allowed a consistent amount of authority in selecting that employee. The supervisory role should include, subject to carefully drawn ground rules, the authority to hire and fire. Too often in the past the authority to hire was retained by "higher ups" (although the supervisor may have been left to do the firing when things did not work out). As supervisors, however, we need to recognize that although hiring is a sometimes difficult and time-consuming process, it is nevertheless an essential part of the job. To be blunt, if we are not capable of hiring people then we should not be supervisors.

## CANDIDATES: OUTSIDE AND INSIDE

Job applicants often come to your organization in response to employment advertising specific to certain personnel needs. Many also come, not in response to specific recruiting efforts, but unsolicited; they fill out employment applications in the hope of finding work. Both solicited and unsolicited applicants reach the attention of the interviewing supervisor following screening interviews in which human resources determines that the applicants are qualified to fill some specific need.

Most organizations operate job-posting systems and have policies governing employee transfers, so a number of candidates for any particular position may also come from within the present work force. The more specialized a need, the more likely the supervisor is to see a preponderance of external candidates (benefits specialist, electrician, pharmacist, radiation therapy technologist, and so on); the more generalized a need, the more likely the supervisor is to see a preponderance of internal candidates (secretary, building service worker, kitchen helper, transport aide, and so on). In more than a few cases, in filling a particular position you will be able to choose from among a pool that includes both external and internal candidates.

Most organizations likewise espouse a philosophy of development from within the organization by way of either lateral or promotional transfers. It should be stressed that this notion of development from within is more likely to be philosophy than policy. No astute top management will absolutely require the supervisor to select an internal candidate in any particular situation. (Unless, of course, there are extenuating circumstances, for example, a valued employee returning from a lengthy absence needs placement or an individual must be placed or moved to avoid a legal problem, prompting higher manager to "request" the selection of a particular person.) To do so without extraordinarily good cause would put the supervisor in a position of sometimes having to take a candidate who is less desirable than the apparently best available. But even though the notion of development from within may not be inviolable policy, you should nevertheless incorporate it into practice whenever reasonably possible.

One organizational characteristic that strongly encourages employee retention is the existence of a real opportunity for varied work experience and for promotion and growth. If lower-level employees continually see all the "better" positions—primarily the promotional opportunities—going to external candidates, the organization will gradually lose those lower-level employees who are capable of growing and are interested in promotion.

As supervisor, you will undoubtedly make most of your hiring decisions with your immediate departmental needs in mind. However, you should also hire in consideration of the longer-range needs of the organization and its employees. These needs suggest that a certain amount of your personnel needs should be filled from within the organization. Neither "always outside" nor "always inside" is appropriate. When you are presented with two or more equally qualified candidates for a given position, there is every good reason for giving preference to the internal candidate.

## PREPARING FOR THE INTERVIEW

### The Job Description

In preparing to interview a job applicant you first need to become fully conversant with the job description. There is nothing wrong with having the job description in front of you for occasional reference during the interview, but you should be prepared to speak knowledgeably about the position without frequent reference to paper, especially since the position is probably one that you supervise.

You should be in a position to discuss the following about the requirements of the position when interviewing a job applicant:

- specific knowledge and skills required
- background and experience required
- formal education required
- necessary familiarity with specific equipment or processes
- job duties, including what is expected in the way of quality and output
- responsibility for supervision of others, if applicable
- responsibility for safety of others, if applicable
- potential loss due to error
- confidentiality requirements
- contacts and relationships with others (customers, vendors, the public, etc.)
- physical demands (lifting, pushing, pulling, and the weights involved)
- visual, auditory, and other sensory requirements
- potential stressors (pace, pressure, etc.)
- closeness of supervision or relative independence of the position
- working conditions (hours, locations, hazards, travel, etc.)

- compensation and benefits
- future potential

Jobs change over time, and often a job description does not accurately reflect the present requirements of a position. Therefore, the pre-interview review of a job description presents a good opportunity to update the job description. The applicant deserves current accurate information about the job at the time of the interview.

## The Employment Application

With the requirements of the position in mind, the next step in preparing for a selection interview should consist of careful review of the individual's employment application (or résumé, if applicable, or both). You need this information in advance of the interview; do not allow yourself to be put in the position of having to read the application for the first time as the applicant sits before you. Should this ever occur, do what you can to discourage the employment recruiters from sending you applicants with applications in hand. You need time to familiarize yourself with information about the job applicant. Otherwise you may make the applicant uncomfortable by reading when you should be listening or speaking, or you may miss something important and ask questions that have already been answered on paper.

There is a great deal the employment application will not tell you. Employment applications of years past called for much information that cannot now be legally requested. Assuming that you are likely to have no control over what is asked on the application, we will not go into detail concerning what can or cannot be requested on an employment application. However, we will shortly discuss some kinds of questions you cannot or should not ask during an interview, and it should go without saying that these same questions cannot be asked on an application. Many of today's employment applications are necessarily sketchy compared with those of years ago.

Chances are that if you have worked for your present employer for a few years, the application you originally completed might today be considered illegal or at least questionable in some way. If you have worked at the same place since 1980 or earlier, the application you originally submitted would today be decidedly illegal in a number of respects.

## Other Considerations

It may also be useful to have a few sample questions prepared in advance of the interview. You are likely to discover that the most valuable questions emerge while you are in conversation with the applicant, but you may well need some starter questions to enable you to get the conversation going. Prepare yourself to guide the applicant and listen, never losing sight of your basic purpose: to learn as much as possible about the applicant.

Make sure the interview takes place in private and in relatively comfortable surroundings. If you have a private office, use it unless you are sure to experience constant interruptions. If necessary, borrow someone else's office, make use of an open conference room or other available space, or use interview space in the human resources department. Your ability to learn about the applicant is severely impaired by interruptions, and interruptions are often unsettling to the applicant.

Be aware of the likely state of mind of the job applicant. Even though the person is not yet and may in fact never become an employee, you are already in a position of authority relative to the person looking for a job. To a potential employee you are an employer; you enter the interview situation at a definite psychological advantage.

Look at the interview situation from the applicant's point of view. You automatically have the upper hand; yet the applicant has far more at stake than you have. The applicant is looking for a job; you not only have a job but you are an authority figure as well. Often the applicant, if truly serious about finding work, will be determined to make a good impression—and may be nervous.

Insofar as possible, be familiar with Equal Employment and other legal considerations. Use this familiarity to guide your interview behavior, but resist the temptation to "play lawyer" and render your own interpretations in questionable areas. When you are able to do so, get advice from human resources and other knowledgeable people in the organization. If you follow the questioning guidelines offered in this chapter, you should encounter few difficulties. However, if you find you have serious doubts about a particular question that occurs to you, do not ask it of the applicant.

## GUIDELINES FOR QUESTIONING

Although common courtesy should prevail in your interview behavior at all times, courtesy by itself is not enough. You must be constantly aware of questions or comments that could be taken as discriminatory in some way although not intended as such. An applicant may volunteer information related to the following precautions, but you may not ask for this information.

### Questions to Avoid

You may not ask any question that requires the applicant to reveal *age, date of birth, race, religion, or national origin*. The direct questions—"When were you born?"—should be easy to avoid. Watch out, however, for indirect questions through which a person can claim you were "fishing" for specific information. For instance, a question that is not allowed is one such as: "I'd say we've both been around about the same length of time—both early baby boomers, perhaps?"

The matter of age has become a particularly sensitive area in recent years, calling for heightened awareness on the part of the supervisor. Although the Age Discrimination in Employment Act (ADEA) has been in place since 1967, it was given added scope and influence by the Age Discrimination in Employment Amendments Act of 1986, effective January 1, 1987. Although it is mostly the concern of the human resources department, this law nevertheless has implications for the supervisor.

The 1986 act prohibits mandatory retirement for most employees and removes the age 70 limit on ADEA protection. Therefore, stay away from all questions related to an applicant's long-term intentions, such as, "How long would you plan on working before thinking about retirement?" because of the age-related inferences that one might draw.

There is no safe question that the supervisor can ask about age, except to inquire whether an apparently young person is of legal age to enter full-time employment under the circumstances required of the job in question (in most instances, at least 18 years of age). Avoid all questions that either directly or indirectly require age-related responses. Also, you need to assure yourself that all the qualifications you are seeking are truly related to the job. Evaluate individual applicants on their individual capabilities and qualifications, not on your general beliefs or personal preferences ("An older person just couldn't keep up," or "Someone her age would resist new technology," or "I want someone who's more likely to stay 10 or 20 years").

Similar to concerns about age, there are few if any safe questions the supervisor can ask about *disability*, whether a job candidate's disability is evident or not. The Americans with Disabilities Act (ADA) of 1990 provides a national mandate barring bias against persons with disabilities. This act calls for supportive and accommodating behavior by employers in maintaining persons with disabilities in the work force. Concerning the employment selection interview and the person with disabilities, the supervisor should ask questions about the applicant's qualifications and experience that focus strictly on the essential functions of the job. The job's peripheral activities that have no bearing on its essential functions—for example, occasional filing or report delivery related to the position of a billing clerk—are subject to "reasonable accommodation" by the organization and have no bearing on the person's capabilities as a billing clerk. More about the ADA appears in Chapter 27.

You may not ask if the applicant has a *recommendation* from a present employer. This may be taken as discriminatory, since it may be difficult for the applicant to secure such a recommendation because of reasons other than job performance (e.g., race, religion, political affiliation).

You can no longer ask the identity of the person's *nearest relative or "next of kin,"* even for the simple purpose of having someone to contact in case of illness or accident. This can be taken as probing into the existence of spouse or family, which you cannot do. Even asking about "the person to be notified in case of illness or accident" should be avoided until the applicant is actually employed.

It is generally permissible to ask if an applicant is a *U.S. citizen or is legally eligible for employment.* However, this should not be an active concern of the supervisor if human resources is fulfilling its proper role in complying with the Immigration Reform and Control Act of 1986 (IRCA). This law requires employers to hire only U.S. citizens and lawfully authorized alien workers, and provides penalties and sanctions for employers who knowingly hire or continue to employ illegal aliens or persons who fail to verify legal eligibility for employment (see Chapter 27).

In compliance with IRCA, human resources must require an applicant to produce certain proofs of identity and employment eligibility within 3 working days *after* an offer of employment is made. For your part in helping the organization comply with IRCA, you should resist the temptation to prevail on human resources to allow a much-needed new employee to begin work before the necessary proofs are produced.

Immigration reform has provided the work organization with a set of risks and pitfalls of a kind never previously experienced, and these risks and pitfalls cannot be avoided by backing away from the problem. The supervisor who might seek to avoid IRCA problems by not considering an applicant because of foreign appearance or language can face discrimination charges as defined by other laws.

In asking about the applicant's *military service*, you may inquire only into the training and experience involved. You may not ask the character of the person's discharge or separation. Whether the discharge was honorable, dishonorable, general, or otherwise remains privileged information, which the applicant may reveal voluntarily but which you may not request.

You may not ask the *marital status* of the applicant at the time of the interview. Particular sensitivity has developed along these lines in recent years. Many women have been able to claim, with considerable success, that they were denied employment because of marital status. Employers often proceeded on the assumptions, sometimes statistically substantiated, that

- young women recently engaged often quit shortly after they get married
- young, recently married women may leave after a year or two to begin families
- unmarried women with small children tend on the average to have poorer attendance records than other workers

Even if an applicant, male or female, has willingly revealed marriage on a résumé, you are not permitted to ask what the spouse does for a living. In the case of a married female applicant, you are also forbidden to ask her maiden name because this question can be interpreted as probing for clues to national origin.

You may not ask if the applicant *owns a home or a car.* This may be interpreted as seeking to test affluence, which may in turn be taken as discriminatory against certain minorities. You may, however, ask if the applicant has a driver's license—if driving is a *bona fide occupational qualification* (BFOQ), that is, a requirement of the job. (Generally, you are on your soundest footing when all questions of a personal nature relate to BFOQs.)

You may not ask if the applicant's *wages were ever attached or garnished* or if the individual has outstanding loans or other financial obligations. Credit information is privileged information; it may be volunteered by the applicant but not requested by the prospective employer.

You may not directly ask any applicant's *height or weight.* Neither of these factors should have a bearing on the applicant's suitability for the job unless there is a specific job-related requirement (BFOQ) that is uniformly applied to all applicants.

Beware of requesting an applicant to take *qualification tests.* Preemployment tests have long been under fire as discriminatory in matters of age, race, and economic background. Preemployment testing is best left to professionals who design tests that are specifically related to the requirements of the job, statistically validated as nondiscriminatory, administered consistently and in good faith, and evaluated impartially.

There are also pitfalls to be encountered in asking an applicant's *educational level*, such as completion of high school or possession of a college degree. An employer may require specific educational levels when these are directly related to job performance (again, BFOQs). Otherwise, it may be possible to show a pattern of employment discrimination. You can require, for instance, a nurse to possess a diploma or degree and a state license since these are essential to the performance of the job as it is structured. However, you cannot require a housekeeping maid or kitchen helper to have a high school diploma since it is possible to demonstrate that people in these job categories may perform equally well with or without the diploma. Effective human resources employment procedures should take most of the burden off the interviewer in this matter.

You cannot ask if an applicant has ever been *arrested*. An arrest is simply a charge, not a conviction. It has even become risky to ask if a person has ever been convicted of a crime. Most courts have ruled that after a few years have passed following conviction and correction, the individual need not be called on to reveal this information. Unless the job is clearly related to safeguarding money or security (a BFOQ), it is best to refrain from this line of questioning.

You may not ask whether an applicant is or has been a member of a union or has been involved in organizing or other union activities.

You may not ask any obviously older applicants if they are receiving *Social Security* benefits. It has been demonstrated concerning older persons applying for part-time work that some employers have discriminated in favor of applicants receiving Social Security payments, since a person receiving a combined income may be more likely to remain on the job longer than one to whom the part-time job is the sole means of support.

### Questions to Ask

The questions you are permitted to ask are broad and in many instances open ended. This is as it should be; remember, you are interested in learning as much as you can about the applicant in a limited amount of time and the way to do this is to listen to the person talk. Try the following questions in conversation with the applicant:

- What are your career goals? What would you like to be doing 5 or 10 years from now? How would you like to spend the rest of your career?
- Who have been your prior employers, and why did you leave your previous positions?
- What did you like or dislike about the work in your previous positions?
- Who recommended you to our institution? How did you hear about this job opening?
- What is your educational background? What lines of study did you pursue? (Be careful, however, of attempting to delve into specifics as cautioned in the list of questions to avoid.)

- What do you believe are your strong points? What do you see as your weaknesses?
- Have you granted permission for us to check references with former employers (see following section)?

If human resources has not already done so, ask the applicant to explain any gaps of more than a few weeks' duration that appear in the résumé or application. Some applicants will omit mention of unsuccessful job experiences or other involvements that they believe might reflect negatively on their chances of being hired. As the hiring supervisor you should be in a position to make a fully informed decision based on more than just selected pieces of a candidate's background. Also, you share a responsibility for ensuring that the organization is protected from possible negligent hiring charges should an employee who was hired without reasonable background verification cause harm.

### "Potential Interview Questions?" Revisited

Returning to the opening exercise, following is a determination of whether each is lawful or unlawful, and the reason for each response.

1. Lawful. You can ask about "a different name" because the organization is entitled to knowledge of one's previous employment with them.
2. Unlawful. It asks about marital status.
3. Unlawful. Asking for place of origin can be construed as fishing for other personal information (national origin, economic status, etc.).
4. Lawful. The employer is entitled to ask about the applicant's ability to fulfill the significant requirements of the position.
5. Lawful. This can be information pertinent to experience, which you have a right to inquire into.
6. Unlawful. The legal way to address this issue is by way of question number 4.
7. Unlawful. This can be interpreted as asking about nationality.
8. Unlawful. A question concerning who (not specifically a relative) to notify in an emergency can be asked after hire.
9. Lawful. It asks for language capability without fishing for national origin.
10. Lawful. It does not probe for personal information.
11. Unlawful. It could be taken as a request for information about national origin.
12. Lawful. There is no problem in asking for schools at which one was educated.
13. Unlawful. It implies inquiry about economic status.
14. Unlawful. The same reason given in number 13 applies.
15. Lawful. Requesting professional references is permissible (and usually a good idea).
16. Unlawful. It asks about marital status and dependents.

17. Lawful. This is simply a way of asking if the applicant can get to work when he or she is expected to be there.
18. Lawful. Many organizations have policies that forbid employing relatives in the same department or in a supervisor-subordinate relationship in any chain of command, and this is a legitimate consideration.
19. Unlawful. All that can be safely asked about one's military service is the nature of the person's experience.
20. Lawful. It is usually a helpful question to ask.
21. Unlawful. It can be interpreted as fishing for information about ethnic background, economic status, etc.
22. Unlawful. It inquires into economic status.
23. Lawful. It is an appropriate question to ask.
24. Lawful. It requests information to which you are entitled.
25. Unlawful. It can be taken as probing for information about ethnic background, religion, and such.

## Employment References

The whole topic of employment references represents a quagmire of potential legal traps for both the supervisor and the human resources department. Ideally, human resources should have secured the applicant's signed permission to check references as part of the screening interview, calling for a specific signed release for each former employer. For good reasons, many applicants indicate that their present employers not be approached for reference information, but they ordinarily grant permission to check with most—but not always with all—previous employers. No reference checks should be performed by anyone in the absence of an applicant's signed authorization to do so. Even if a signed release is presented, reference checking should be left to the human resources department. Under no circumstances should an interviewing supervisor endeavor to check an applicant's references personally.

References must be checked systematically in accordance with strict guidelines governing the kinds of information requested and the kinds of responses to expect. In these litigious times, many unsuccessful applicants are quick to charge that they were not hired because of defamatory information acquired from previous employers. It is therefore important for all references to be checked by persons who do so regularly enough to be sensitive to the legal pitfalls that can be encountered. For example, an applicant might claim to have been defamed in being labeled on a reference check as "uncooperative and unreliable"—and can succeed in pursuing such a claim if there is insufficient information in the individual's past employment record to prove such contentions. Reference information used in making a decision not to hire needs to be substantiated in the past employment record. For instance, to stand up as valid if challenged, a reference of "poor attendance" should be backed up (in the personnel file maintained by the employer supplying the reference) with attendance records or with records of disciplinary actions dealing with attendance.

Because of the possibility of legal problems, many organizations have backed away from supplying much pertinent reference information, limiting themselves, by policy, to verifying job title and dates of employment and giving out nothing else. In recent years, however, an increasing number of organizations have been subject to charges of negligent hiring because of harm done by employees who were hired with little or no effort expended to check their employment histories. Although many prior employers may respond with dates and titles only or with no information at all, your human resource department should make certain it is able to demonstrate that the organization made a good-faith effort to check references.

Regardless, the details and actual performance of reference checking should remain with human resources. Should you be in a position to use personal contacts such as your colleagues in other organizations to check on potential new employees, in no way should you ever actively use information so obtained in justifying a decision not to hire a particular person. All reference information used in making employment decisions should be objective (always fact based, never opinion based) and verifiable in the records of the organization providing the information.

## THE ACTUAL INTERVIEW

Assume you have reached the point where you are well aware of questions you should avoid and well advised of the kinds of questions you should ask. In addition, assume that you and an applicant are now face-to-face in private and that you are mindful of the edge you hold in this interchange and of the possibly uncomfortable position of the applicant. Having reached this stage, proceed according to the guidelines below.

### Put the Applicant at Ease

At the beginning of the conversation you need to put the individual at ease and instill a degree of confidence. You might want to try several different topics at the start of the interview—for instance, the weather, the ease with which the person may have found your office, or an invitation to enjoy a cup of coffee—to get the person talking and take you a step toward conversational rapport. Whatever opener you employ—and usually it need be only brief—it will get you off to a far better start than the shock of something like: "Good morning. Why do you want to work here?"

During these first few critical minutes try to avoid making judgments and freezing a picture of the applicant in your mind. First impressions are often difficult to shed, and when formed while the person is not yet at ease they can be unfair. Rather, reserve judgment until you have been able to explore the person's skills and abilities.

### Avoid Short-Answer Questions

Avoid asking questions in such a way that they can be answered in one or two words, and especially avoid questions that can be answered simply "yes" or "no." For instance, a question such as: "How long did you work for County General Hospital?" might simply be answered: "Three years." This gives you very little information. Rather, a request on the order of "Please tell me about the work you did at County General Hospital" requires the person to use more than just a couple of words in response. Your purpose is to learn about the applicant, and you can do so only by getting the person to talk.

However, you should avoid permitting the applicant to wander off the subject for minutes at a time. When this occurs, interrupt (as politely as possible) with another question or a request for clarification intended to draw the conversation back to the focus of the interview.

### Avoid Leading or "Loaded" Questions

Avoid questions that lead the applicant toward some predetermined response. For instance, if you ask: "You left County General because the pay raises weren't coming along, is that right?" you are channeling the applicant toward a response that you may have already decided is correct. It is far better to ask, "Why did you leave County General?"

Leading questions can be a particular hazard when you are talking with someone who is shaping up favorably in your eyes. In the process of unconsciously deciding you like this person, you may begin to bend the rest of your questions in a fashion that calls for the answers you would like to hear. Most people are sensitive to leading questions and, depending on the nature of the questions, will feel either forced or encouraged to deliver the answers that seem to be wanted.

### Ask One Question at a Time

Avoid hitting the applicant with something like: "What kind of work did you do there and why did you leave?" This is in fact two questions, and although they may well be properly asked one after the other the person should be given the opportunity to deal with them individually. Combining or pyramiding questions tends to throw some people off balance; a person prepared to deal with a single question is suddenly confronted with two or three at once. It is always preferable to limit your questioning to one clear, concise question at a time.

### Keep Your Writing to a Minimum

Try not to take voluminous notes while the prospective employee is talking. This can be disconcerting to the individual, creating the impression that everything that is said is being taken down in writing. Also, it is distracting to you. Writing and listening are both communication skills subject to their own particular ground rules and neither can be done with maximum effectiveness if you are trying to do the other at the same time. The more note taking you attempt, the more it detracts from your listening capacity. Take down a few key words if you must, but focus most of your attention on listening to the applicant. If you need or desire a written report of the interview, generate this report immediately after the applicant leaves and the conversation is still fresh in your mind.

## Use Appropriate Language

At all times deliver your questions and comments in language appropriate to the apparent level of education, knowledge, and understanding of the prospective employee. If you are a nursing supervisor interviewing an experienced registered nurse, you will likely talk on a level at which you would ordinarily expect to communicate with a registered nurse. However, if you happen to be interviewing for the position of unit clerk, talking with a person who has never worked in a hospital, you should alter your language accordingly. Always assume a reasonable degree of intelligence—you wish to avoid talking down to the person—but do not dazzle or confuse the applicant with unfamiliar terminology.

## Do More Listening Than Talking

Throughout the interview be interested and attentive, never impatient or critical. Avoid talking too much about yourself or the institution. Remember, you are not selling yourself to the applicant—it is supposed to be the other way around. Also, you are not necessarily selling the institution to the applicant, although if the interview moves far enough in constructive directions you may wish to answer the applicant's questions about the institution. However, even on this score there are precautions to note: specifics of certain features of employment like insurance, retirement, and other benefits for which you may not have all the details should be left to the personnel department and broached only when you are ready to extend an offer of employment and the individual needs this information to aid in making the decision.

## Indicate Some Type of Follow-Up

Conclude the interview with a reasonable statement of what the applicant may expect to happen next. It is true you generally cannot (and probably should not) make a definite statement at this time, but you should suggest what may be expected and when it might occur. For instance, you can always say something like: "We'll let you know our decision after we've finished all scheduled interviews, say within a week or 10 days," or "You should be getting a letter from us next week," or perhaps simply "We'll call you by Friday." In any case, conclude the interview with some simple indication of impending follow-up. Never let the applicant go away feeling that he or she has just been told "Don't call us—we'll call you."

Exhibit 8–1 provides a summary listing of guidelines for the supervisor to apply for effective employment interviewing.

## FOLLOW-UP

Follow-up is no problem when you decide to extend a job offer to an applicant—you will extend the offer and the person will either accept or decline the job. In either case the interview process has been taken full circle.

**Exhibit 8–1**  For Effective Employment Interviewing

- Ensure privacy. Knowing your conversation can be overheard is unsettling—and unfair—to the applicant.
- Do not permit interruptions. The applicant deserves your undivided attention.
- Put the person at ease before jumping into questioning.
- Do not read an application, résumé, or job description in the applicant's presence.
- Avoid short-answer questions—you learn little or nothing from them.
- Avoid leading questions—you want the applicant's answers, not yours.
- Ask one clear question at a time.
- Use language appropriate to the applicant's education and background.
- Keep note taking to a bare minimum—you cannot listen effectively while writing.
- Overall, do much more listening than talking.
- Leave benefits details to be covered by human resources.
- Promise timely follow-up—and see that it happens.

However, even in instances when you do not wish to extend a job offer you should follow up and complete the interview cycle. Follow-up by the institution is a simple but deserved courtesy; although the applicant was looking for a job, you were also looking for an employee, and this particular individual traveled to meet you and gave you a certain amount of time.

Appropriate follow-up takes very little time. Once you have decided you do not wish to extend a job offer, a short, polite letter to that effect is appropriate. Also, you can use this same approach to let individuals know that although you cannot extend a job offer at the present time you would like to keep their applications on file for future consideration. Depending on your organization's employment system these letters might originate with you or they might go out from the human resources department. In most organizations the employment section of the human resources department will take care of applicant communication, but it is within the realm of reason for you to follow up with personnel to make sure this communication has occurred. In any case, and even for the most clearly unqualified of applicants, you should conclude the interview process with an answer. It is a courtesy due the applicant, and it serves to protect the image of the institution as an employer in the community.

The employee selection interview is a hazardous process filled with opportunities for miscalculation and misjudgment. It offers no guarantees that you will always locate the right person for the job. However, the interview is the best available way of gaining information about prospective new employees. As such it will continue to remain one of the most important kinds of personal contact for the supervisor.

## REVIEW QUESTIONS

1. What is the benefit to the organization of ensuring that a significant proportion of attractive job openings are filled from within the organization?

2. Why is it said that the most effective interviewing involves more listening than talking?

3. Why are you not permitted to ask an applicant whether he or she has a recommendation from a present employer?

4. How can you briefly describe essentially all of the questions that can be asked of a job applicant?

5. Why is it advisable to faithfully avoid short-answer questions in an employment interview?

6. What is the rationale for limiting employment reference checking to the human resources department only?

## ROLE-PLAY: WOULD YOU HIRE THIS PERSON?

### Interviewer: Business Manager

You are the business manager for a small hospital. You are interviewing for a junior accountant. In your department you have two accountants, both qualified, reasonably effective individuals, one junior accountant, one open position for a junior accountant, and two clerks.

The employment manager is sending you the second and third job candidates to interview. The first you rejected as overqualified and looking for more money than the junior position would warrant. It is your understanding that the stream of job applicants dried up after candidates 2 and 3 submitted their applications. You feel strongly about the necessity to fill this position in the near future and will have this foremost in mind when you interview candidates 2 and 3. You do, however, have an alternative—you can hold the job open for a longer time and wait for the ideal candidate to appear.

After the initial review of applications you contacted some people you know to get an idea of the character of candidate 3. You learned that he has been with his present employer only 4 months but has not missed a day's work nor come in late. You did not check on the other applicant (2) because his application indicated he preferred you not contact his present employer.

### Candidate 2

You are 42 years old and you have approximately 15 years of routine bookkeeping experience in a large commercial organization. You believe you are probably older than most persons who would be expected to apply for this position, and you have done approximately the same level of work for about 10 years.

You are still employed but you are not especially happy with your job. You have realized that you will probably go no higher in the organization, so you decided to look for something better.

### Candidate 3

You are a 23-year-old high school graduate from another state. You did factory work for a year before taking 1 year of liberal arts courses at a community college. You then spent 3 years in the military service and after being discharged settled in this area, married, and took a laborer's job in a local cotton mill.

You are not hesitant to reveal that you have been looking for a new job since the day you were hired at the mill. You generally agree that your background seems not to qualify you for accounting work but you have embarked on a crash program of learning basic accounting on your own, primarily by acquiring books and practice sets and getting assistance from an acquaintance who is an accountant.

### Instructions

This is an exercise appropriate for groups of six or more people.

Divide all participants into three smaller groups of approximately equal size. Assign one of the three roles to each group. Each small group should designate a spokesperson to play the role assigned to the group.

The business manager group should prepare its "interviewer" by developing a tentative line of questioning for the interviews. It should be this group's intention to learn as much as possible about each candidate—following acceptable lines of questioning—in a brief simulated interview.

The groups representing candidates 2 and 3 should prepare their spokespersons by considering the kinds of questions they might expect to be asked. It is up to the "candidates" to respond to questioning, making reasonable assumptions as necessary, and to "sell themselves" to the "interviewer."

Devote approximately 10 minutes to group preparation; then allow about 5 to 7 minutes for each interview. Those participants not involved in the exercise as spokespersons should critique the interviews according to the interviewing guidelines provided in the chapter.

Discuss the conduct of the interviews.

## CHAPTER 9

# The One-to-One Relationship

*I know that you believe you understand what you think I said,*
*but I am not sure you realize that what you heard is not what I meant.*
*—Anonymous*

## CHAPTER OBJECTIVES

☛ Emphasize the importance of establishing an effective one-to-one communicating relationship with each employee.

☛ Stress the essential two-way character of interpersonal communication.

☛ Highlight the common barriers to effective communication, and suggest how they can be avoided or overcome.

☛ Offer guidelines for improving your listening capacity.

☛ Introduce cultural diversity considerations as they affect employee communication.

☛ Suggest guidelines for effective interpersonal communication in the supervisor-employee relationship.

## SITUATION: THE CASE OF THE EMPLOYEE WHO IS "NEVER WRONG"

"I know what I heard, and that's that," Staff Nurse Janice McCoy said in the no-nonsense tone that Head Nurse Wilma Pauley had come to know so well.

"Dr. Borden says otherwise, Janice," said Wilma. "He told me in no uncertain terms that the instructions he gave you were just the opposite of what you did."

"He's wrong," snapped Janice.

"He says that you were wrong, and he seemed quite sure about it." Wilma paused thoughtfully before adding, "He took the trouble to explain the whole situation to me, and I have to say that I understood his instructions. At least I was able to give them back in my own words so he was satisfied that I understood."

Janice scowled, then shrugged and said, "Then Dr. Borden changed his story."

"You're suggesting that he lied to me?"

"I didn't say that. I'm just saying that he told me one thing and then apparently told you something else. Maybe he didn't understand what he was telling me. You know how he just kind of rattles off something quickly and runs away."

Wilma sighed and said, "Janice, did you consider the possibility that you didn't understand? It isn't hard to misinterpret when everything happens so fast and—"

"I know what I heard," interrupted Janice. "When I know I'm wrong I'll say so. If I even think I may be wrong I'll say so. But in this case I know I'm right. It's not even remotely possible that I could have misinterpreted Dr. Borden."

144

Feeling that Janice had given her cause to say something that had been nagging at her for quite some time, Wilma said, "It seems to me that you're never wrong, Janice."

Janice McCoy glared at her supervisor. "What do you mean by that?" she asked.

Wilma took a deep breath and plunged in: "I've been head nurse of this unit for 3 years, and in those 3 years I've never known you to admit to being wrong about anything. This business with Dr. Borden is just one more example. You always turn everything around so you come up clean. Is it so necessary that you be right about everything?"

Janice's tone, already cool, became colder. "As I said, I'll admit when I'm wrong—but only when I *am* wrong. And I want to know the other times you're talking about, the times when I supposedly 'turned everything around.'"

Wilma began, "Well, there was—." She stopped, shook her head, and said, "No, that was something else. In any case, you ought to know what I'm talking about. Think about it, and you'll know what I'm saying. You've got an answer for everything, an answer that always places you in the right."

"You can't think of any specific incidents because there haven't been any," said Janice. She rose from her chair and continued, "You may be my supervisor, but I don't have to listen to this. Is there anything else you wanted to say about Dr. Borden's problem?" She glared down at Wilma.

Wilma rose to her feet. "Just that the incident is not to be considered closed. Dr. Borden insists that it be written up for disciplinary dialogue—an oral warning."

"I'll protest, of course," said Janice. "I won't sign a warning I don't deserve, and I won't say I'm wrong when I know I'm right."

When Janice left the office Wilma began to regret having spoken to Janice as she did. She was convinced, however, that she had to try to get through to Janice about her apparent need to be "right" about everything.

*Instructions*

As you proceed through this chapter, consider the following questions:

1. When Wilma "took the plunge" and left the specific incident to talk about Janice's overall conduct, she made a mistake that is embodied in the statement "You always turn everything around so you come up clean." What was Wilma's mistake?

2. How would you recommend attempting to determine the cause for the misunderstanding involving Janice McCoy and Dr. Borden?

3. How could you propose to deal with the employee who is "never wrong" in the future?

## THE TRANSFER OF MEANING

On any given day the largest part of a supervisor's job is likely to consist of interpersonal contact with other employees of the institution; these employees are primarily those who report directly to the supervisor. In recognition of the supervisor's constant contact with employees to get things accomplished through them, in this chapter we will concentrate on face-to-face communication specifically within the context of the supervisor-employee relationship.

A simple beginning for a complex subject that goes far beyond the limits of this chapter might be to describe communication as "the transfer of meaning." In an organizational sense, communication involves the transmission of information and instructions from person to person in such a way as to accomplish mutual understanding on the part of both the sender and the receiver of every message. The goal of communication is always a complete and accurate transfer of meaning resulting in assurance that the understanding of the person who received the message is identical to that of the person who originated the message.

Regarding the supervisor-employee relationship, we can say at the outset of this discussion that there is no single absolutely "correct" way of dealing with employees. All of your employees are different from each other, and they are all different from you. What works well in your relationship with employee A may not work at all in your relationship with employee B, and vice versa. We can go so far as to say that in your relations with your employees there may be fully as many "correct" ways of dealing with employees as you have employees.

An effective relationship with each employee is not something that can simply be established and assumed to exist forever. No such relationship between two people is ever completely "established," and the relationship must be constantly nurtured and conscientiously maintained if it is to serve appropriately the needs of the people involved and the organization.

Although interpersonal relations constitute a large part of the supervisor's job, it is not always easy to concentrate on people and their problems and needs. There are hidden pressures that encourage us to focus on things rather than people. After all, things cannot hurt, disappoint, frustrate, influence, disagree, or misunderstand. There is a measure of safety and security in things. However, the supervisor must learn to overcome the tendency to seek reduced vulnerability and look in the direction of the job's true demands.

The effective supervisor is called on to acquire and practice empathy—the capacity to put oneself in another's place and respond accordingly. Not many people are naturally attuned to the feelings and needs of those around them, but empathic sensitivity can be developed through conscious effort. Although we tend to take our communication capacity for granted, we are not really very good communicators by nature. We can, however, learn to communicate effectively. To do so we first need to appreciate the difficulties inherent in human communication, and we need to recognize one critical tendency in ourselves: the tendency to believe that we are better communicators than we in fact really are.

We use our primary tools of communication, words, to express meaning; yet a tremendous gap exists between the thoughts or feelings we experience inside and the words we use to direct them toward another person. Likewise, a similarly large gap exists between the words taken in by the other person and the thoughts or feelings experienced as a result of those words. Rarely is it possible, except in the most inconsequential situations, truly to transfer meaning to another person in every precise dimension in which it was experienced.

We are all unique individuals. Countless factors and influences in your upbringing, background, education, and life experience make you the unique person you are. Because of our differences, we relate to the world in our own particular ways. Individual experiences are never identical, and our uniqueness affects our ability to communicate with each other. Whenever we communicate with others we are attempting to describe what has happened within us as a result of experiences coming from outside of us. As long as each of us can sense with only a single mind—our own—the process will remain imperfect. We have no control over the mind of another; rather than directly transferring a thought or feeling, the best we can do is put it into words and hope those words create a similar thought or feeling in someone else.

Interpersonal communication frequently fails because of the imperfections in the process. Too often communication fails simply because we assume the person we are talking with knows and understands what we happen to be talking about—after all, *we* know what we are talking about. Also, the process is fully as susceptible to failure when viewed from the other side; we assume we know what the other person means without taking steps to make certain this is so. The greatest number of communication failures probably occurs in simple interchanges between people: You say something to another person and the two of you part, each with a meaning in mind. You believe you have been understood, and the other person believes he or she understands; yet you have parted with completely different meanings in mind.

## THE TWO-WAY STREET

Communication within the supervisor-employee relationship must be a two-way street heavily traveled in both directions. You are the supervisor; the authority of your position and the number of people with whom you must be concerned will limit the amount of communication flowing from employees to you. Therefore, it is generally up to you consistently to go more than halfway in the communication process.

One-way communication—the simple delivery of orders and instructions in authoritarian fashion with no information flowing the other way—is not communication at all. Admittedly there are occasions when one-way communication seems to work effectively. Consider the giving of orders in a military situation or the snapping-out of instructions in a medical emergency. However, these one-way transactions work only because they have been preceded by a significant amount of two-way communication in the form of instruction, training, and practice.

There are pressures, sometimes of undeniable proportions, that encourage managers to communicate in a one-way fashion, that is, simply to deliver orders or instructions in a few words before moving on to other problems. The pressures of time are often upon us, and it is always faster to deliver an instruction (even a seemingly well-thought-out one) than it is to engage in discussion or encourage a few simple words of feedback. One-way communication is clean and neat—at least it seems that way, until the misunderstanding begins to surface—and seems to be accomplished without wasting time or words.

One-way communication is often the refuge of the insecure manager. It discourages feedback and suppresses discussion, and the manager is considerably less likely to be challenged and therefore cannot be found "wrong." One-way communication is also the province of an authoritarian manager, the individual who behaves as though all meaning must flow from the "boss" downward and that nothing valid can be expected to flow in the opposite direction. True two-way communication, on the other hand, takes time, often considerably more time than a corresponding one-way contact would have taken. It is a simple trade-off: more time is invested for the sake of achieving greater accuracy in the transfer of meaning.

Consider the originator of a message in a two-way communication situation. The "sender" of the message experiences a certain vulnerability by virtue of being open to feedback and thus open to question, discussion, and perhaps disagreement. This position of vulnerability is not acceptable to all people in their communicating relationships, but feedback is the all-important element in two-way communication. It is feedback that helps clarify what has been said and ultimately determines whether the message has been correctly received.

## BARRIERS TO EFFECTIVE COMMUNICATION

### Semantics

Words, our most actively used tools of communication, are in truth quite inadequate for the role we make them play. We expect far too much of these small bits of language. A word is simply a symbol we use to stand for something; it is not the thing itself. The only true meanings words have are the meanings we give them through active use.

Words are inconsistent in so-called meaning; many of them possess a variety of definitions. In fact, the 500 most frequently used words in the English language have a total of nearly 15,000 dictionary definitions. This suggests that the "average" word, if we can say there is such a thing, can have 30 definitions, some quite similar to each other but some extremely different from all others.

Words are also likely to mean different things to different people. For instance, how long or short a span of time does prompt mean to you? Some words can even mean different things to the same person at different times or under different circumstances. For example, fix may mean one thing if you happen to be repairing an automobile and something else entirely if your immediate interest is locating a reference point for navigation purposes.

We have words in our language that can be described only as fuzzy in terms of meaning and usage. Take a good look at a few of the words that fill our organizational communication sometimes to the point of overflowing. Again, we have prompt. We also have sufficient, appropriate, adequate, and other similarly vague terms. What meaning are you going to get if the last sentence of the memorandum you just received says: "You are requested to take prompt action, employing adequate measures to ensure appropriate response sufficient to the situation"?

You can sample many of the problems of semantics by pondering your reaction to a simple question long used in discussions on this subject: How tall is a tall man? More than 6 feet tall? Six feet 6 inches tall or taller? Five feet 9 inches tall or taller? We can suggest that your answer depends in part on how tall you are, and that ultimately the answer to the question depends entirely on who is doing the judging.

## Emotion

Words often carry emotional overtones that vary from person to person and create additional barriers to interpersonal communication. Words that register neutrally or perhaps favorably on some people are likely to hit "sore spots" in other people. Aside from the obvious—profanity, obscenity, ethnic slurs, and downright insults—many words used without malicious intent will trigger negative emotional responses in listeners. Perhaps the word stubborn does not bother you, but the person you are talking with may resent being referred to as stubborn. Perhaps your boss places a favorable connotation on the term "eager beaver" and applies this to you; however, you may resent the term as suggesting you are trying too hard or bordering on being annoying. (You would prefer to be called a "loyal and energetic employee.")

No matter how inoffensive you try to keep your language you are likely (perhaps frequently) to touch one of someone's sore spots and trigger an emotional reaction. Consider the times you may have turned away from a conversation with the impression that you have somehow hurt, offended, or angered the other person, and you honestly did not have the slightest idea of what you might have said to cause that reaction. You do this unintentionally, and it is not likely that you will ever be able to eliminate this from your communication entirely. However, what you can do is be aware that this occurs with all people in interpersonal situations and, exercising empathy, try to understand the other person's position. Also, since you may hurt, offend, or anger someone unintentionally, always extend to the other person the benefit of the doubt. Remember that when someone touches one of your little sore spots and you are hurt, offended, or angered, chances are it was completely accidental and no injury was intended.

Positive emotions can be good to some extent in interpersonal communication. However, even positive emotions (e.g., joy or enthusiasm) can cloud individual judgment and impair communication when they are experienced to a degree that the feelings themselves become more important than the message being communicated.

The negative emotions—hurt and anger and all their variations—definitely tend to impair effective communication. Generally, the higher the negative emotional level of one or both parties to an interpersonal exchange the less are the chances of meaningful communication. When emotion threatens to turn a discussion into an argument, it is time to back away from the situation as diplomatically as possible and try again when tempers have abated.

Emotion in interpersonal exchange also tends to polarize views and drive participants toward opposite positions. Anger or any of its variations are also likely to be evident in the behavior of someone who has been put on the defensive and is using emotion unconsciously to cover a weakness or shield a position from attack.

It would be easy, but quite useless, for us to say we should not allow ourselves to be hurt or angry. You cannot help experiencing a feeling, and feelings themselves are neither right nor wrong—they are just there. However, be aware of the destructive potential of negative feelings.

In all dealings with your employees and others, be reasonably careful of the words you use, remain normally polite and friendly, and do not hesitate to be conciliatory if it appears necessary or helpful. Although you happen to be the manager and occupy a so-called position of authority, never consider yourself too important to apologize when you err in your interpersonal communication.

In all dealings with other persons, and especially in dealing with employees on critical issues and points of difference, avoid sweeping generalizations that are by their nature untrue. Two of the worst words you can use are always and never, as in "You're always late," or "You never submit it correctly." Rarely are always and never strictly true, but both are usually inflammatory.

## IS ANYONE REALLY "NEVER WRONG"?

It is doubtful that any of us could identify a single person, present or past, who is or was never wrong. Yet we all know that we occasionally encounter people who find it difficult, if not impossible, to admit to being wrong about anything.

In the "Situation" posed at the beginning of the chapter, when she said, "You always turn everything around so you come up clean," Wilma abandoned specifics and started to generalize about Janice's behavior. Time and again, always and never show themselves to be two of the most troublesome words in the English language. They are certainly two of the worst words to use in delivering criticism. Rarely is either absolutely true, but both are all-inclusive terms. They simply solidify the position of one party or the other and expand the opportunity for disagreement.

Also, in delivering criticism it is a critical mistake to generalize. All criticism should be specific to a particular problem and should be constructive; that is, it should include the means of correction or at least some guidance in that direction. In order to be valid, criticism has to go beyond identifying what is wrong and include advice about how to make it right. Even if there have been a number of specific instances of a certain kind of undesirable behavior, it is still best to cite them individually rather than to generalize them.

The relationships in "The Case of the Employee Who Is 'Never Wrong'" are also affected by emotion to some extent. A certain amount of anger on the physician's part is implied. The employee, Janice, is reacting to criticism with extreme defensiveness; the manager, Wilma, soon finds herself at least partly driven by frustration. The presence of these emotional reactions is bound to impede communication.

The best way to get to the cause of the misunderstanding involves bringing the disagreeing parties together. It may, of course, be extremely difficult, if not impossible, to get the physician to agree to a meeting, but Wilma should at least make the attempt. If Wilma tries to resolve the matter by shuttling between the two parties, then she will likely accomplish little or nothing.

The relationship between Janice and Wilma could be difficult for a considerable time to come. The best advice we could give Wilma in dealing with the employee who is never wrong would be to pay extra attention to detail and consistently to be as timely as possible and as specific as possible in addressing problems as they arise. Also, Wilma should be creating clear, concise documentation of every instance in which she must deal with Janice's behavior. Though she might be tempted to let some of Janice's behavior go unaddressed because she knows what to expect from Janice, she should avoid doing so. An unfavorable situation left unaddressed rarely gets better by itself, and more often than not it gets worse.

## LISTENING

The following words of wisdom once occupied a prominent place on an office wall: "How come it takes 2 years to learn to talk and 60 or 70 to learn to be quiet?" How much of the talking do you do in any interchange with an employee? This is a valid question because you cannot truly listen while you are talking.

Of our four verbal means of communication—writing, reading, speaking, and listening—listening, when effectively practiced, requires most of our communication time. Yet listening is the single verbal communication skill for which the least amount of solid, practical help is available. Writing, reading, and speaking are all active processes; to engage in any of these it is necessary to decide to do so and take the appropriate action. Too often, however, listening is treated as passive; one can *hear* without conscious effort, but without the deliberate application of such effort true listening cannot occur.

Although listening skills are not easy to describe or define, these skills can nevertheless be learned. Conscientious attention to the following suggestions and precautions can make you a better listener.

### Be Attentive

Force yourself to concentrate on what the other person is saying. Do not turn off the speaker as uninteresting or reject close attention to the subject because you "know it already." Some people speak in ways that fail to grab and hold your attention automatically, and if you are really to listen to what is being said, then you will find it necessary to apply some conscious effort. Knowing that your forced attention may be required is often more than half the battle; the remainder becomes a matter of actually applying your undivided attention. Also, keep in mind that even though a topic may not seem interesting or important to you it usually is important to the person doing the speaking.

### Wait before Responding

All but trained listeners are likely to rush their responses by reacting to only a portion of what is being said. The temptation is great; you hear a few words that trigger a response in you and your mind begins to race ahead and form the comment you will deliver as soon as the other person pauses. Resist this temptation. While your mind is busy forming your response, your listening capacity is reduced, sometimes to the point where you will interrupt the other person. Instead, deal with one complete thought or idea at a time, hearing the person out completely before offering a response.

### Get the Whole Message

Many people have a habit of listening only for "facts"—specific bits of information. Facts are useful, of course, but their usefulness is diminished if they are not considered within the context of the entire message. Listen to the whole message before making decisions or rendering judgments.

### Keep Interruptions to a Minimum

If you can possibly avoid doing so, try not to interrupt the other person to offer a correction of something you think has been improperly stated. Certainly avoid interrupting to offer advice or to scold or otherwise criticize. This is especially important in face-to-face communication within the supervisor-employee relationship. Generally, interruptions are in order only if you make them to ask for expansion or clarification of something that has been said or to ask related questions intended to encourage more relevant comments.

### Be Aware of Your Emotional Sore Spots

While you are listening, be aware of the possibility of emotional reactions within you. As discussed earlier, it is possible that the other person will unintentionally trigger an emotional reaction in you. Give the other person the benefit of the doubt and force yourself to concentrate on the message as being distinctly separate from its emotional overtones. You cannot help what you feel, but you can control what you do with those feelings. If you allow negative feelings to come to the foreground and dominate your reaction, your listening capacity will be sharply reduced.

Summary guidelines for effective listening appear in Exhibit 9–1.

## DIVERSITY IN THE ONE-TO-ONE RELATIONSHIP

### An Inevitable Concern

Chances are that the majority of people who presently are or will become health care managers will manage increasingly diverse work groups. The diversities encountered in the work force may be rooted in ethnicity, religion, race, gender, or social differences, but in the work organization we have essen-

**Exhibit 9–1**  For Effective Listening

- Remain attentive; deliberately concentrate on what is being said.
- Wait before responding; hear the person out before judging or answering.
- Listen for the whole message, context as well as facts and data.
- Take in not only words, but also vocal tone, facial expression, and body language; these non-verbal cues are often the largest part of the message.
- Interrupt as little as possible, then only to ask for needed clarification.
- Know your emotional "hot spots" and keep your temper under control regardless of what you hear.
- Keep note-taking to a bare minimum; writing detracts from listening capacity.
- At the end of the other person's message, or periodically throughout a lengthy interchange, feed back what the other party has said in your own words and seek agreement or clarification.

---

tially gathered all of these areas of difference under the single term cultural diversity. This term suggests a broad range of differences, also implying, for example, differences in values, assumptions, expectations, and needs.

Labor projections offered several years ago told us that during the first decade or two of this new millennium the majority of new entrants into the work force would likely be women, minorities, and immigrants. In fact this is already the case in a number of areas of health care.

It is reasonable to assume that the majority of people are most at ease around people who look, think, and act as they do. However, these days rarely do people of a single cultural group populate an entire function, department, or organization. Rather, it is common to find most employee populations culturally mixed to some extent. It is lack of understanding of the differences between and among cultures that gives rise to difficulties for the manager.

Workplace tensions often arise from failure to recognize or understand cultural differences, and these tensions can cause interpersonal conflict, reduced productivity, absenteeism, turnover, and even charges of discrimination and other legal complaints. In addition, communication problems arise from language and literacy concerns related to individual background, and other concerns develop from lack of cultural awareness and respect.

In the work force in general it is now and will become increasingly more necessary to interact with people who hold different values and believe in different ways. Increasing diversity in the work force is unavoidable, especially in health care. In health care, diversity exists at all levels (for example, a significant percentage of licensed physicians are foreign-born). But in health care, cultural diversity is greatest in the lower-paying or entry-level jobs such as housekeeping workers, nursing assistants, and food service staff, among others.

## Recognizing Our Differences

In the absence of knowledge of cultures other than our own we incline toward stereotypes in our thinking about others. Although stereotypes are usually superficial or simply wrong, they nevertheless tend to influence our thinking and decision-making.

A manager should be able to respect each employee as an individual and hold all employees to the same standard of job performance. Yet in the one-to-one relationship between manager and employee, the manager must recognize individual differences that are culturally based. A few examples of differences you may encounter as a manager follow:

- In some cultures prolonged, direct eye contact is acceptable; in others it is considered rude and improper.
- People from some cultural backgrounds believe it is disrespectful to offer opinions or suggestions to a superior (potentially quite frustrating to the manager who wants employee input).
- Workers from some cultural backgrounds are uncomfortable with being singled out in any way, even for praise.
- Workers from some backgrounds will point out their own successes with pride while others will remain silent no matter how successful; to them, self-praise or self-promotion is not acceptable behavior.
- In some cultures physical touching or entering another's close personal space is acceptable, but in some it is not.
- Some male workers from certain cultures may be extremely ill at ease reporting to a female supervisor.

The foregoing and more add up to numerous individual differences that a manager may have to account for in relating to each individual member of a work group.

## In the One-to-One Relationship

All employees should be expected to adapt to the reasonable requirements of the job and the workplace as necessary, but they will always bring their individualism to the job as well. The effective manager will always remain aware of individual differences and respect these differences in the relationship with each employee.

It is also to the manager's advantage to become familiar with applicable aspects of antidiscrimination laws. In reacting to culturally based individual differences, it is sometimes possible to unintentionally enter into discriminatory practices out of ignorance of the law.

Every health care manager would stand to benefit by attending a sound cultural diversity program and making a determined effort to learn about the cultures prevalent in the department or organization. The manager must not only successfully relate to each employee, but also must manage the interactions between and among employees to ensure that equal treatment, opportunity, and respect exist for all.

Over the coming few decades the more effective organizations—health care and otherwise—will be those that successfully manage work force diversity and tap the maximum potential that each employee has to offer.

## GUIDELINES FOR EFFECTIVE INTERPERSONAL COMMUNICATION

### When You Are Doing the Talking

- Before speaking up, put some effort into structuring the communication you are about to deliver. First think out the what and the why of the communication, then when you know what you are going to say and what you are trying to accomplish, you can consider how best to communicate it.
- Consider your listener's needs, interests, and attitudes. Try to exercise empathy at all times, constantly judging what you are saying from your listener's point of view.
- Deliver your comments in language properly suited to the level of knowledge, education, and experience of your listener. Never talk down to or over the head of the other person.
- Except in the direst of emergencies (and even in emergencies, when you are not convinced that your listener is prepared to respond appropriately) follow up your communication immediately with a request for feedback. Ask to have the message played back to you in the listener's own words. This could be as simple as: "How would you describe what I've just asked you to do?" Ideally, your approach should not be one that suggests you are trying to find out if the other person understood you—although that is a major purpose—but rather that you are trying to assure yourself that you communicated your thoughts clearly and fully.

### When You Are Doing the Listening

- Pay attention. Really listen—your undivided attention conquers many potential obstacles.
- Listen always for meaning, striving constantly to determine what is being said and why it is being said.
- Consider the whole person, searching out attitudes and feelings as well as meanings. Keep in mind that words and other signs—the nonverbal signals given out by the other person—cannot be fully separated from attitudes and feelings.
- Be as patient as necessary to encourage the individual to try to communicate fully.
- Be prepared to compromise as necessary to achieve agreement or understanding, and consider yielding completely on minor points or unimportant details. Compromise is not the dirty word it is regarded to be by some; rather, reasonable compromise is often the most important step in establishing mutual understanding.

- Return the message to the speaker in your own words, using discussion to iron out differences until you both agree that the message sent and the message received are the same.

## THE OPEN-DOOR ATTITUDE

Every manager has probably said at one time or another, "My door is always open." This is an easy statement to make, but it takes effort to ensure that these words reflect more of an honest attitude than a timeworn platitude.

Your job is to help your employees get their work done. In addition to guiding and directing their overall efforts you must answer questions, deal with problems, silence rumors, and put fears and suspicions to rest. Remember that your employees do not work for you as much as they work *with* you and that a large part of your function is to "run interference" for your employees so that they can accomplish their work as efficiently as possible. To do all of this you must be visible and readily available to your employees, and you must have an always-growing one-to-one relationship with each employee. It is your responsibility honestly to consider the employee as a whole person, not simply as just a producer. To do so often requires you to be a person first and a manager second. Successful supervision requires human sensitivity. Without sensitivity, a supervisor has only rules, policies, and procedures, which are useful but which by themselves are grossly inadequate for the complete fulfillment of the supervisory role.

Effective one-to-one communication with each employee is the basis for mutual understanding between supervisor and employee. A healthy attitude for the supervisor assumes a Golden Rule approach to communication: Deal with others as you would wish to be dealt with yourself.

Your one-to-one relationship with each employee is critical to the institution as a whole. The way each employee sees you—available, friendly, caring, and helpful, or perhaps the opposite—so may he or she come to see the entire organization. As a member of management you represent the organization to the employee. The impression you create as a person will contribute, for good or ill, to the individual employee's impression of the organization as a whole.

---

## REVIEW QUESTIONS

1. Why is so-called one-way communication actually not communication at all? What is the missing essential ingredient?
2. What are the more common results of the presence of negative emotions (anger, etc.) in interpersonal communication?
3. Explain the statement: The same words can mean different things to different people at the same time.
4. Explain the difference between the open-door policy and the open-door attitude.

5. Describe the role of and necessity for feedback in interpersonal communication.

---

## CASE: WHAT'S IN A PHRASE?

Don Harrison accepted the position of director of materials management at County General Hospital.

In his middle 30s, Don had considerable experience in related work in hospitals. Years before, following his graduation with a degree in general business, he was central supply supervisor in a small hospital. After 5 years in that capacity he moved on to become manager of purchasing at a 400-bed hospital. Now, after 8 years, he had just moved to the 1,000-bed County General Hospital.

Don reported to Arthur Phillips, an associate administrator. Don was impressed with Phillips, who seemed to have his finger on everything within his organization. He was likewise impressed by the tempo, tone, and general enthusiasm of the County General organization. It was a significant change from the relaxed environment from which he had come.

Don joined County General during an extremely busy period. Not only did he have the expected task of getting to know the people in his various groups, but there was also the problem of relocating his department's largest storeroom to a newly completed area. Also, it was the time of annual budget preparation and Don's first week was the one in which each department's initial drafts were assembled.

On Monday, Don's first day, he received considerable orientation from Arthur Phillips along with several instructions concerning things he was expected to do. The last item Phillips covered was the matter of the budget. As Phillips put it to Don, "I realize you are new but you've walked right into the annual budget exercise. All other directors are expected to have their first-cut budgets to me on Wednesday. You're going to be involved enough as it is, so let's say I'll expect to have your first rough cut as soon as you can do it but no later than noon Friday."

Later that day Don began assembling preliminary numbers for the budget draft. He took it home with him and did a small amount of work on it.

On Tuesday some severe problems developed with the transfer of goods to the enlarged storage area and Don found himself deeply involved. At the same time, he was pursuing a series of face-to-face meetings with employees. By midweek Don was thinking that never in several years on his past job had the work come at such an unexpected pace.

Shortly after noon on Friday Don was seated at his desk handling a few items of correspondence when his phone rang. It was Phillips, who asked, "Don, where is that draft budget?"

Don suddenly realized that he had not touched the budget since Monday evening. Recalling (or believing he recalled) Phillips's words he said, somewhat defensively, "You told me to get it to you as soon as I could. I've been buried; I just haven't been able to get at it."

"I did say as soon as possible," Phillips replied. "I could have used it Wednesday. I also said 'no later than Friday noon.' It's now Friday, past noon, and I don't have your draft."

Don said, "I'm sorry I let it slip. I'll get it to you as soon as—" he stopped and caught himself for he had almost said, "as soon as I can." Instead he said, "I'll get it to you as quickly as I can put it together."

After a few seconds of silence on the other end of the line Phillips said, "I'll be here straight through until 10 or 11 o'clock tonight. I expect your budget draft on my desk before I go home."

Don cleared his desk and prepared to work on the budget, thinking somewhat glumly, "First week on the job and I'm already on the list." He also could not help thinking that his boss on his previous job would never have expected a new employee to get up and running so rapidly.

## Instructions

Isolate the particular words or phrases that got Don into trouble. Explore the likely reason why trouble resulted from a few seemingly innocent words.
What does this tell you about:

- the context within which a message is delivered?
- the apparent meanings of simple words?

## CHAPTER 10

# Leadership: Style and Substance

*Real leaders are ordinary people with extraordinary determinations.*
*—John Seaman Garns*

## CHAPTER OBJECTIVES

☞ Describe patterns of leadership, or leadership "styles," ranging from rigid (autocratic) to open (participative).

☞ Review opposing sets of assumptions about people that give rise to different leadership styles.

☞ Establish the necessity for sufficient flexibility in leadership to vary style according to circumstances.

☞ Determine the primary characteristic of effective leadership.

☞ Relate the employees' view of the supervisor to critical elements of leadership performance.

## SITUATION: ONE BOSS TOO MANY

The engineering and maintenance groups at Memorial Hospital are managed by three first-line supervisors. These supervisors and a department secretary report directly to a manager of engineering and maintenance who, in turn, reports to the director of environmental services.

The institution is in the midst of a prolonged period of growth and expansion owing mostly to merger and acquisition. Almost weekly some organizational unit or another is being located to new quarters or drastically rearranged within its original area. The institution promises to be in a chronic state of change for some time to come, with much extra effort required by engineering and maintenance as numerous areas are opened, renovated, or rearranged.

The position of director of environmental services was created at the start of this period of major change. The incumbent was hired specifically for his apparent ability to get a new operation up and running through active involvement of personnel at all levels.

The director was quick to discover that his immediate subordinate, the manager of engineering and maintenance, came across as a man of considerable inertia who moved slowly, was reluctant to change, and usually defended "the way we've always done things."

Although the manager had long-standing relationships with the three supervisors, the director began avoiding the manager and dealing directly with the first-line supervisors. Most matters, however, found their way back to the manager who would then take action or give instructions contrary to what the director had done.

After several weeks in this mode of operation, one of the first-line supervisors summed up their circumstances as follows: "We now have two bosses, and they're opposed to each other on everything. What one decides, the other reverses; what one puts together, the other tears apart. They can't even agree on anything as basic as an obvious need for disciplinary action. How do we go about maintaining effectiveness in dealing with our employees, and how do we prevent morale and efficiency from going straight down the drain?"

*Instructions*

As you proceed through this chapter, consider the case. Based on what you believe to be sound management practice, develop an approach the three supervisors might take. State any assumption you may have to make, and be prepared to explain the reasons for your recommended approach.

## INTRODUCING LEADERSHIP

A great many people have some potential for leadership, although in some individuals this potential may be limited. The essential difference between the leader and the nonleader is determined by the degree to which a person succeeds in learning about leadership and applying what has been learned.

Leadership is like many other human endeavors—talent helps, but it is not necessary to be extraordinarily talented to be successful. You may not be a natural leader; you may not be able to run a large organization or get hundreds of people to follow you in some undertaking. However, you stand at least an average chance of being able to furnish true leadership to the employees in a department or other work group.

Since there are vast differences in perceptions of what characterizes a leader and how a leader should behave, this discussion of leadership will begin with the consideration of style—the patterns of behavior projected by leaders as they work. And although it is tempting to talk about leadership on a grand scale (since most of the great leaders we learn about led armies, nations, churches, or corporations), we will better serve our needs by limiting the discussion to the context of the supervisor's environment.

## PATTERNS OF LEADERSHIP

Leadership styles range along a continuous scale from purely authoritarian at one extreme to fully participative at the other. In the scale in Figure 10–1 from left to right the following styles are delineated:

- Exploitative autocracy describes the harshest style of leadership. The exploitative autocrat not only wields absolute power over the people in the group but also uses the group primarily to serve personal interests. This type of leader literally exploits the followers.
- Benevolent autocracy is when the leader wields absolute power, often with an iron hand, but is generally sincere in believing that the behavior of those in the group must be closely ordered and regulated for the good of the organization. References to autocratic leadership throughout the remainder of this chapter will refer generally to this particular leadership pattern.

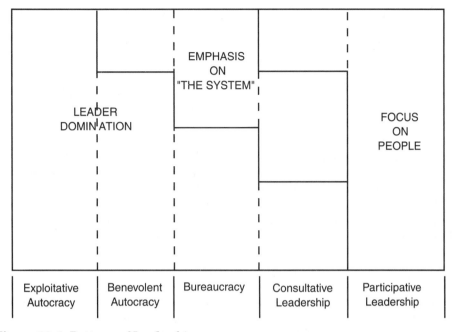

Exploitative Autocracy | Benevolent Autocracy | Bureaucracy | Consultative Leadership | Participative Leadership

**Figure 10–1** Patterns of Leadership

- Bureaucracy is a term that immediately raises visions of massive federal and state government agencies (especially where health care is concerned). As a leadership pattern it refers to the primary emphasis on rules and regulations. The bureaucratic leader goes by the book, creating new rules and regulations as new situations arise, to such an extent that the "book" itself often becomes more important than the purpose it is intended to serve.

- Consultative leadership is exhibited when the leader remains open to input from members of the group, but, by pronouncement, attitude, or practice, retains full decision-making authority. In many instances consultative leadership is appropriate (as even autocratic leadership of the benevolent kind is sometimes appropriate), but often consultative leadership is practiced under a participative label. Some supervisors claim they are open to participation, but in practice they are "open" only as long as the employees come up with the same decisions they would have made themselves.

- Full participative leadership exists when plans or decisions are made by all of the department's employees as a group or team. The supervisor is a key member of the group, providing advice, information, and assistance in any way possible but in advance has made a decision to accept the outcome of the group process.

With the exception of exploitative autocracy, no particular leadership pattern can always be labeled "wrong." What is right for one department may be wrong for another; what is right in one particular situation may be wrong under a different set of circumstances. And what was right at some time in the past may be wrong today.

Time and changing social conditions have lessened the need for autocratic leadership over the years; yet autocratic leadership patterns prevail in many organizations. Gone are the days when the average worker was uneducated and completely dependent on orders from above. Autocratic leadership was the rule when the average worker was illiterate, or at best, semiliterate, but even today many outmoded organizational assumptions prevail and autocratic and bureaucratic leadership hold forth when they should have given way to more consultative and participative styles.

We must briefly examine some of the assumptions on which so-called modern organizations are based, limiting this discussion to the extent necessary to allow us to continue exploring leadership. More complete consideration of the reasons why people work is provided in the discussion of motivation in Chapter 11.

## SOME ASSUMPTIONS ABOUT PEOPLE

Douglas McGregor, in his landmark work "The Human Side of Enterprise,"[1] wrote of two opposing approaches to management: Theory X and Theory Y. Theory X in its pure state is what we have been calling autocratic leadership. Pure Theory Y is participative leadership. Each of these management theories is based on a number of assumptions, only the first of which, relating to management in general, is common to both. That common assumption, valid in any case, is that management remains responsible for organizing the elements of all productive activity, that is, bringing together the money, people, equipment, and supplies needed to accomplish the organization's goals. Beyond this assumption, however, the two theories proceed in opposite directions. Theory X assumes the following:

- People must be actively managed. They must be directed and motivated, and their actions must be controlled and their behavior modified to fit the needs of the organization. Without this active intervention by management, people would be passive and even resistant to organizational needs. Therefore, people must be persuaded, controlled, rewarded, or punished as necessary to accomplish the aims of the organization.

- The average person is, by nature indolent, working as little as possible. The average person lacks ambition, shuns responsibility, and in general prefers to be led.

- The average person is inherently self-centered, resistant to change, and indifferent to the needs of the organization.

Theory Y, on the other hand, is predicated on the following assumptions:

- People are not naturally passive or resistant to organizational needs. If they appear to have become so, this condition is the result of experience in organizations.

- Motivation, development potential, willingness to assume responsibility, and readiness to work toward organizational goals are present in most people. It is management's responsibility to make it possible for people to recognize and develop these characteristics for themselves.

- The essential task of management is to arrange organizational conditions and methods of operation so people can best achieve their own goals by directing their efforts toward the goals of the organization.

## STYLE AND CIRCUMSTANCES

If you are an autocratic leader, you are operating under Theory X assumptions. You choose to make all the decisions and hand them down as orders and instructions. If you are a participative leader, you are generally ascribing to Theory Y assumptions and encouraging your employees to participate in joint decisions.

You have a choice of leadership styles available to you ranging from extremely closed to fully open. The trick is to know which style to apply and when to apply it. You may have some "Theory X people" in your department; they will likely be a minority—those few who actually prefer to be led and have their thinking done for them. However, you may also have a number of "Theory Y people" who are self-motivated and capable of significant self-direction. This is especially likely in departments employing large numbers of professionals, such as nursing service. Although the same "rules" (meaning personnel policies) apply uniformly to all employees, you will deal differently with individuals in other ways. Some you will consult and invite their participation; others you will simply direct.

Avoid making assumptions about people. Know your employees and try to understand each one as both a producer and a person. By working with people over a period of time, and especially by working at the business of getting to know them, you can learn a great deal about individual likes and dislikes and capabilities. Learn about your people as individuals and when necessary lead accordingly. If you are convinced that a certain employee genuinely prefers orders and instructions and this attitude is not inconsistent with job requirements, then use orders and instructions. Although many employees of health care organizations seem to prefer participative leadership, not everyone will desire this same consideration. Maintain sufficient flexibility to accommodate the employee who wants or requires authoritarian supervision. It is fully as unfair to expect people to become what they do not want to be as it is to allow a rigid structure to stifle those other employees who feel they have something more to contribute.

There is no single style of leadership that is appropriate to all people and situations at all times. Now, however, there is more reason than ever before to believe that consultative and participative leadership is most appropriate to modern organizations and today's educated workers.

A final word about style: Some supervisors and managers expend a fair amount of effort telling employees what style of management they practice. For instance, it is not uncommon for a manager who is new to the organization to make statements like, "I practice employee empowerment," "My door is always open," "I want your input," or "I believe in total quality management." There are hazards in presenting one's self in this manner. First, in the words of a wise, anonymous observer, "It's Management 101—using the buzzwords, saying what you think you should be saying." Second, and a far greater hazard, is the risk of being trapped by employee perception.

It takes only one or two perceived contradictions of your self-described style to create dissonance. As soon as you are seen unilaterally (although necessarily) making a decision or as soon as someone finds you unavailable although you have said the door is always open, you have created a conflict between your words and your actions. It is probably best to say as little as necessary about your own management style and let your actions convey your style. In other words, instead of telling them what you are, let your actions show them.

## OUTMODED VIEWS

In addition to harboring erroneous assumptions about people, many managers cling to outmoded notions of how a manager should behave. They see, with all good intentions, the leader as being a "boss"—the essential giver of orders: "I'm the boss. I'm paid to make decisions and I'm responsible for the results of those decisions, so I will make those decisions." In brief, some managers see participative leadership as "passing the buck" or "spreading the blame" and in general view participative leadership as a shirking of responsibilities.

However, participative leadership is anything but abrogation of responsibility. Recall from the material on delegation that although you can parcel out your management authority and spread it among a number of employees, you remain responsible for the decisions and actions of your employees. The true participative leader, willingly remaining responsible for the decisions of the group, is displaying considerably more courage than the autocrat who simply decides and gives orders. To trust your employees with a share of your authority while you retain full responsibility is a sign of strength, not a sign of weakness.

Another outmoded view of leadership is reflected in the belief that the leader should always know best, that employees look to the leader to "tell them how to do it." The true function of the leader is to help the employees find the best way to do it themselves. The leader does not take up a position at the rear of the pack and shove. Neither does the leader move in front of the crew and urge them to follow. Rather, the leader is somewhere in the pack—a facilitator, a remover of obstacles, and in general a catalytic agent that causes the entire group to move forward in the proper direction. The true leader is not the master of a department but rather its busiest, most responsible servant.

## LEADERSHIP'S PRIMARY CHARACTERISTIC

Many attempts have been made at creating detailed listings of qualities that characterize leaders. It is done all the time; great lists are generated that include standard noble but intangible characteristics such as honesty, integrity, and initiative and slightly more measurable criteria such as academic qualifications. People who write hiring requirements for managerial positions do it all the time, creating job specifications as full of noble characteristics as the Boy Scout Law. However, there is hardly a characteristic we can name—education, experience, integrity, communication ability, energy, conscientiousness—that we cannot find to be completely lacking in some supposedly successful leaders. In short, you cannot make a list, even a brief list, and truly say that a leader must have these characteristics.

Consider, then: is there anything that always and truly defines a leader? A leader is certainly not defined by organizational appointment or by the simple conferring of a management title. A title may describe a position but not a person; a great many so-called leadership positions are occupied by people who are anything but leaders in the true sense of the word.

The single factor that defines or characterizes a true leader is the *acceptance by the followers*. This means acceptance of the individual as a leader, not simply acceptance of obedience to the position the individual occupies. You have undoubtedly known managers who were not especially respected, were perhaps even ridiculed or joked about when not present, but were nevertheless obeyed. Obedience, although it may be grudging, will often be extended to the position because of the authority of the position itself. However, willing obedience will be extended consistently only by those employees who have accepted the supervisor's leadership.

Acceptance by one's followers cannot be mandated; it must be earned. Without this acceptance, a supervisor is a manager in title only and a leader not at all.

## WORD PLAY: LEADERSHIP VERSUS MANAGEMENT

Leadership has been attracting a great deal of attention and acquiring newer shades of meaning in the total quality management (TQM) movement. As empowerment is "in" and delegation attracts little concern—although empowerment is no more than proper delegation with a slick new finish on it (see Chapter 5)—so is leadership "in" at present and likely to remain that way for the coming several years. Many concerned with the quality movement speak of the need for "not management, but leadership."

With this highly positive connotation placed on the word leadership, we are left with an eroded connotation of management, conveying the impression that somehow mere management does not measure up to leadership. However, management and leadership remain two words that are generally synonymous and freely interchangeable in many uses.

As suggested above, someone can be a manager—or supervisor, director, coordinator, administrator, chief executive officer, or whatever—in title without being a true leader. However, this in no way renders management as a whole anything less than, nor anything significantly different from, leadership. There is poor management and there is good management; there is poor leadership and there is good leadership. One can be a manager in title without being a leader, but in terms of function one cannot manage without leading and cannot lead without managing. Good leadership and good management go together, as do poor leadership and poor management.

We frequently hear management described as both art and science. We might say the same about leadership, but we are usually ready to consider leadership more as art. Leadership is more likely to inspire thoughts of the human element, whereas management conjures up images of "techniques" and "tools." Whether we are speaking of management or leadership, however, we are dealing with the process of accomplishing goals through the efforts of people. Only so much of this process can be quantified and reduced to rules and techniques; the remainder will come from the heart and the gut. It can be developed from within but it can never be instilled from without. Whether leadership or management, it is this unquantifiable, frequently elusive "soft" side that puts the word "good" or another adjective in front of management or leadership. And leadership and management cannot be justly compared without the use of qualifying adjectives.

## CAN YOU LEAD "BY THE BOOK"?

The previous section made mention of the so-called art of leadership and the perceived techniques and tools of management. If we accept the contention that good leadership (or good management) is both art and science, we can perhaps reason that leading or managing "by the book" is only partially possible. However, one of the errors commonly committed by struggling leaders is over-reliance on what we might refer to as cookie-cutter management. Cookie-cutter management is what occurs when we attempt to apply specifically named management techniques or kinds of management often cynically described as "flavors of the month."

Think of what occurs when you roll out a batch of cookie dough and apply a cookie cutter. You obtain a desired shape, but you also get leftover material. Even if you roll out the leftover dough and cut another time or two, you are still left with a remaining lump of dough that fails to fit the required shape.

Whenever effort is applied to produce a desired shape from some form of input, some material is squeezed into the desired shape. Like the dough left outside of the cookie cutter, the extra material that falls away during the shaping process is ignored, for all practical purposes lost to consideration. This is what occurs when we attempt to apply "formula" management.

It is reasonable for us to seek order in our work. However, we tend at times to look beyond simple order and seek formula approaches, recipes for doing this or that task or handling particular kinds of problems. We look for cookie cutters, unconsciously willing to settle for the neat boundaries created by the instrument and equally willing to ignore what falls outside. However, management's problems cannot be consistently and adequately addressed by processes that by their very nature attempt to force issues into certain configurations.

Cookie-cutter management is especially prevalent in management literature. A number of management authors have named their own approaches to management using labels that each fervently hopes will catch on and become the next flavor of the month. This sells books, attracts speaking engagements, and enhances an author's value as a consultant.

Consider, for example, the "excellence" movement inspired by *In Search of Excellence* by Peters and Waterman.[2] While this extremely enlightening book did not itself espouse a cookie-cutter approach to management, the concepts it advanced were taken up by others who did exactly that—created dozens of cookie-cutter approaches as they attempted to formularize and proceduralize these concepts into "excellence programs." Much the same happened years earlier with management by objectives (MBO). The entire MBO concept sprang from a single chapter of an excellent book written by Peter F. Drucker in the 1950s.[3] As presented by Drucker, MBO was largely honesty and common sense; it was not the periodic exercise with forms and notebooks that it became for so many managers. Drucker himself even cautioned against allowing such a process to become a paper mill, yet many of those who picked up on his work and ran with it turned it into one of the biggest wastes of time and paper with which managers have ever had to contend.

We have likewise been offered cookie-cutter approaches in the forms of quality circles and many of the permutations of the principles of TQM. There also have been many less notable approaches that have come and gone as successive authors have attempted to originate the next flavor of the month, or to be the one to launch the next MBO or TQM.

The good news about cookie cutters is that they all include concepts of potential value to managers at all levels. The bad news is that none of the cookie cutters includes everything that a manager might need to know because by its very nature the cookie cutter always leaves some material outside. Also, none of the cookie cutters can instill in the individual the qualities and characteristics of a successful leader. Common sense, honesty, integrity, insight, pride, enthusiasm, and the belief in every employee's value and potential contribution cannot be proceduralized; these qualities are among the elements that fuel the art of leadership. If they are not there in sufficient quantity to inspire people to follow willingly, the best that can ever be obtained from the latest cookie-cutter approach is a brief burst of success—perhaps real, perhaps only perceived—to be washed away in a returning tide of cynicism. You cannot lead or manage by the book; the book provides only the science, but the art springs from the capabilities and actions of the individual manager.

## AN EMPLOYEE'S VIEW

Not all the employees in a department will view the supervisor in the same light or develop the same impression of the supervisor as a leader. Each of your employees will experience your leadership "style" in bits and pieces that add up to a total impression. As long as you are convinced you are doing the best job you know how to do, there is little to be gained from worrying about the opinions your employees hold of you. However, it pays to remember that your view of yourself as a leader is rarely the same as the view of you that your employees hold. What you see as your strengths may not be seen as strong points by your employees. Conversely, what your employees see as your strong points may not even have occurred to you as significant characteristics of your style.

There are several aspects of supervisory performance that are likely to influence your employees' assessment of you. Your employees may not use the same terms we use to describe these aspects of performance, and neither may they use labels such as "autocratic," "authoritarian," or "participative." However, the view your employees form of you is usually related to the way you come across in regard to some or all of the following:

- Do you communicate openly, sharing all necessary or helpful information with the employee group? Openness to communication is associated more with consultative or participative leadership, and a closed communication posture is associated more with autocratic leadership.
- Do you display awareness of people's problems and needs? The participative leader tends more toward awareness of individual problems while the autocratic leader often appears unaware or even uncaring.
- Do you display trust and confidence in employees? The autocratic leader displays little trust or confidence, relying mostly on close supervision. The true participative leader is able to extend trust and confidence.
- What means do you use to motivate employees? The autocratic leader frequently relies on fear and punishment to move people forward. The participative leader motivates through involvement and reward whenever possible.
- Do you provide support to employees? The employees of the autocratic leader often find they stand alone when things go wrong and they need the supervisor's backing. Support for employees and their decisions and actions is a hallmark of the participative leader.
- Do you request input on job problems? The autocratic leader tends to go it alone, but the consultative or participative leader is generally open to input from the work group.

## THE VISIBLE SUPERVISOR

Supervisors experience many pressures that encourage them to "face upward" in the organization toward higher management. After all, the supervisor's praise, reward, and recognition come from this upward direction. It is natural for supervisors who seek career growth to recognize that advancement is often facilitated by the extent to which they are organizationally visible outside of their own areas of responsibility.

In facing upward, however, the supervisor runs the risk of losing sight of the rank-and-file members of the department. In the long run the employees and their day-to-day performance have the greatest effect on the performance of the supervisor, but it is all too easy for supervisors to be so busy facing upward—meeting with the boss, serving on committees, attending outside functions, and such—that they lose touch with the people who can truly make or break supervisors by how they perform.

To provide true leadership to the work group, the supervisor must be seen as an integral part of the work unit and must in fact be such a part of the work unit. To get things done effectively through employees, as supervisor you should (1) be visible and available, spending most of your time where you are really needed; (2) show concern for the employees' problems; (3) maintain a true open-door attitude so that your employees can always reach you when they need you; and (4) rely on immediate feedback to let all of your employees know exactly where they stand. Much of true leadership is provided by visible example, and the more visible you are to your employees, the greater the chance of your gaining their acceptance.

## LEADING BY DEFAULT

The supervisor who is frequently neither visible nor available is often put in a position of "leading" by default. When the supervisor cannot be found or does not act, different employees will proceed—or not proceed, as the case may be—in different ways. In the absence of direction some employees will bite the bullet and use their own best judgment in taking action. Some, however, will do nothing and allow events to follow their normal course, which may lead just as easily to disaster as to inconsequential results.

The majority of defaults occur because allowing them to do so is the supervisor's course of least resistance. Because one soon discovers that default is frequently neutral and occasionally even helpful, there develops a temptation to often just let things go until they resolve themselves. Given the crush of activities many supervisors are regularly drawn into, it can be extremely tempting to sometimes let events follow their own course.

However, default management will not long be seen as representative of real leadership. Your employees should, of course, be encouraged to work independently as much as reasonable under the circumstances, but it is important for them to know that you are readily available when needed and that you will not default on them.

## TRUE LEADERSHIP

We have already mentioned that in the last analysis the only factor that truly defines a leader is the acceptance of leadership by the followers. It has been further suggested that a style that leans toward participative leadership is more likely to be found acceptable by the majority of today's workers than a style that leans toward autocratic behavior. However, no single pattern of leadership behavior is appropriate to all situations at all times. If your employees are largely health care professionals and paraprofessionals you may lean toward participative leadership most of the time. However, there still may be times when the situation calls for autocratic behavior—you need to be able to make a decision, issue an order, and expect results. Also, there may be times when bureaucratic behavior (strict interpretation and application of the rules and regulations) may be required. True leadership is flexible; it responds to both individual and organizational needs and is shaped to fit the needs of the moment.

## RETURN TO: "ONE BOSS TOO MANY"

Concerning the "Situation" presented at the start of this chapter, a great deal of time could be expended exploring possible reasons for the resistance of the manager of engineering and maintenance. Suffice it to say that this manager now has a superior, the director of environmental services, where no superior previously existed, and that this superior and the long-time manager are in constant conflict. Unfortunately, the three first-line supervisors and their staffs are adversely affected by the conflict between their managers.

A suggestion—the next time the director bypasses the manager and delivers an important instruction to the supervisors, the supervisors should stop the director, tell him what they have been experiencing, and ask for a joint meeting of the director, the manager, and the three of them. The issue of conflicting instructions—and especially of one manager's reversal of another manager's instructions, if that has indeed been happening—needs to be out in the open in front of all concerned. As long as the supervisors are bounced from director to manager and back again, they remain victims of a tug-of-war between two higher-ups.

If not blessed with an immediate meeting to iron out differences, the supervisors are left in a position of having to decide whom to obey. In the absence of any other assistance, they are probably better off paying more attention to the director, the higher of the higher-ups, than to the manager, simply because of position in the chain of command.

If every effort to correct the situation by dealing directly and jointly with manager and director is made and conditions fail to change, the supervisors might consider following the chain of command upward and requesting a meeting with the person to whom the director reports. This is of course a frequently risky step, and it is one that should never be taken without first making every reasonable effort to solve the problem at the level at which it occurs.

The primary responsibility for the existence of this problem lies with the director. The manager is, after all, the director's subordinate. Properly and thoroughly advised of what is occurring, the director may well address the problem before it has to go further.

## REVIEW QUESTIONS

1. Describe the essential difference between *consultative leadership* and *participative leadership*.

2. Why do we so often speak of *bureaucracy* in terms of frustration and annoyance?

3. Can you think of circumstances under which *autocratic leadership* (although not exploitative) could be appropriate? Provide an example and your rationale.

4. Cite an example of a Theory X working environment and an example of a Theory Y environment, and cite two or three characteristics of a hypothetical environment midway between X and Y.

5. How would you describe the concept referred to as *situational leadership*? (This concept is not named in the chapter but is implied in two of the chapter's sections.)

## EXERCISE: A VIEW OF YOU AS A LEADER

This exercise may be difficult for you—not difficult to accomplish, but difficult to accept what you learn from it. However, it can be helpful in suggesting areas in which your employees' view of your leadership style differs from your view.

The six questions appearing below are taken from the six points discussed in the chapter section titled "An Employee's View." Each is provided with its own scale, extending from 0 (fully autocratic) to 10 (completely participative).

1. Do I communicate fully and openly?

   0   1   2   3   4   5   6   7   8   9   10

   (0 = Not at all; 10 = Completely)

2. Am I aware of people's problems and needs?

   0   1   2   3   4   5   6   7   8   9   10

   (0 = Unaware; 10 = Fully aware)

3. Do I display trust and confidence?

   0   1   2   3   4   5   6   7   8   9   10

   (0 = Not at all; 10 = Fully)

4. Do I motivate using fear and punishment or appreciation and reward?

   0   1   2   3   4   5   6   7   8   9   10

   (Fear and punishment = 0; Appreciation and reward = 10)

5. Do I furnish backing and support in a pinch?

   0   1   2   3   4   5   6   7   8   9   10

   (Never = 0; Always = 10)

6. Am I open to employees' input on problems?

   0   1   2   3   4   5   6   7   8   9   10

   (Rarely, if ever = 0; Usually = 10)

Prepare a simple handout sheet including the questions and the scales as they appear above and a few lines of instructions. You need only instruct employees on how to use the scales, explaining that you are seeking—related to a management development exercise, if you wish—an employee view of the department's leader. Stress that completing the form is optional, and they should not use their names. Provide a drop-off point so you will be unable to determine who did or did not complete a form.

Before you receive any completed forms, rate yourself on the same six questions using the same form.

After you receive the completed forms, compare the employee ratings with your own, both individually and by taking an average rating offered by all employees on each question.

You and your employees may not see your strong or weak points in the same light. If you are unhappy with a particular response, remember that a poor rating does not mean you *are* that way, but it can mean that you *are viewed* that way because it is how you are coming across to people. The results may suggest aspects of your style that could use your attention.

---

**NOTES**

1. D. M. McGregor, "The Human Side of Enterprise," *Management Review* 46, no. 11 (1957): 22–28, 88–92.
2. T. Peters and R. H. Waterman Jr., *In Search of Excellence* (New York: Warner Books, 1982).
3. P. F. Drucker, *The Practice of Management* (New York: Harper & Row, 1954).

## CHAPTER 11

# Motivation: Intangible Forces and Slippery Rules

*The only way to motivate an employee is to give him challenging work in
which he can assume responsibility.*
*—Frederick R. Herzberg*

## CHAPTER OBJECTIVES

☛ Establish a perspective on what employees want from the organizations they work for.

☛ Review the basic forces at work in human motivation and suggest the varying influences of different forces on employees in today's organizations.

☛ Identify the significant effects of the changing health care delivery environment on employee motivation.

☛ Examine the value of material rewards as motivators.

☛ Describe the supervisor's role in creating the environment in which employees will become self-motivated.

## SITUATION: ALWAYS THE LAST TO KNOW

Like some other hospitals in the state, the John James Memorial Hospital found itself subject to decreasing rates of bed utilization in obstetrics/gynecology and pediatrics. In fact, for more than 2 years the hospital had been operating these services at lower levels than those specified as limits below which full cost would not be reimbursed.

The newspapers in the community carried occasional stories about the efforts of Regional Health Planning to regulate total bed availability for various services. More than one of these articles had suggested some institutions would probably be asked to either curtail or abandon obstetrics/gynecology or pediatrics, or both.

A number of employees at John James Memorial, especially those who had been in obstetrics and pediatrics a long time, were concerned about the future. One of these was Mrs. Mary Sawyer, who had been the obstetrics supervisor at John James Memorial for 14 years.

More than once Mrs. Sawyer had expressed her concern to the director of nursing as well as to various members of administration. She received no answers from the director, who seemed to know little more about the future than Mrs. Sawyer. From administration she received only references to published documents describing how the percentage utilization limits would be applied and what some of the implications might be. These references only raised more questions in her mind because they suggested some of their services would have to be reduced or cut out entirely.

One afternoon when Mrs. Sawyer visited a food market after work she encountered a neighbor. They talked a few minutes before the neighbor said,

173

"Oh, that thing about the hospital in the paper today—what is it going to do to your job?"

Mrs. Sawyer was puzzled, but rather than display her lack of specific knowledge she said, "Oh, I don't really know yet. We'll have to wait and see."

Upon reaching home Mrs. Sawyer picked up the newspaper; the story was featured on the front page. Regional Health Planning had made some far-reaching recommendations for regional distribution of beds in various services, and after many compromise-filled sessions the majority of the hospitals in the region had agreed to most of the adjustments. Among the adjustments were the following:

- Reduce pediatrics at John James Memorial from 34 beds to 18 beds.
- Eliminate obstetrics/gynecology at John James Memorial, with this service to be combined with that of County General Hospital 6 miles away.

The next day when Mrs. Sawyer went to work she noted a number of solemn faces among obstetrics/gynecology personnel. Before the morning was over she discovered that several of her best nurses were already talking about applying at County General.

Mrs. Sawyer met briefly with the director of nursing service, who indicated she had no prior knowledge of the change. She further suggested that Mary Sawyer was under consideration for an upcoming opening as assistant director of nursing service, but even this news had little effect on Mrs. Sawyer's disposition.

*Instructions*

Consider the following questions while proceeding through the chapter:

1. What are some of the possible short-range effects on the morale, performance, and individual effectiveness of the obstetrics/gynecology personnel?
2. What morale factors are most affected by the impending changes at the hospital?
3. Keeping in mind that the employees' need to be included in on things must be balanced against the institution's inability to know exactly what is happening in the external environment, how might this matter have been approached so as to minimize negative reaction among employees?

## SATISFACTION IN WORK

We can describe motivation as the initiative or drive causing a person to direct behavior toward satisfaction of some personal need. Each of us has needs, and many of these needs are the reasons why we work. Depending on how well our needs are met through our employment, we may be more or less satisfied with our role in the organization.

At this early stage of the discussion, please accept the premise that in the long run the satisfied employee will more likely be a better producer than the employee who is generally dissatisfied. A satisfied employee is usually more enthusiastic, more willing to work, and more of a self-starter.

Unfortunately, traditional organizations have done much to assure that a fair amount of dissatisfaction will exist at many organizational levels. We find that so much work has been structured, subdivided, and systematized that human factors beyond mere job performance are ignored and the inherent challenge of work as a normal human activity is diluted or dissipated. People respond to work in terms of personal needs and desires, so productive efficiency turns out to be not especially satisfying in itself. It becomes necessary, then, for management to seek ways and means of allowing employees to satisfy basic personal needs through work.

## DEMANDS ON THE ORGANIZATION

People want the organizations they work for to supply them with a number of things. We cannot list them in any particular order; what is important to one person may matter very little to another. Generally, however, we should find that the following list encompasses most of what employees expect of their employers:

- capable leadership that can be respected and admired
- decent working conditions—surroundings that promote safety and physical well-being
- acceptance as a member of a group
- recognition as an individual or partner, not simply as a servant of the system
- fair treatment relative to that received by others
- a reasonable degree of job security
- knowledge of the results of individual efforts
- knowledge of the organization's policies, rules, and regulations
- recognition for special effort or good performance
- respect for individual religious, moral, and political beliefs
- assurance that all others are doing their share of the work
- fair monetary compensation

## MOTIVATING FORCES: THE BASIC NEEDS

Before continuing we should say something about a small word we have been throwing about almost carelessly since the beginning of the chapter. The word is *needs*. It is necessary, in considering human motivation, to take as broad a view of this term as possible. If someone is pursuing a promotion or other reward, you might be tempted to say that the person does not really need this—considering a need as something essential—but rather may simply want it. However, we are not speaking of needs in such a way that we are forced into defining absolute essentials and separating them from other things we could call wants, desires, wishes, or aims. Rather, we are referring to those things you pursue simply because they represent fulfillment to you. In this sense they are indeed "needs" because we see them as essential to our fulfillment as individuals.

## A Classical Theory of Motivation

In his well-known "need hierarchy," A. H. Maslow described the basic human needs as follows[1]:

- Physiological needs—These are the most fundamental needs—those things we require to sustain life, such as food and shelter.
- Safety needs—These include our need to feel reasonably free from harm from others and reasonably free from economic deprivation (call this "job security").
- Love needs—These include our need to be liked by others and to be accepted as part of a group—be it a work group, family, or social group. Needs at this level involve a sense of belonging.
- Esteem needs—At this level in the hierarchy we experience needs for recognition, approval, and assurance that what we are doing is appreciated.
- Self-actualization—According to Maslow, the need for self-actualization represents "a pressure toward unity of personality, toward spontaneous expressiveness—toward being creative, toward being good, and a lot else."[1]

Maslow states that we proceed through the need hierarchy from the most fundamental needs toward the highest-order needs. Once a need is satisfied, another arises to take its place, and thus we experience needs of increasingly higher order. If we are in need of food, clothing, and shelter, then the basic physiological and safety needs are motivating our behavior. Relating these needs to work, when we experience unmet physiological and safety needs, then factors like job satisfaction and interesting work experiences will not mean a great deal to us. At that level we are most interested in generating an income with which to buy the basics of life. However, once these lower-order needs have been satisfied to a reasonable extent, we begin to experience the love needs, look for acceptance, and attempt to take our places in various groups. Thus, we progress through the hierarchy until we find that ultimately we are motivated by the need for self-actualization.

The need hierarchy has been rather firmly established, but there are vast differences among people as to individual needs and thus corresponding differences in what is required to satisfy those needs. For instance, one person's need for assurance of reasonable job security may be filled by the knowledge that the job will last at least another 3 months, while another person may feel uneasy unless assured the job will last until retirement. Also, love needs and esteem needs may be quite powerful in an individual who requires constant reassurance of worth and capability, while another person may experience much lesser needs at this level simply because of the presence of a higher degree of confidence and more sense of self-worth. Regardless, however, of the needs actually experienced by any given individual, the matter of progression through the need hierarchy holds true: as a need is reasonably satisfied, another, higher-order need arises to take its place.

People have vastly different reasons for working. As it was in our country years ago, today in some of the underdeveloped countries people concentrate most of their energies on simply remaining fed, clothed, and sheltered at a minimal level; they rarely go beyond the satisfaction of basic physiological and safety needs. In our modern industrial society, however, these lower-order needs are satisfied for most people most of the time. We then experience higher-order needs and proceed to seek satisfaction. Even the person who feels continually driven by the same goal—for instance, money—will be doing so for changing reasons. Once reasonable economic security is no longer a concern, money may be seen as the means of securing leisure time, social acceptability, status, prestige, and perhaps even power and influence, all expressions of higher-order needs.

### Motivating Factors and Environmental Factors

The Maslow theory alone does not supply all of the supervisor's answers but it is especially helpful when considered along with other approaches. Most helpful for further consideration is the motivation-hygiene theory of Frederick Herzberg.[2]

Rather than starting with human needs, Herzberg looked at factors comprising the job and surrounding the job. He concluded that the true motivators are inherent in the work itself and that hygiene factors (those circumstances making up the environment in which the work is done) are not motivators but rather are potential dissatisfiers. Herzberg's work suggests that managers must focus on jobs and their content as central to the motivation to work and then look at salaries, benefits, working conditions, and such as factors in the environment that must be reinforced periodically to stave off dissatisfaction. Herzberg's approach is occasionally presented in the management literature as simply the "two-factor motivation theory," the two primary factors simply being *dissatisfiers* and *motivators*.

Therefore, the factors having a bearing on a person's relationship with the work can be divided into two groups: motivating factors and environmental factors. The motivating factors can and do truly motivate a person to perform. The environmental factors, although they are not motivators, have influence for better or worse on employee satisfaction.

As Herzberg suggested, the true motivating factors are inherent in the work. The key word to use in describing these factors is opportunity. The sources of motivation are the opportunities to

- achieve
- learn and acquire new knowledge
- perform interesting and challenging work
- do meaningful work
- assume responsibility
- become involved in determining how the work is done

The environmental factors, on the other hand, exist in all aspects of the employee's relationship to the organization. Even if these factors are all acceptable, they do not necessarily motivate. However, if they are not acceptable, they can lead to employee dissatisfaction. The environmental factors may be grouped under the following five general headings:

1. communication in all of its forms, including performance feedback, knowledge of where the organization is heading, and employee confidentiality
2. growth and advancement potential
3. personnel policies or how an employee is treated both as an individual and relative to others
4. salary administration or the perceived overall fairness of salary and benefits
5. working conditions and the extent to which they promote employee well-being relative to what is expected

The foregoing suggests that although the environmental factors may receive regular attention, they will not, by themselves, move employees to greater performance. If not maintained, however, they can cause dissatisfaction that interferes with performance.

## Other Perspectives on Employee Motivation

We might say without much fear of contradiction that the "big three" of classical motivation theory are A. H. Maslow and Frederick Herzberg, whose work was discussed in the preceding paragraphs, and Douglas M. McGregor, whose Theory X and Theory Y were cited in the chapter on leadership.[3] McGregor's Theory X, which he essentially rejects, is based on the premise that employees must be pushed to perform; his Theory Y, which he supports, holds that under humane and enlightened management employees are self-motivating. McGregor's need hierarchy is very nearly identical to Maslow's, proceeding from physiological needs through safety needs, social needs, and ego needs, eventually arriving at self-fulfillment needs.

Coming at the whys and wherefores of employee motivation from a slightly different perspective but with the same essential core beliefs as the Maslow, Herzberg, and McGregor theories is that of Theory Z. First advanced in a 1981 book by William G. Ouchi, Theory Z addresses what had come to be known as Japanese management.[4] The essence of Theory Z is that involved workers are the key to increased productivity. The same message of employee involvement can be inferred from Maslow's work and is directly implied in the theories of Herzberg and McGregor. The Theory Z approach, which must be considered primarily in light of the cultural climate of Japan, emphasizes an extremely close relationship between an individual's work life and personal life. Although Theory Z is similar to other approaches in calling, for example, for participation in decision making and other aspects of management, it differs in that one of its critical elements is life-long careers with the same organization. The rationale behind this relatively unattainable and impractical "motivator" seems to be the belief that one will be a more willing and effective worker if employment security is assured.

Management expert and prolific author Peter F. Drucker took the question of employee motivation beyond the classical concept of need satisfaction. He stated: "Responsibility—not satisfaction—is the only thing that will serve. One can be satisfied with what somebody else is doing, but to perform one has to take responsibility for one's own actions and their impact. To perform, one has, in fact, to be dissatisfied, to want to do better."[4(p.303)]

There has been a great deal written about employee motivation, and surely employee motivation is acknowledged as one of management's primary concerns in health care and all other industry settings. A few who have written works concerned with management theory have even identified motivating as one of the several basic management functions. However, the overwhelming proportion of published work about employee motivation either cites or is directly built on the work of Maslow, Herzberg, and, to some extent, McGregor.

## WHAT MAKES THEM PERFORM?

In a four-decades-old survey conducted by the U.S. Chamber of Commerce, the first-line supervisors in 24 organizations were asked to rate ten so-called morale factors in the order in which they believed these factors would be important to their employees.[5] In short, they were asked to rank these factors as motivating forces. A second phase of the survey then required all the employees of the same supervisors to rank the same ten factors in order of importance to them as individual workers.

The supervisors guessed that the ten factors would appeal to their employees in order of importance as follows:

1. good wages
2. job security
3. opportunity for promotion and growth
4. good working conditions
5. interesting work
6. organizational loyalty to employees
7. tactful disciplining
8. full appreciation of work done
9. understanding of personal problems
10. being included in on things

The employees placed the same morale factors in the following order of importance:

1. full appreciation of work done
2. being included in on things
3. understanding of personal problems
4. job security
5. good wages
6. interesting work
7. opportunity for promotion and growth
8. organizational loyalty to workers
9. good working conditions
10. tactful disciplining

Note that the order of importance expressed by the employees places primary emphasis on satisfaction of higher-order needs rather than those usually associated with purely materialistic factors. Certain economic motives such as wages and job security were considered important; they do in fact appear in the upper middle portion of the employees' list. However, to these people who were employed and had normal expectations of remaining employed, the economically related factors did not appeal to them as primary expectations of their work.

In addition to the difference in position of the economic motives on the two lists, note also that the three factors rated highest by the employees were rated lowest by the supervisors. This raises some obvious questions about the importance of higher-order needs and job satisfaction and about the relative value of money as a motivator.

Although the study cited above is sufficiently old to be considered "history," its conclusions remain generally applicable. A survey on a much smaller scale than that described, yet using the same ten morale factors, was conducted with supervisors and employees of a number of upstate New York hospitals.[6] There were some differences in results, ascribable at least in part to the characteristics of the population surveyed. In the original survey as well as in the updates, the list of "supervisor's guesses" remained nearly the same. With the supervisors, "good wages" and "job security" remained the top two items, but in 1995 "job security" edged into first place over "good wages" and remained in first place in 2000 by a slightly greater margin. This seems to reflect supervisors' awareness of changes in health care. Another change coming to light in the 1995 update: on the employees' list, "job security" rose from fourth place to third place narrowly behind "being included in on things," and in the 2000 update was in second position by a narrow margin. Regardless, however, "full appreciation of work done" remained in first place overall.

The foregoing continues to suggest that supervisors tend to see economic factors as stronger than the employees see them. However, this also suggests that environmental circumstances influence the strength of any particular factor at any specific time. That is, "job security" becomes more important to employees as the perception of job security is eroded by circumstances.

Readers who are in a position to do so are invited to conduct surveys of their own using the ten factors identified above. Results may vary according to the relative stability of the environment in which the survey participants are working; for example, the participants in the limited 1995 and 2000 updates were for the most part employed in an environment that was perceived as anything but stable owing to mergers, acquisitions, closures, and cost-cutting activities, so "job security" rated understandably high because of widespread feelings of insecurity. Nevertheless it will still likely be found that psychological factors such as "full appreciation of work done" will remain at or near the top of the employees' list.

## MONEY AS A MOTIVATOR

We can no doubt all agree that money is an important reason for working. However, it has frequently been shown that money does not necessarily motivate people to work more effectively. Yet many managers continue to regard money as the principal key to motivation.

Money is important; not many of us would be against receiving more money for doing what we do now. However, money's main functions are primarily to help us avoid pain or discomfort. Our salaries help us avoid the feeling of economic deprivation we experience when we "don't have enough to live on" as we see that need and help assure us—given that we are being paid equitably relative to others doing the same kind of work—that we are not being treated unfairly.

Money and those other external factors that relate to money have one desirable characteristic that the true motivating factors do not possess: they can be measured on an objective scale. How do you begin to measure such intangibles as achievement and the feeling of worth resulting from the doing of meaningful work? How do we apportion such "rewards" among the work force? The fact is we cannot. Money, however, can be measured, so it constantly is measured and is frequently regarded as a motivator.

## LEARN WHAT MOTIVATES YOUR EMPLOYEES: LOOK TO YOURSELF

### More Alike Than Different

As already established in this chapter, many managers tend to feel that their employees are motivated largely by material concerns. However, these same managers, also employees of the organization, tend to behave more as employees when considering their own motivations in that they usually cite higher-order needs as their principal driving forces. Managers seek appreciation, managers wish to be included, managers want to do interesting work, and managers want to learn and grow.

Compared with the rank-and-file employees, the supervisor earns more money and bears more responsibility. Yet the supervisor of the workers is just another employee. As far as issues of employee motivation are concerned, it would behoove every manager to think: *My employees and I are more alike than unlike, and for the most part we are motivated by the same forces. Chances are that what I wish to obtain from my employment is much the same as what they wish to obtain. Therefore, I can enhance my employees' motivation by helping them obtain from their work the same things I wish to obtain from my work.*

### Motivate Another Person?

The answer to the question, "Can we motivate others?" is an unqualified *no*. However, the answer to the question, "Can I motivate myself?" is a definite *yes*. Motivation consummated—a need satisfied through the actions of an individual reacting to a drive or desire—is individual and personal. True motivation is self-motivation.

We have often heard, "You can lead a horse to water but you can't make him drink." That is, you can provide all of the appropriate conditions but you cannot instill that all-important drive or desire required to complete the process. That drive or desire, or its absence, lies within the person who has to act to complete the process.

You cannot motivate another human being. You can, however, seek ways in which to attempt matching the motivations of the individuals with needs you are attempting to meet. Motivation is internal to the individual, so the best we can ever do is create circumstances in which people will become self-motivated. Therefore, when we speak of employee motivation we are talking about arranging conditions so that people react to them in a positive manner.

## Key Principles of Motivation

There are some motivational principles that seem to prevail. Whether we ascribe to Maslow's theory, Herzberg's approach, or the work of still others, some constants consistently emerge from actual behavior.[7] These constants are as follows:

- Reinforcement of behavior encourages its repetition. Reward or praise for work well done will encourage more of the same; failure to provide encouragement will eventually be countered with declining performance.

- The faster the response to behavior, the stronger the effect on future behavior. Reinforcement delayed is reinforcement weakened. A "thank you" delivered for today's effort today is far more effective than the "thank you" saved up for performance appraisal time.

- Positives are always better incentives than negatives. Although people will often perform in the short run to avoid unpleasant consequences, they will do so with resentment and usually with less than their best effort.

- The importance of any specific motivational factor is subjective. What is important to one person may not be of equal importance to another, so workers in the same group can be vastly different from each other in terms of what they need from the work organization.

## A Rule for the Supervisor

The behavior of the manager to whom you report can serve as a most effective model for your own behavior in both a positive and a negative sense. We may not always be conscious of doing so, but as managers we frequently emulate the behavior of those who manage us. It is up to each of us to incorporate and pass along the appropriate behavior we learn from our role models, and avoid passing along the inappropriate behavior. This can become one of the most difficult parts of the supervisory role—treating your employees with every human consideration even though you may be subject to mistreatment from above.

The rule is: You can do no wrong by deciding to treat your employees in the manner in which you would like always to be treated by higher management. Fair, respectful, and humane treatment of your direct-reporting employees goes a long way toward enhancing their willingness to perform for you and thus encourages self-motivation.

## WHY THE LAST TO KNOW?

Returning to the "Situation" that opened the chapter, it is not difficult to believe that the events described could have a significant negative impact on employee motivation at just about all levels of the organization.

The possible short-range effects on morale, performance, and individual effectiveness of the department's personnel include reduced morale because of uncertainty and insecurity, as well as diminished productivity, sagging performance, and reduced individual effectiveness. There may be increased turnover as employees begin to "bail out" of what they may already perceive as a losing situation. There also can be a noticeable increase in disciplinary problems and an increase in absenteeism. Most of the staff will be worried. Some will be angry, and perhaps some will be sad. Some staff will spend more time complaining or discussing their plight than working. Overall the group will soon become less productive than before and will be more difficult to manage than before.

All of the "morale factors" (see the section titled What Makes Them Perform?) are affected to some extent. First and foremost are "job security," giving way to sudden feelings of insecurity, and "organizational loyalty to employees," which some will feel is now nonexistent. Job security so threatened places satisfaction of some of the other factors—"good wages," "opportunity for promotion and growth," "good working conditions," "interesting work"—at risk, since it is now felt that these could readily vanish. Some employees will feel unappreciated, and some will feel that they have been excluded from important information.

"Being included in on things" is undeniably important to many employees. However, a great many managers do not communicate with employees as often as they should because they feel they have nothing substantive to share. But even a complete lack of substantive information or hard news should not preclude regular communication with employees. When it comes to employee communication we might suggest to every working manager: Even when you have nothing to say, say it anyway. Periodically remind people that although nothing firm has been decided, you will let them know as soon as something occurs. Be especially willing to wander the organization and meet informally or formally with groups of all sizes. Listen to employees and solicit their questions and concerns; respond as best as you can. Take advantage of every opportunity to dispel rumors; in the "Situation," you can bet that someone has heard that "John James Memorial Hospital is closing." Overall, talking with people, squelching the rumors, dealing with what few facts are available, and above all listening to the employees will help minimize negative reactions.

## MOTIVATION AND THE FIRST-LINE MANAGER

The age-old carrot-and-stick approach, alternating reward and punishment for certain behavior, simply refuses to work once people have reached an adequate subsistence level and are motivated primarily by higher-order needs. The supervisor could do well to remember that economic rewards are but a portion of the total reward the employee works for.

Leadership and employee motivation are directly related to each other. The quality of supervision will generally have a significant bearing on the willingness with which employees perform. Leadership that employees can respect and admire is far more likely to produce positive performance than leadership that employees see as harsh, arbitrary, or unethical.

All of your employees are unique individuals and their motives are actually fairly stable personality characteristics that each brings to work. Some may be ambitious and desire money and leadership positions, some may be fulfilled largely by helping others, and some may satisfy their needs through overcoming obstacles to accomplish difficult tasks. These drives remain much the same within each person, so what you are actually attempting to influence in your employees is "aroused motivation." You wish to awaken in them the drive to seek fulfillment of certain needs.

Generally, we provide aroused motivation by doing the following:

- valuing employees as individuals and treating each as such
- providing challenge in the work situation whenever possible
- increasing or varying job responsibilities when possible
- helping employees to grow in such ways as to benefit both them and the organization

Although it is not always possible to provide a great deal of challenge in certain jobs or provide certain workers with increased responsibility, it is always possible to bring one or two of the prominent motivating forces into play in any situation. A simple "you did a good job" can be a powerful motivator, and a "thank you" can be valued compensation for someone's efforts. Ultimately you will discover that you cannot "motivate" an individual as such. Rather, you can only create the climate within which the person will become self-motivated.

## REVIEW QUESTIONS

1. Referring to the section "Demands on the Organization," identify those "wants" on the list that represent largely sociological needs.

2. In the motivation-hygiene theory of Herzberg, what is necessary to prevent the potential dissatisfiers from becoming actual dissatisfiers?

3. Why is a seemingly important factor such as the opportunity for promotion and growth of obviously greater importance to some employees than to others?

4. Once sufficient money has been assured to sufficiently fulfill all of their psychological and safety needs, why do some people seem to remain driven by the pursuit of material reward?

5. Referring to the section "What Makes Them Perform?" explain why supervisors and workers could hold different views of what is important to the workers.

## CASE: THE PROMOTION

With considerable advance notice, your hospital's director of medical records resigned to take a similar position in a hospital in another state. Within the department it was assumed that you, the assistant director, would be appointed director. However, a month after your boss's departure the department was still running without a director. Day-to-day operations apparently had been left in your hands ("apparently," because nothing had been said to you), but the hospital's assistant administrator had begun to make some of the administrative decisions affecting medical records.

After another month had passed you learned through the grapevine that the hospital had interviewed several candidates for the position of director of medical records. Nobody had been hired, however.

During the next several weeks you tried several times to discuss your uncertain status with the assistant administrator. Each time you tried you were put off; once you were told simply to "keep doing what you're now doing."

Four months after the director's departure you were promoted to director of medical records. The first instruction you received from the assistant administrator was to abolish the position of assistant director.

### Questions

1. What can you say about the likely state of your ability to motivate yourself in your "new" position? What can you say about your level of confidence in the relative stability of your position, and how might this affect your performance?

2. At the time you assume the director's position officially, what is likely to be the motivational state of your staff? Why?

**NOTES**

1. A. H. Maslow, "A Theory of Human Motivation," *Psychological Review* 50 (1943): 370–396.
2. F. Herzberg et al., *The Motivation To Work* (New York: Wiley, 1969).
3. D. M. McGregor, "The Human Side of Enterprise," *Management Review* 46, no. 11 (1957): 22–28, 88–92.
4. W. G. Ouchi, *Theory Z: How American Business Can Meet the Japanese Challenge* (Reading MA: Addison-Wesley Publishing Company, Inc., 1981).
5. P. F. Drucker, *The Practice of Management* (New York: Harper & Row, 1986).
6. Chamber of Commerce of the United States, *Washington Review*, 1966.
7. C. R. McConnell, *What Makes Them Perform?* (Unpublished Survey, 1975; updated 1985, 1995, 2000).
8. E. J. Brennan, *Performance Management Workbook* (Englewood Cliffs, NJ: Prentice Hall, 1989).

## CHAPTER 12

# Performance Appraisal: Cornerstone of Employee Development

*The privilege of encouragement is one that may be exercised by every executive and supervisor and it should be cultivated, not so much as a working tool to be employed objectively, but as an act of deserved kindness and intelligent leadership.*
*—Anonymous*

## CHAPTER OBJECTIVES

☛ Establish the objectives of performance appraisal as a management technique.

☛ Identify and review common approaches to employee performance appraisal.

☛ Assess common appraisal problems and suggest why many appraisal programs fail.

☛ Outline the requirements of an effective performance appraisal system.

☛ Highlight the requirements or characteristics necessary to make the organization's performance appraisal system as legally defensible as possible.

☛ Introduce standard-based appraisal as a desirable long-range consideration in improving the organization's evaluation process.

☛ Introduce the concept of "constructive performance appraisal."

☛ Suggest how the supervisor can make any existing appraisal method better serve the true objectives of performance appraisal.

## SITUATION: "IT'S REVIEW TIME AGAIN"

"Well, Jack, I'm sure you know why you're here—it's performance appraisal time again.

"I want you to know that I've seen a lot of good work coming from you these past 12 months—14 months, really, since we're a little off schedule as usual. I appreciate it, and I'm sure administration appreciates it, too. There's always room for improvement, of course, but let me hit the good stuff first.

"Your output has been great, and I'm especially satisfied with the way you tackled the energy management program. You showed plenty of good judgment in the decisions you made and in the formal recommendations you prepared.

"There are a couple of things that bother me, however. But I know I can speak straight from the shoulder. Your aggressiveness is still something of a problem—I can think of two, maybe three times when I've had to handhold Morrison to get him calmed down after you'd ruffled his info systems crew. I'm sure you'll agree that tact and diplomacy aren't your strong suits. I point this out because your lack of political sensitivity isn't going to do you any good if you're thinking about moving up someday.

"And another thing. . . ."

186

*Instructions*

As you proceed through this chapter, prepare to critique the foregoing "opener" of Jack's annual appraisal interview. Be especially sensitive to the following:

- apparent "system" weaknesses
- the rendering of personality judgments
- the treatment of the causes and results of behavior

## APPRAISAL AND THE MANAGER

The evaluation of employee performance through the application of some formal system of performance appraisal is ordinarily an important part of the job of every manager who directly supervises employees. And if it is not so, it should be; nobody other than an employee's immediate supervisor should be the primary evaluator of the employee. Yet as common as the requirement for performance appraisal may be, managers often dread the appraisal process and all that goes with it. Nevertheless, in most modern health care organizations employee appraisal remains a basic responsibility of all persons who direct the work of others.

Even in those increasingly rare organizations in which there is no formal requirement for performance appraisal, supervisors must still occasionally pass judgment on employee performance. The supervisor who reprimands an employee for a breach of policy is, in effect, appraising performance. Likewise, the supervisor who compliments an employee for a task well done or who criticizes an employee for committing an error and provides the employee with directions for correcting the error or avoiding its recurrence is also appraising performance. Thus any instance of criticism or praise, whether offered within or outside the context of a formal performance appraisal system, constitutes employee evaluation.

Pursued within the context of a formal, mandated system, as it is in most health care organizations, performance appraisal requires a great deal of the supervisor's time and attention. Most supervisors have had occasion to discover that there is often not enough time to do everything they must do, so appraisal is left to compete with numerous other activities for the available time. Since appraisal requires information that the supervisor must accumulate over an extended period of time, elements of the appraisal process are always competing for space on the supervisor's list of priorities. This is the case for performance appraisal overall, since it appears to have no direct impact on the accomplishment of the day-to-day work in the department. Therefore, it often gravitates to the lower part of the supervisor's priority list until attention is required.

Some appraisal systems call for the evaluation of all employees at the same time, ordinarily once each year or perhaps even once every 6 months. Under the all-at-once approach, the supervisor often views the performance appraisal task as overwhelming; other essential tasks may suffer because appraisals must be done. Under the pressure created by the knowledge that important work is being left undone, the supervisor may fail to do justice to the appraisals. If the supervisor has a large number of appraisals to do, perhaps the ones undertaken first receive the most care while the latter appraisals receive diminishing time and attention. Because the requirement to do a number of appraisals within a specified number of days or weeks is placed on them at what is usually an inappropriate time (and rarely is there an appropriate time for a task that intrudes so deeply into the daily routine), many supervisors come to regard appraisal as, at best, a necessary evil or, at worst, an unnecessary and resented intrusion.

However, not all appraisal systems call for the evaluation of all employees at the same time. A significant number of systems call for the appraisal of employees on their employment anniversary dates. Although many prefer this approach rather than the all-at-once approach, it too can have its problems. The supervisor who must evaluate every employee at once may be extremely busy for a few weeks, but this supervisor knows that once the appraisals are finished the process will, for all practical purposes, go away for the greatest part of the year. However, when appraisals are done on employees' anniversary dates, the manager still has the same number of appraisals to do but they are staggered throughout the year. Under this approach, appraisals are never "caught up" and the process hangs over the supervisor as a nagging task that, through its constant presence, places subtle but steady pressure on the supervisor.

Not all of the pressures associated with performance appraisal are nearly as subtle as those created by the anniversary-date appraisal approach. There are also direct pressures that come from higher management, usually by way of the human resources function, aimed at getting appraisals accomplished according to some schedule. Because the human resources people must invariably remind evaluators of due dates and must otherwise ride herd on the process, many supervisors come to view appraisal in a decidedly unfavorable light as "human resources' system" or "just more personnel paperwork."

A considerable amount of discomfort with performance appraisal also arises from the understandable reaction of many supervisors to the uncertainties inherent in the appraisal process. Supervisors may be well aware that they are expected to advance opinions and render judgments, and they are made uncomfortable by the necessity to do so. Supervisors are also well aware that if they are to pursue the process to any truly conscientious extent, they may have to discuss unfavorable judgments with employees. Thus, in addition to reacting negatively to what they see as a requirement imposed on them from above, supervisors also often tend to react negatively to what they see as a highly subjective process in which their opinions and judgments may ultimately be indefensible.

In short, in many organizations the supervisors tend to view performance appraisal primarily as a requirement of the system rather than as a key element of the essential supervisor-employee relationship.

## THE OBJECTIVES OF APPRAISAL

The primary objectives of performance appraisal should be:

- to encourage improved performance in the job each employee presently holds
- to provide growth opportunity for those employees who wish to pursue possibilities for promotion, and, conversely, provide the organization with people qualified for promotion to more responsible positions

In general, the true objectives of appraisal are not always well served. An appalling number of appraisal systems are oriented almost entirely toward criticism and faultfinding. Certainly these systems were not intended to be used in this fashion, but their weaknesses, primarily their focus on the past, have brought about their general misuse. Rather than simply looking at the past and stopping there, an effective performance appraisal system should seek to utilize the past only as a starting point from which to move into the future. When the appraisal interview becomes history and the form finds a home in the personnel file, the employee should be able to reasonably answer these two questions:

1. How am I doing in the eyes of my supervisor (and thus in the eyes of the organization)?
2. What are my future possibilities?

In this brief review of performance appraisal we will describe the common approaches to employee evaluation, consider some reasons why appraisal programs frequently fail, comment on the need for performance appraisal, and consider ways of more fully utilizing performance appraisal as an effective management technique.

## TRADITIONAL APPRAISAL METHODS

Over the years a number of appraisal systems have evolved, some depending on a greater or lesser amount of structure than others. Generally there have been continuing efforts to make appraisal systems more objective, more reliable, and less dependent on the unsupported judgment of the people doing the evaluating. The major approaches to performance appraisal are discussed below.

### Rating Scales

Rating scales, the oldest and most widely used appraisal procedures, are of two general types.

In continuous scales, in reference to a particular evaluation characteristic, the evaluator places a mark somewhere along a continuous scale (Figure 12–1). The evaluator is ordinarily aware of some position on the scale that constitutes "average" or "satisfactory" performance.

In discrete scales, each characteristic is associated with a number of descriptions covering the possible range of employee performance. The evaluator simply checks the box, or perhaps the column, accompanying the most appropriate description (Figure 12–2).

Factor: Quality of Work

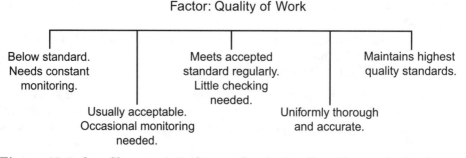

Figure 12–1 One Characteristic from a Continuous-Type Rating Scale. *Source: Author.*

Rating scale methods are easy to understand and easy to use, at least in a superficial manner. They permit numerical tabulation of scores in terms of measures of average tendency, skewness (the tendency of a group of employees to cluster on either side of a so-called average), and dispersion.

Rating scales are relatively easy to construct, and they permit ready comparison of scores among employees. However, rating scales have several severe disadvantages. Do total scores of 78 for Jane and 83 for Harriet really mean anything significant? These systems are also subject to assumptions of the ability of a high score on one characteristic to compensate for a low score on another. For instance, if an employee scores low relative to quantity of work produced, can this really be counterbalanced by high scores for attendance, attitude, and job knowledge?

Ratings frequently tend to cluster on the high side when rating scales are used. Supervisors may tend to rate their employees high because they want them to receive their fair share of pay raises and feel good about themselves, and also because it is easier to praise than it is to leave oneself open to the appearance of being critical. Also, different supervisors tend to rate differ-

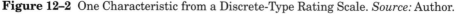

Factor: Quantity of Work

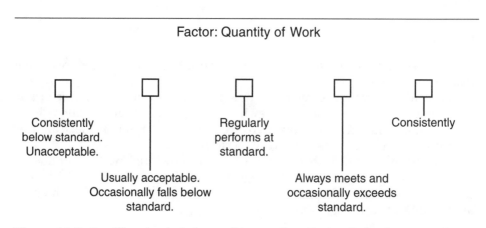

Figure 12–2 One Characteristic from a Discrete-Type Rating Scale. *Source:* Author.

ently. Some consider average as precisely that—average acceptable work, nothing to be ashamed of. However, other supervisors seem to think of average as something of a dirty word and thus tend to rate most employees on the high side of the scale.

## Employee Comparison

Employee comparison methods were developed to overcome certain disadvantages of the rating scale approaches. Employee comparison may involve the ranking method or the forced distribution method.

### Ranking

The ranking method forces the supervisor to rate all employees on an overall basis according to their job performance and value to the institution. One approach is simply to look at your work group and decide initially who is the best and who is the poorest performer and then to pick the second and next-to-last persons in your rank order by applying the same judgment to the remaining employees. This is simple enough to accomplish, but the process is highly judgmental and strongly influenced by personality factors. Also, some employee must end up as low person on the totem pole, and this may not be a fair assessment overall.

### Forced Distribution

The forced distribution method prevents the supervisor from clustering all employees in any particular part of the scale. It requires the evaluator to distribute the ratings in a pattern conforming to a normal frequency distribution. The supervisor must place, for instance, 10 percent of the employees in the top category, 20 percent in the next higher category, 40 percent in the middle bracket, and so on (Figure 12–3). The objective of this technique is to spread out the evaluations. However, while it is true that the general population may be distributed according to a normal curve, in an organization we are dealing with a select group of persons. If employees have been properly trained and probationary periods correctly used to eliminate the genuine misfits, then the true distribution of abilities and performance in the work group should be decidedly skewed. That is, your group's "average" should be better than the general average assumed by the so-called normal distribution (Figure 12–4).

## Checklists

### Weighted Checklist

The weighted checklist consists of a number of statements that describe various modes and levels of behavior for a particular job or category of jobs. Every statement has a weight or scale value associated with it, and when rating an employee the supervisor checks those statements that most closely describe the behavior exhibited by the individual. Some evaluation characteristics are worth more or less than others. Often in checklist evaluation systems the weights are intentionally kept secret from the supervisor. This is done supposedly to avoid deliberate bias on the part of the supervisor; it is not

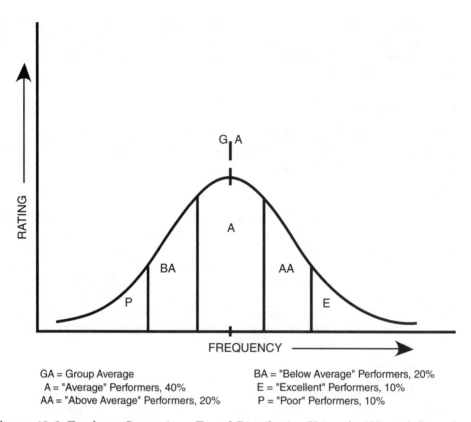

GA = Group Average
A = "Average" Performers, 40%
AA = "Above Average" Performers, 20%

BA = "Below Average" Performers, 20%
E = "Excellent" Performers, 10%
P = "Poor" Performers, 10%

**Figure 12–3** Employee Comparison: Forced Distribution Using the "Normal *Curve.*"
*Source:* Author.

possible to "slant" a rating to make the final score come out in some predetermined manner.

*Forced Choice*

Like the pure checklist approach, the forced choice method requires the development of a significant number of statements describing various types of behavior for a particular job or family of jobs. These statements are arranged in groups of four or five each, and within each group the evaluator must check the one statement that is most descriptive of the performance of the employee and the one statement that is least descriptive of the employee's performance. The groups are so designed that each will contain two statements that appear favorable and two that appear unfavorable. A set of five statements from among which the supervisor must make the choice just described is shown in Exhibit 12–1. While statements A and B both appear favorable, only statement B actually differentiates between high- and low-performance employees. Statement C is actually descriptive of low-performance employees. Although E also appears to be unfavorable, it is inconsequential in this set because of the presence of C. Statement D is neutral. Once again, the actual value or weight of the statements is kept secret from the supervisor.

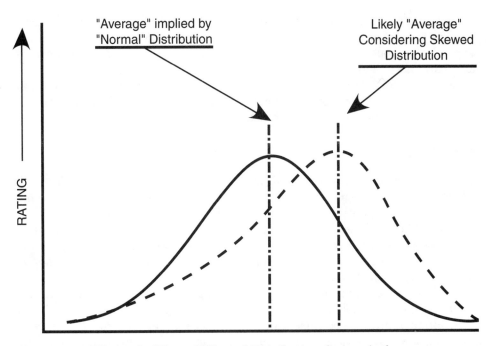

**Figure 12–4**  Effects of a "Skewed" Normal Distribution. *Source:* Author.

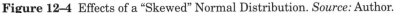

## Critical Incident

The critical incident method requires a supervisor to adopt the practice of recording in a notebook all those significant incidents in each employee's behavior that indicate either effective or successful action or ineffective action or poor behavior. The notebook itself is designed to provide reminders of performance characteristics under which various incidents can be recorded. For instance, if an employee saved the day by spotting an urgent problem and taking bold and imaginative action, you might record the incident under "initiative."

**Exhibit 12–1**  Illustrative Group of Statements from a Forced-Choice Appraisal

---

Circle the letter for the statement that is most descriptive of the employee's performance and the letter for the statement that is least descriptive of the employee's performance:

*Most*     *Least*

| | | |
|---|---|---|
| A | A | Makes mistakes only infrequently |
| B | B | Is respected by fellow employees |
| C | C | Fails to follow instructions completely |
| D | D | Feels own job is more important than other jobs |
| E | E | Does not exhibit self-reliance when expressing own views |

There is a severe hazard in the use of the critical incident method. Supervisors are busy people, and often everything that should be recorded does not reach the notebook. However, negative incidents, because of their "seriousness," are more likely to reach the pages of the book than are many occasions of positive performance. Also, this approach can lead to employees feeling that the supervisor is watching over their shoulders and that everything they do will be written down in the "little black book."

### Field Review

Under the field review appraisal method the supervisor has no forms to fill out. Rather, the supervisor is interviewed by a representative of the human resources department who asks questions about the performance of each employee. The interviewer writes up the results of the interview in narrative form and reviews them with the supervisor for suggestions, modifications, and approval. No rating forms or factors or degrees or weights are involved; rather, simple overall ratings are obtained.

The field review approach relieves the supervisor of paperwork. It also assures a greater likelihood that supervisors will give adequate and timely attention to appraisals because human resources largely controls the process. However, the process takes the valuable time of two management representatives (the supervisor and the human resources interviewer), and it requires the presence of far more human resources staff than most institutions feel they can afford.

### Free-Form Essay

This method requires the supervisor to write down impressions about the employee in essay fashion. If desired by the organization, comments can be grouped under headings such as job performance, job knowledge, and goals for future consideration, for example. To do a creditable job under this method, the supervisor must devote considerable time and thought to the evaluation. On the plus side, this process encourages the supervisor to become more observant and analytical. On the other hand, the free-form essay approach generally demands more time than the average supervisor is willing or able to spend. Also, appraisals generated by this method are often more reflective of the skill and effort of the writer than of the true performance of the employees.

### Group Appraisal

Under this approach an employee is evaluated at the same time by the immediate supervisor plus three or four other supervisors who have knowledge of that employee's work performance. The virtue of this method is its thoroughness. It is also possible for multiple evaluators to modify or cancel out bias displayed by the immediate supervisor. However, the drawbacks of this approach are such that it is rarely used: it is extremely time consuming, tying up perhaps four or five members of management to evaluate a single employee, and it is often inapplicable because there may be few if any managers beyond the immediate supervisor who are sufficiently familiar with the employee's performance.

## COMMON APPRAISAL PROBLEMS

A common problem encountered in performance evaluation is the "halo effect." This refers to the tendency of an evaluator to allow the rating assigned to one or more characteristics to influence excessively the rating on other performance characteristics. The rating scale methods are particularly susceptible to the halo effect. For instance, if you have declared an employee to be excellent in terms of "initiative" and "dependability," so might you be inclined to rate high relative to "judgment" and "adaptability." Since it is extremely difficult to force oneself to separate completely the consideration of each performance factor from the others (many performance characteristics actually include shades of others), there is no guaranteed way of eliminating the halo effect.

Mentioned earlier, and repeated because it is a common problem in most rating systems, is the tendency of many supervisors to be liberal in their evaluations, that is, to give their employees consistently high ratings. Most approaches to rating are partially based on the assumption that the majority of the work force will be average performers. However, many people (supervisors included) do not like to be considered "only average."

Central tendency or clustering is another problem, one that some of the rating methods just described have attempted to overcome. Some supervisors are reluctant to evaluate people in terms of the outer ends of the scale. To many supervisors it is "safest" to evaluate all employees consistently. This often leads to a situation in which everyone is average, contrary to the likelihood that in a work group of any considerable size there are, in fact, performers who are both better and worse than the so-called average.

Interpersonal relationships pose a considerable problem in performance evaluation. The supervisor cannot help but be influenced, even if only unconsciously, by personal likes and dislikes. Often a significant part of an evaluation will be based on how well the supervisor likes the employee rather than how well the employee actually performs.

## WHY APPRAISAL PROGRAMS OFTEN FAIL

Many performance appraisal programs fail outright or at least partially fail to do the jobs they were intended to do. A number of the reasons for appraisal program failure stem from weaknesses in the systems as already described, and some result from deeper-seated reasons, which will be discussed in the following paragraphs.

Appraisal programs often fail because they require the supervisor to render personality judgments. Consider the difficulty of truly evaluating a number of employees relative to each other as they relate to their work in terms of "characteristics" that are often actually personality characteristics. There are many appraisal systems in which the performance characteristics defy objective assessment (Exhibit 12–2). How can a supervisor truly rate someone on a characteristic such as "adaptability"? The problems are compounded by problems of semantics—what in fact is "initiative," "judgment," and so on?

Another reason for failure is that supervisors are unqualified to judge personality characteristics. Very few people are qualified to render personality judgments, yet supervisors are put into a position of having to do so time and time again.

Related to pressures toward the making of personality judgments, many systems fail to allow for distinguishing between the cause and results of behavior. For instance, an employee who comes across as irritable and constantly argues with others is likely to get marked down on "attitude." However, the results of the behavior (the clashes with other people) are the only real evidence the supervisor has to go on. To say that these interpersonal clashes result from a poor attitude is to try to assign a cause to the behavior. This assignment of cause to result is an unqualified leap for the supervisor; it is inappropriate to call an employee who appears unwilling to adapt to your ideas "stubborn," but our appraisal systems constantly require us to second-guess cause in this fashion.

Programs also fail because of the uncomfortable position of the person doing the evaluating. It is an extremely serious matter to probe the personality of an employee in a fashion that results in a permanent record in the employee's personnel file. The supervisor is put into a position of power over the employee's potential for promotion and pay increases and perhaps even the ability to obtain favorable references in the future. Many supervisors dislike being put into this position and compensate by keeping all their evaluations high or at least harmless.

Some systems fail mechanically, owing to poor system administration. Perhaps appraisal forms and notices are not distributed on time, are not followed up, do not get discussed with employees, or perhaps do not get completed at all. The mechanics of any appraisal system must be such that a system is kept moving; because of natural resistance to the uncomfortable task of appraisal, a system can die of its own weight unless it is continually nudged along.

Poor follow-up on appraisals can weaken a program, if not cause the program to fail entirely. This suggests, as mentioned at the beginning of the chapter, that an appraisal should not be an evaluation of the past to be filed away and forgotten. Since it should ideally be a guide to future action, a performance appraisal should be reflected in an active document that is used in the

---

**Exhibit 12–2** Listing of Rating Characteristics from an Actual "Appraisal" Form

| | |
|---|---|
| 1. Quality of work | 6. Initiative |
| 2. Volume of work | 7. Dependability |
| 3. Effectiveness | 8. Attitude |
| 4. Job knowledge | 9. Attendance |
| 5. Adaptability | |

employee-supervisor relationship during the months to come. In many systems, unfortunately, the only time the last performance appraisal is pulled out of the file is when the next appraisal is due.

## WHAT ABOUT JACK'S EVALUATION?

In the "Situation" presented at the beginning of the chapter, our hypothetical employee, Jack, has reason to be wary when he hears that it's review time again.

An immediately recognizable system weakness is timing. If the evaluation is two months late, with this condition described as "a little off schedule as usual," it suggests that timing of appraisal is not considered especially important and that delays are normal and acceptable. However, evaluation timing delays can creep; two months becomes three months becomes six months. Delay alone can kill an appraisal system.

The evaluator's opening includes personality judgments. Jack's alleged aggressiveness, his supposed lack of tact and diplomacy, and his alleged lack of political sensitivity are all unwarranted judgments that focus on Jack the person rather than on Jack's performance.

In claiming the problem with the information systems crew was due to Jack's aggressiveness, the evaluator was making an unwarranted leap from observed results of behavior to the alleged cause of that behavior. However, it is not the role of the evaluator to attempt to deal with causes. The evaluator must focus on the results of behavior, and if those results are inappropriate the emphasis should then become how to change behavior to make the results appropriate—and never to simply attach a cause to results.

Overall the two paragraphs constitute a weak beginning to an appraisal interview. It has set the stage for employee defensiveness and distrust before any substantive information is introduced. It is highly likely that Jack, although he may remain outwardly calm, will internally experience emotional reactions that will reduce his capacity for effective listening throughout the remainder of the appraisal interview.

## WHY APPRAISE AT ALL?

As discussed in Chapter 11, most employees are not very well motivated by just the rewards that exist as part of the organizational setting. Those "environmental factors" (such as salary, fringe benefits, and working conditions) are not the only things that employees work for.

Recall the position of "full appreciation of work done" as a potentially powerful motivator of employee performance. People who are doing good work need to know they are doing good work, and they need to know that what they do is appreciated. This knowledge and appreciation are essential parts of the "psychic income" that every employee needs to receive in some measure in addition to the real income associated with the position.

In addition to knowing they are doing well and that their work is appreciated, employees need to know when they are not doing particularly well and what they can do to correct their behavior. Criticism itself, even so-called constructive criticism, does not bring about long-lasting behavioral change. It is one thing to criticize; however, it is something else entirely to criticize and be able to supply alternatives for behavioral change and improvement.

Performance appraisal is needed because all employees deserve to know where they stand in the eyes of the supervisor and the organization. Beyond this, however, the employees need to know where they stand so as to be able to do something positive about future performance.

## REQUIREMENTS OF AN EFFECTIVE APPRAISAL SYSTEM

For a performance appraisal system to have a realistic chance of being effective, it must meet a number of conditions. If it does not satisfy these conditions, it will do less than it should be expected to do. However, even if the system does meet all the conditions, success is not necessarily guaranteed. To be fully effective, a system requires thorough, conscientious application by managers who believe in the value of performance appraisal. Careless or indifferent application can kill even the best systems or turn them into mere paper exercises. The requirements of an effective performance appraisal system are discussed below.

### System Objectives

Overall, the system must serve the true objectives of performance appraisal as previously described.

### Appropriateness of Criteria

System criteria—those requirements upon which the employees are evaluated—must be as closely related as possible to the kinds of work being evaluated. Never does a single approach fit all of the jobs to be evaluated within a single organization, especially a health care organization with its many and varied occupations.

### Standards of Performance

The majority of the evaluations of any individual employee should reflect specific standards of performance that are established based on the employee's job description. These standards of performance should be set in terms of objective measurements; that is, the manager should be able, for a significant number of evaluation criteria, to come up with a numerical measure of results that may be compared with an established standard.

### Employee Knowledge of Criteria

Employees must know, well in advance of being evaluated, the criteria on which they will be evaluated. Employees must be fully aware of the job description tasks as they are presently known to the manager, and they should be fully aware of all applicable job standards.

## Management Education

Managers should be thoroughly oriented in the use of the system and thoroughly trained organization-wide in the consistent application of the process.

## A Working Tool

Once it is completed, an evaluation should serve as a live, working record to be used as a starting point for monitoring progress. This is especially important for unfavorable evaluations, which should be sufficiently complete as to spell out specific steps and time frames to be involved in correction and improvement.

## Appraisal Interview

The appraisal interview should be a reality; it should not be avoided because the manager is uncomfortable nor should it be treated once-over-lightly and disposed of quickly simply because the manager feels the pressures of time. The appraisal interview should be a true two-way exchange and receive the manager's full attention for whatever time is required.

## Self-Contained Record

Once it is placed in the employee's personnel file, a completed performance appraisal should stand on its own. Cross-reference to an appraisal manual, evaluation key, or list of explanations should not be necessary in determining what any particular rating means.

## System Administration

Appropriate system administration must be maintained. All scheduled review dates must be observed. Managers must receive appraisal forms and reminders a reasonable amount of time before appraisals are due, and they must receive interim reminders as necessary to assure that appraisals are not allowed to run late. In short, someone needs to pay constant attention to the process of keeping the system moving.

## THE CHANGING LANGUAGE OF APPRAISAL

Within this chapter and throughout the language of performance appraisal, there are numerous references to evaluation "criteria." Criteria are, of course, the bases for evaluation, those demonstrations of performance that we actually rate for their correctness and effectiveness. In all appropriate appraisal systems, written criteria are expressions of the job description; they relate what the employee is expected to do in performance of the job. Criteria may in turn have "standards" associated with them, expressions of quantity or quality that describe how well criteria have been met.

For a number of years we have spoken of criteria-based evaluation as the legitimate successor to inappropriate and outmoded personality-based appraisal (attitude, initiative, etc.). This is true of all present expectations of the appraisal process—that it be based on the individual's job description. For some time the language of health care utilized the phrase criteria-based evaluation fairly broadly.

In recent years, however, at least in organizations accredited by the Joint Commission on Accreditation of Healthcare Organizations (JCAHO), the term "criteria" has given way to "competencies." Joint Commission standards call for competence assessment for staff on an annual basis, essentially meaning the assessment of each employee's ability to achieve job expectations as stated in his or her specific job description.

In today's terms, competencies are demonstrations of actual practice in a designated setting consistent with established standards, and competence assessment is synonymous with performance appraisal. Competencies are, in brief, the expectations of job performance. In different appraisal systems or at times in the past, we may have spoken of rating characteristics, rating factors, evaluation criteria, or performance expectations, or we may have used any of several other labels. The language of evaluation, or at least of accreditation, seems to change every few years. However, competence assessment is no different from properly implemented criteria-based performance evaluation.

## MAKING PERFORMANCE APPRAISAL LEGALLY DEFENSIBLE

Performance appraisal now carries with it a growing number of potential legal traps. An increasing number of wrongful termination lawsuits are an outgrowth of inadequate performance appraisal procedures. If an employee is let go for any performance-related reason but the evaluations on file show "good" or "standard" or "satisfactory" performance, the stage is set for a wrongful discharge complaint.

Performance appraisal information is also playing an increasingly active role in complaints filed under the Age Discrimination in Employment Act (ADEA). Such actions most commonly involve complaints concerning promotions, retirements or layoffs, and discharges.[1] In all of these kinds of actions there are questions of employee performance, and regardless of what the defendant organizations say about the performance of the individuals who complain they were discriminated against, the courts generally rely on the documentation of performance found in the personnel file—that is, the written appraisals of performance.

The biggest trap in performance appraisal, referred to earlier in this chapter, is now coming back to haunt many appraisers. That trap is the lenient appraisal—stating on the record that the individual's work is acceptable when in truth it is unsatisfactory in some respect.

Drawing on how performance appraisal has fared in the legal system through a significant number of cases, we can make some reasonable conclusions as to the characteristics of a legally defensible system. All embodied within the requirements of an effective appraisal system reviewed in the preceding pages, the critical elements of a legally defensible system are as follows:

1. The system is based on the job, with the appraisal criteria arising from an analysis of the legitimate requirements of the position. This is the embodiment of the oft-repeated admonition to focus on the job itself and not the person who does the job.

2. Performance is assessed using objective criteria as much as possible given the unique requirements of the job. There must be reasons behind the assessments rendered amounting to more than simply the unsupported subjective assessment of the appraiser.

3. The appraisers have been trained in the use of the system and possess written instructions on how the appraisal is to be completed. This establishes that any appraiser is as reasonably capable of evaluating performance as any other appraiser using the same system, and that the system can be expected to be applied as intended.

4. The results of each appraisal are reviewed and discussed with the employee. This is a major concern. Documentation of performance problems and efforts to correct them are necessary if an employee fails to improve and must be let go, but it is also necessary to prove that the employee knew about the difficulties. The legally defensible appraisal system can be used to demonstrate that the employee knew of the problems and was given the opportunity to correct them.[2]

## STANDARD-BASED APPRAISAL: A LONG-RANGE TARGET

The difficulty often encountered in the setting of performance standards and the sheer volume of work sometimes involved in this process should not be taken lightly. Going to the standard-based appraisal on an organization-wide basis requires that performance standards be developed for the majority of the task lines on every active job description in the organization. More often than not, this first requires that the organization's job descriptions be updated and revised so that most of the individual task descriptions lend themselves to the development of standards. It also means that the organization must adopt—which usually means install from scratch—some form of work measurement system. However, with sufficient effort, it is usually possible, for any specific position, to come up with several measures that are applicable to various aspects of each employee's work.

Effective job standards ordinarily reflect a concern for four major dimensions of an employee's work: (1) quantity, (2) quality, (3) use of time, and (4) use of financial resources (cost). These four areas are, of course, interrelated—time is money, quantity is related to time, and so on—but it is nevertheless possible to focus performance standards in each of these four key areas. An employee performance standard may take any of the following general forms:

1. Quantity
   - Number of patients served or cases handled (usually per unit of time such as per hour, per day, or per week)
   - Number of items processed
   - Number or percentage of occurrences

2. Quality
   - Error rate
   - Number of repeats or rejections
   - Percentage of down time
   - Employee turnover rate (as would apply in evaluating a supervisor)

3. Time
   - Deadlines missed, turnaround time (actual as compared with desired)
   - Acceptable work accomplished within a time unit

4. Cost
   - Cost per case or per contact
   - Cost per item
   - Amount of cost savings
   - Budget variance, both bottom line and line item (again applying to the appraisal of supervisors)

Consider an example of a performance standard that relates to quality of work. Suppose an acceptable error rate for a particular activity has been determined to be four mistakes per month (each necessitating, of course, rework or repeat) and further that the normal anticipated range of error has been determined to be three to five mistakes per month. The performance standard for the particular activity is set at three to five errors per month, so the individual who generated three, four, or five errors in a month for this activity may be said to have met the standard.

Consider another example, one of the very few that may be applicable to all employees in an organization. Assume that an organization that allows its employees up to 12.0 paid sick days a year has generated a long-run average of 7.2 sick days used per employee per year. Further, suppose that this organization, wishing to provide modest incentive to reduce sick time usage, establishes (perhaps arbitrarily but certainly realistically) that 6 days per year would be an acceptable level of sick time usage. Again, allowing some flexibility about the desired performance target, it might be decided that 5 to 7 sick days represents standard performance relative to sick time usage, less than 5 days' sick time implies that the standard has been exceeded, and more than 7 days' sick time indicates that the standard has not been met.

It will not always be possible to attach a measurable standard of performance to every last task on an employee's job description. For most employees, however, it will in fact be possible to come up with performance standards that measure most of the major tasks an employee performs.

It should be noted that the preceding simple examples used only three outcomes in comparing performance with a standard. The employee either failed to meet the standard, met the standard, or exceeded the standard. Little else is needed, least of all the judgmental variations suggested by the rating-scale approach and several of the appraisal ratings appearing in Exhibit 12–2. Rarely are more than three simple outcomes required, and often it is possible to rely on only two outcomes; many employees have job responsibilities, the fulfillment of which can be assessed simply by noting whether they did or did not get accomplished. In some cases there are only two outcomes—yes or no.

The essential intent in using standards of performance in appraisal is to quantify the outcomes of performance as much as possible and thus reduce the necessity for managerial judgment to the lowest possible level. This can be accomplished only when appraisal is not based on general personality or performance characteristics but is based rather on specific job responsibilities and standards of performance for the fulfillment of those responsibilities.

## CONSTRUCTIVE APPRAISAL

There is another performance appraisal method available in addition to those already discussed. It is not a specific system but rather a broad approach that may be used in place of a more formal system under certain circumstances or perhaps used as part of or in support of an existing system.

The constructive approach to performance appraisal involves those employees who are capable of setting goals for themselves and thus helping determine the basis on which they will be evaluated. This approach is workable in most health care institutions, since it is highly applicable to managerial, professional, and technical personnel. It is also applicable to most other employees who have a reasonable degree of self-determination or control over their immediate work environment and the order and manner of performance of their tasks. For instance, many medical record workers, business office and finance employees, and even many secretaries and clerks can be appropriately evaluated using the approach.

The four elements of constructive appraisal include:

1. Job description analysis. To set the stage for future activity, the employee is asked to analyze the job description independently and indicate where it should be expanded, contracted, or altered in any way. While the employee is doing this, the supervisor should also be reviewing the job description. When a supervisor and employee have thoroughly reviewed the job as it exists on paper, both meet to discuss all elements of the job and work on correcting or modifying the job description until they jointly agree on job content and on the relative emphasis each part of the job should receive. This step allows supervisor and employee to come to agreement on what the employee should be doing. As a byproduct of this process, the department is assured of having job descriptions that are as current as they can reasonably be made.

2. Employee performance objectives. Working independently, the employee develops a few simple targets or objectives covering some key aspects of the job. Within reason, these objectives should be: manageable—attainable through the employee's own effort and not dependent in any way on forces beyond the employee's control; realistic—attainable within a reasonable period of time; and challenging—representing at least a modest improvement over past performance. These objectives should be expressed in a few simple statements that cover several aspects of the employee's job but do not necessarily try to cover everything. They

should simply constitute a modest plan of improvement that the employee will pursue while still concentrating primarily on day-to-day activities. The objectives suggested by the employee should be as specific as possible. Ideally an objective will embody statements of what, how much, and when. For instance, an objective formulated by a senior billing clerk in the business office may look like: "To reduce billing errors coming from my section (what) by at least 50 percent (how much) before the end of the year (when)."

3. Negotiate objectives. Once the employee has developed the objectives, these should be discussed with the supervisor. The supervisor should make no effort to impose any personal objectives on the employee. Rather, it is the supervisor's job to help the employee keep the objectives realistic, manageable, and challenging, while also assuring they remain consistent with the overall objectives of the department and the organization. Once the supervisor and employee have agreed on a program of objectives, this program should be committed to writing, perhaps in a separate memorandum or possibly in a space available on the employee appraisal form.

4. Discuss results. Periodically the supervisor and employee should meet to discuss where the employee is in terms of progress toward the objectives. This will not necessarily occur at the time of the next scheduled performance appraisal; some objectives may be realizable within 2 or 3 months, and some may take 2 or 3 years to attain. This approach usually requires the supervisor and employee to get together on the subject of employee performance more often than a rigid performance appraisal program would require.

Certainly the employee will not always achieve the objectives set. Some objectives will be exceeded; some will barely be approached. However, the most important facet of this appraisal approach is the total process of involving the employee in setting objectives, working to attain them, and working with the supervisor to analyze the differences between planned performance and actual results.

Under the constructive appraisal approach, the employee knows well in advance the basis for evaluation. Having participated in establishing the objectives, the employee is better able to understand the goal to be attained. Also, having participated in establishing the objectives, the employee is usually more willing to work for improvement.

This appraisal approach also encourages the employee and supervisor to come to complete agreement on the content of the employee's job—no small accomplishment in many departments. Without such agreement, it often appears that a job exists in three distinctly different forms: (1) the supervisor envisions the job in one fashion, (2) the employee sees it another way, and (3) it exists "on paper" in perhaps a somewhat different form.

Most important, constructive appraisal takes place entirely within the context of the supervisor-employee relationship and can serve only to strengthen that relationship. More opportunities for growth and job satisfaction are created, and appraisal's most valuable function is being performed in that it is helping to create the climate necessary to support open communication between supervisor and employee.

The more often constructive appraisal contacts occur between employee and supervisor, the stronger the supervisor-employee relationship becomes. When the ideal employee-supervisor relationship exists, performance appraisal becomes a mere formality, because under these conditions both supervisor and employee know fully where the employee stands at any given time.

## THE APPRAISAL INTERVIEW

Much of what was said about the mechanics of interviewing in Chapter 8 is pertinent to the formal performance appraisal interview. The appraisal interview should occur on time, that is, when it was scheduled to occur or when the employee was told it would occur. The setting should be one that allows for privacy, freedom from interruptions, and free and open discussion. The appraisal interview should focus on joint problem solving.

## LIVING WITH AN EXISTING SYSTEM

More often than not the particular approach to performance appraisal used in your organization is decided elsewhere. You may be using an appraisal method that was in place before you arrived in the organization, or you may be required to use an appraisal system that was designed and implemented by others (usually personnel administration).

The vast majority of performance appraisal systems make use of some variation of the rating scale method. Therefore, accept what we have said about the pitfalls of such scales and checklists (especially those that require you to render personality judgments) and appreciate that you are required to operate in risky territory. Try to make the best use possible of the system you are required to use. Use the system because you must, but make every effort to use it wisely and fairly. Awareness of the pitfalls of standard appraisal approaches, such as the halo effect, central tendency, the making of unqualified judgments, and others, is a large part of the protection you need to keep you from falling into these traps.

Regardless of the system used, make every effort to emphasize performance or production (i.e., results) rather than personality traits.

Even within the confines of an existing system it is possible for you to get away from scales and boxes at least partly by going beyond checklist requirements. With supervisory and professional employees it is possible to use constructive appraisal along with the checklist method. Even with lower-rated employees, those doing repetitive, manual jobs, it is possible to open the appraisal process to some degree of input. Consider asking some of your employees one or both of the following questions:

1. What do you do now that you believe you could do better?
2. How would you change your job if you could?

You may get nothing in response to your questions, but at least you will have made the effort to let someone know you are interested. However, you may get far more than you could ever hope for in terms of positive suggestions. Some of the best suggestions for improving performance in the so-called menial tasks come from the people who do the jobs day in and day out. After all, regardless of how you, the supervisor, may view the job from the outside, when it comes to the inside details there is no one who knows more about the job than the person who does it.

Consider also the use of self-appraisal along with your existing performance appraisal system. Give the employee a blank copy of the appraisal form, and ask for a self-rating to be brought to the appraisal interview (so you do not see it prior to generating your own evaluation of the employee).

There are, of course, some weaknesses in self-appraisal. Some employees use the opportunity to "ego trip," giving themselves high marks in many areas. However, you will find that in practice most employees tend to be more critical of themselves than you are. In any case, the process will help you gain some insight into an employee's self-concept.

Self-appraisal also gives you insight into employee strengths and weaknesses, both as observed by you and perceived by the employee. The process can also suggest where you and the employee might best concentrate your efforts at joint problem solving. For instance, if your rating system calls for assessment of the employee on 12 characteristics and if you and the employee are reasonably close together in your independent assessment of 9 or 10 of these characteristics, then you know that the 2 or 3 characteristics on which you are far apart constitute the most potentially productive starting ground for joint problem solving.

The organization's performance appraisal system and how you use it will often relate directly to the general philosophy of leadership in the organization. Autocratic leadership will usually perpetuate the use of a highly structured, rigid appraisal system, leaving little room for constructive appraisal or employee input in any form. Conversely, a more participative leadership style will encourage appraisal methods that are correspondingly more open to employee input and involvement. Regardless of the organization's formal appraisal system, however, within your own department you generally have the freedom to back up the system with some constructive steps of your own and turn appraisal into a more growth-producing process.

## A SIMPLE OBJECTIVE

At the beginning of this chapter the objectives of performance appraisal were stated. It is indeed true that appraisal is intended to improve performance in the job the employee now holds and to develop the employee for possible promotion. However, consider an employee who performs, and perhaps has been performing for years, a simple job in quite acceptable fashion, leaving little room for improvement and no opportunity for growth or advancement. Even in this limited set of circumstances performance appraisal has a simple but still extremely important objective: to encourage the employee to continue delivering the same acceptable performance.

Thus, performance appraisal is essential to employees at all levels. Proper appraisal stimulates improvement, encourages growth and advancement, and conveys your appreciation of individual effort.

## REVIEW QUESTIONS

1. What should be the objective of appraisal as applied to an employee who is acceptably productive, apparently happy, and has neither the ambition nor the qualifications to advance?

2. Select two "Traditional Appraisal Methods" and give two advantages and two disadvantages of each.

3. Define and describe the oft-cited "halo effect." Why is it necessary to be aware of this effect?

4. Explain how appraisal system administration can make or break an appraisal system.

5. What would be your reaction to being evaluated primarily on your adaptability, your cooperativeness, and your attitude?

6. What are *standards of performance?*

## ROLE-PLAY: MS. WINSTON'S APPRAISAL

Ms. Cole, an ambitious young nurse, was recently promoted to shift supervisor. Success oriented, she recognizes the importance of running efficient units.

Ms. Cole inherited a subordinate, Ms. Winston, head nurse of a general medical/surgical unit. Having been in her position for 7 years, in recent years Ms. Winston required minimal direct supervision and was considered a competent departmental administrator. Her staff was loyal, stable, and highly motivated; they worked well together and seemed to emphasize quality care properly.

Ms. Winston and her staff were acutely aware of Ms. Cole's promotion. Within a few days there were frequent references to Ms. Cole as "the new kid on the block" and "the snoopervisor." Ms. Winston quickly came to resent the flurry of questions, criticisms, and suggestions that seemed to come out in every discussion with Ms. Cole.

In appraising Ms. Winston, Ms. Cole made some critical comments. While not complaining specifically about Ms. Winston's work, Ms. Cole rendered some harsh judgments concerning "negative attitude." Ms. Winston was referred to as "resistant," "sarcastic," and "irritating." The two women's concepts of supervision clearly differed markedly, and there was reason to conclude that a basic clash of personalities was making itself evident in the subordinate's performance appraisal.

The foregoing information reveals the potential for turning the appraisal interview from the learning situation it should be into a conflict. Your task is to consider the possibility of avoiding the personality clash and viewing the meeting in a way that would facilitate a positive approach to appraisal.

To the person designated as Ms. Cole: You honestly believe that Ms. Winston is automatically resistant to change regardless of the nature of a particular change. She truly strikes you as irritable and generally sarcastic. You realize, however, that some of her behavior may result from a combination of factors, including your "new ideas" and your relative youth.

To the person designated as Ms. Winston: You have been distressed by the steady stream of communications from Ms. Cole, including many items you consider unnecessary, nitpicking, and change merely for the sake of change. You feel you know much about quality patient care and you believe you have much to contribute. You would welcome a setting that gives you the opportunity to present what you know in such a way that it would be considered fairly.

Ms. Cole and Ms. Winston are to assume they have already had one tentative appraisal contact during which many of the aforementioned hard feelings came out. They are ready to try again.

The role-play participants are to conduct an appraisal meeting intended to establish a desirable new beginning for the relationship between Ms. Cole and Ms. Winston. It is suggested that the participants consider the positive approach to appraisal and attempt to reach agreement on two or more sample performance targets. (Participants may use tasks from their own areas of responsibility in the appraisal discussion—and may even move the setting from nursing to some other functional area to accommodate participants' backgrounds—as long as the two primary role players agree in advance on what is or is not included.)

The remaining members of the group should take either side of the appraisal in a discussion. (It works best if group members "choose sides" before starting and do not change during the exercise.) Afterward, all participants should critique the results of the role-play in general discussion.

---

**NOTES**

1. M. H. Schuster and C. S. Miller, "Performance Appraisal and the Age Discrimination in Employment Act," *Personnel Administrator* 29, no. 3 (1984): 48.

2. C. R. McConnell, *The Health Care Manager's Guide to Performance Appraisal* (Gaithersburg, MD: Aspen Publishers, Inc., 1993).

## CHAPTER 13

# Criticism and Discipline: Guts, Tact, and Justice

*Indifference is probably the severest criticism that can be applied to anything.*
*—Ann Schade*

## CHAPTER OBJECTIVES

☞ Establish the need for "rules and regulations" in the operation of any organization.

☞ Suggest some self-improvement guidelines for taking—as well as delivering—criticism.

☞ Introduce the concept of progressive discipline.

☞ Distinguish between problems of conduct and problems of performance and describe how each should be addressed.

☞ Provide guidance for the use of fair and effective disciplinary action.

## SITUATION: DID HE HAVE IT COMING?

"That was a stupid thing to do," said Peter Jackson, associate administrator.

"In what way?" asked the recently hired purchasing supervisor, Dan Smither, flushing noticeably at the words.

"You fiddled around with your price-break calculations so long you stalled us right into a price hike. Thanks to you we'll go about $10,000 over budget on paper products for the year."

"So I made a mistake," Smither retorted.

"Mistake? More like a colossal blunder. Ten thousand bucks! I don't know what ever convinced you that you know the paper market. The way all prices have been going you should know you've got to get in and cut a contract fast." Jackson shook his head and repeated, "Ten thousand!"

Smither stood and glared down at Jackson. "So I slipped, and I know it. In the two months I've been here I've saved twice that in other areas—how come I don't hear about those?"

"Because that's your job," Jackson replied curtly.

"Well maybe I need a new one," Smither said, and stormed out of the office.

*Instructions*

As you proceed through the chapter, prepare to address the following questions:

1. Do you believe Smither "had it coming" or that some criticism was deserved?

2. What essential element is missing from Jackson's criticism of Smither?

3. How might this situation have been approached to minimize the chances of an emotional interchange?

## THE NEED FOR RULES

Rules do not exist solely to benefit the organization, and they are not traps set by management to snare the unwary employee. However, neither are rules, as the old saying might suggest, made to be broken. They exist for good reasons.

Rules outline a general pattern of behavior that we are expected to observe and practice. Generally created with the rights and needs of the majority in mind, rules exist to protect us in a number of ways. In terms of the health care organization, rules exist to safeguard the institution and its patients and employees. They are guidelines for individual and group behavior and action, and as such they represent the organization's expectations of its employees.

Rules should be reasonable both as to their stringency and as to the number of them that exist. When organizations give way to the temptation to write a rule or regulation to cover every last contingency, the result is a bureaucratic structure. Nowhere is this more true than in the health care environment: each institution must operate in a virtual regulatory maze in which it is sometimes impossible to do anything without running afoul of some regulation.

As well as being reasonable in quantity and strictness, rules should attempt to serve the common good without infringing on individual rights and freedoms. Since nothing remains constant for long, rules should be regularly examined for their applicability to present circumstances and conscientiously updated as real needs change. For instance, it would be helpful for the "rules of the organization" (perhaps called the employee handbook or the personnel policy and procedure manual) to be thoroughly reviewed for possible changes at least once each year.

The rules of the organization should be made known to every employee. At the very least the organization should assure that every employee has had the opportunity to become thoroughly familiar with the rules. It may seem unnecessary to mention this, but it has been proven that many employees are not conversant with their own organization's rules. Even in systems that require each new employee to sign a statement indicating receipt and review of the employee handbook, many people will sign without reading the rules.

Rules and their enforcement are but a part of our concern with criticism and discipline. Many forms of behavior, often involving marginal, questionable, or otherwise hazy aspects of job performance, are deserving of criticism. There are few rules for the supervisor to use in criticizing an employee except rules of the broadest possible kind, or rules of reason or judgment. Even rules defining employee conduct, the breaking of which can result in disciplinary action, are not always as clear-cut as we would like to think they are.

## CRITICISM

Anyone who has been a supervisor for any length of time will have found it necessary to criticize someone because of conduct or work performance. Also, persons with experience in supervisory positions will have found they are sometimes targets, rather than sources, of criticism. The first-line supervisor is in the position of having to take criticism from above for everything that's wrong with worker conduct and performance and to take criticism from below for everything that's wrong with the organization and its policies and practices.

Think about the last time you were criticized. Try to remember how you felt, how fair or unfair the criticism seemed to be, and how the critic's attitude and words actually struck you. Then, keeping in mind how you believe the criticism should actually have been handled, try to put yourself in the position of the critic. You are likely to find that criticism is no more pleasant to give than it is to receive.

When you are criticized, learn from it. Learn what you should do and what you should avoid in criticizing others by carefully reviewing how you have been criticized under certain circumstances and how you reacted to that criticism. Learning to take criticism is the first step toward learning how to criticize others appropriately.

## Taking It

When you are criticized, whether by an employee, your supervisor or another member of management, a medical staff member, or someone from outside the institution, remember the guidelines below:

### Keep Your Temper

Make up your mind that no matter what is said you are going to remain calm. Do not jump to conclusions based on the possibly harsh, uncomplimentary, or unfair remarks you may be hearing. If you allow your critic to get to you, you will experience emotional reactions that will serve only to diminish your true listening capacity and hamper your ability to deal effectively with what you are hearing. Whatever you do, stay calm.

### Listen Completely

Often when you are hearing something critical of yourself the temptation to react is so nearly overwhelming that you are busy developing a defensive stance while your critic is still speaking. To strive for an open mind and the ability to listen completely, try imagining yourself in the position of a neutral third party—act as though you were hearing about someone else, not about yourself.

### Consider the Source

The often-given advice to consider the source reached cliché status long ago as a justification for ignoring criticism you simply do not want to hear. However, this expression often retains a degree of validity. Ask yourself the following questions:

- What are the person's credentials? Is this person qualified to criticize in this instance?

- What are this person's motives? Are there any vested interests involved?
- Are the comments valid, or do I just happen to be a convenient target?

Whenever you are criticized, especially by your supervisor or another member of management, try to determine whether the person is genuinely trying to help you improve.

### Evaluate the Criticism

Try to judge whether your critic had all the facts available and whether, quite simply, the criticism made sense. Search for positive suggestions in the criticism, and try to determine whether you will benefit by following your critic's advice.

### Keep it in Perspective

Some people—and it does not pay for a supervisor to be among them—do not take criticism well. They can be absolutely crushed by a few harsh or critical words. Realize, however, that criticism, no matter how harsh or ill directed, is not the end of the world. More often than not it is business as usual and interpersonal relationships drift back toward their original state. Criticism, unless carried to destructive extremes, is simply words strung together. As Mark Twain said, "If criticism had any real power to destroy, the skunk would have been extinct long ago."

### Follow-Up

Having evaluated criticism directed at you, you can do what you wish with it depending on how deserved you believe it was. If you can honestly accept what you have heard, then take steps to change your behavior accordingly. However, if you feel you honestly cannot accept the criticism, that it is perhaps misdirected, undeserved, or unduly harsh, you have still gotten something from it. At the very least, you have learned a bit more about the person who did the criticizing.

## Giving It

Supervisors are often reluctant to criticize employees. This reluctance may be rationalized as owing to our unwillingness to take the chance of hurting others' feelings. However, it is likely that the reluctance to criticize is just as readily attributable to the supervisor's natural resistance to performing an unpleasant task.

Certain kinds of behavior may deserve criticism and may perhaps even be deserving of disciplinary action—criticism plus warning or punishment. The reasons for criticism are generally incidents of misconduct or poor performance or the manifestation of a poor attitude.

Misconduct hinges largely about the existence and application of rules; its presence is often relatively clear-cut. Poor performance, on the other hand, often relates to assessments of quality and other judgments that are at least partly subjective, so the line separating what is deserved from what is undeserved is likely to be indistinct. Problems of employee attitude, especially if not immediately reflected in misconduct or poor performance, are the most difficult to deal with and call for the greatest care on the supervisor's part.

Few of us would deny the value of receiving constructive criticism when it is due. However, criticism is still criticism, and regardless of the sugar coating afforded by the word constructive, it is still likely to have a bit of a sting to it even when it is humanely delivered.

Criticism is necessary, but only if it is truly constructive. First and foremost, criticism should always include guides for correction. Simply telling people what they have done wrong without suggesting how they might do it correctly amounts to no more than placing blame. Criticism should always focus on the problem—on the results of a person's behavior and not on the person who created the problem. Beyond simply suggesting corrective measures, criticism should also allow the supervisor and employee to work together to develop a new approach jointly. Criticism, properly applied, can be used to strengthen the joint problem-solving aspect of the supervisor-employee relationship.

Criticism should also be

- *Timely.* It should be delivered as soon as possible after the behavior occurs or the results are discovered. Saving up criticism for some special upcoming contact (for instance, a performance appraisal interview) is ineffective and quite possibly damaging.
- *Private.* Never criticize an employee in the presence of other people. The words that pass between the two of you are no one else's business. Even when you walk in on a situation in which a number of people are present, after you take whatever steps are necessary to stop what is going on you should meet with the problem employee in private before delivering individual criticism.
- *Rational.* Never criticize in anger. Take the risk of blunting the impact of your criticism by allowing yourself time to cool down and assess the situation calmly before criticizing. Often when your anger has dissipated you will be able to see dimensions of the problem that were previously hidden by your emotional state.

Consider some of the more common causes of incidents, errors, and omissions leading to criticism of employees: lack of adequate job knowledge, poor understanding of management's expectations, inability to perform as expected, and attitude problems. Recognize that each of these causes embodies some reflection of the supervisor's responsibility for the knowledge, understanding, capability, and attitude of the employee. It would be beneficial, then, for the supervisor to begin considering each situation apparently deserving of criticism by asking: Have I fulfilled all of my responsibilities to this employee?

## PERHAPS HE HAD SOMETHING COMING

Having just gone through a discussion about the manner in which criticism is best taken as well as best delivered, it is appropriate at this point to offer some comments pertinent to the "Situation" that opened the chapter.

Certainly Smither deserved some kind of critical feedback concerning his error, but he did not deserve what he received. It is difficult to imagine any circumstances under which an employee deserves the anger, insults, and name-calling Smither received. In opening up angrily, Jackson simply sparked anger, resentment, and defensiveness in Smither. In beginning with "That was a stupid thing to do," Jackson virtually guaranteed an emotional, completely nonproductive interchange.

The essential element missing from Jackson's criticism of Smither is the constructive element. Criticism of an individual's performance is not valid if it is not accompanied by information that will help improve that performance. Criticism alone accuses; it does nothing to inspire or enable correction. Valid criticism also carries with it the means for correction, or at least it points out the direction in which correction may be found.

The interchange could have gone entirely differently if, for example, Jackson had opened up with something like: "Dan, we have what could be a serious problem with the paper-products budget. We need to talk about it." Had Jackson not opened angrily and insultingly, chances are Smither would not have reacted angrily. Of course Dan Smither could have defused the situation by not taking offense when Jackson opened up as he did, but his anger was likely a reaction to being caught completely off guard as he was and we can understand his reaction under the circumstances. The responsibility for this damaging interchange must lie with Jackson.

## DISCIPLINE

A bit of research into the origin of words will reveal that discipline comes from the same root as the word disciple and as such actually means "to teach so as to mold." Originally, teaching was the key to discipline—to shaping or molding the disciple. However, we have come to think of discipline, and thus disciplinary action, as punishment.

The true objective of discipline should not be punishment. It should be correction. Thus, one of the primary requirements of disciplinary action is that the employee be afforded the opportunity to correct the behavior that prompted the action.

### Conduct Versus Performance: Separate Progressive Paths

In all but the few legitimate instances in which immediate termination is appropriate, corrective action must be progressive. That is, it must follow through a number of steps in which subsequent similar infractions are addressed with increasing severity. At each step in the progressive process two pieces of information must be made clear to the employee: what the person must do to correct the problem and what may follow if the problem is not corrected. Throughout the process it is essential to view the sequence of occurrences exactly as it would be viewed—and often is viewed—by an empowered outsider such as an investigator for a civil rights or employee advocacy agency, by asking: Was the employee given every opportunity to correct the offending behavior?

In applying corrective action it is also necessary to make a distinction between problems of conduct and problems of performance. Although traditional progressive disciplinary processes may work well for problems of conduct, such processes are not appropriate for performance problems. The employee who has broken no work rules and violated no policies is not appropriately handled with a progressive disciplinary process for work performance that falls short of standard or expectation.

The supervisor always needs to ask: Is the employee not capable of performing as expected under present circumstances? If the employee cannot, for one reason or another, perform as expected, it is not a discipline problem, and to treat it as a discipline problem is to burden the process with a layer of negativity that serves only to impede correction.

## Conduct Problems: Traditional Progressive Discipline, Plus

### Counseling

The first step taken to address a specific kind of errant behavior should be counseling. One to one, supervisor to employee, the employee should be told what was done that was wrong, why it was wrong, what the organization's rules are concerning this behavior (with specific use of handbooks, policy manuals, and other written references), what the possible consequences of this kind of behavior are, and the period of time within which correction is expected. All of this needs to be accomplished without reference to any kind of "warning"; it is simply an important, job-related discussion between supervisor and employee.

Any such counseling session should be thoroughly documented by the supervisor in notes retained in departmental files.

### Oral Warning

Repeated errant behavior following counseling should be addressed using the more formal early stages of the progressive disciplinary process, specifically the oral warning. It should be stressed that the oral warning stage, often regarded as a "counseling" session, should be utilized only after the employee has failed to respond to counseling.

The oral warning should be documented by the supervisor, preferably on a corporate form created for that purpose. (See Exhibit 13–1 for an example of a simple oral warning form.) If it is documented, is this not actually a written warning? It certainly may seem so, but the difference between a written and oral warning lies in what goes into the employee's personnel file. The record of an oral warning should be retained in department files; it should go into the official personnel files only as part of a subsequent warning for the same kind of behavior.

If it is truly to be an "oral" warning, why document it at all? Because the oral warning is a step in the progressive disciplinary process, and when an employment relationship breaks down and legal problems result, it can become necessary to provide evidence that each step in the process was followed.

**Exhibit 13–1** Record of Oral Warning

Employee Name _____  ID No. _____

Department _____  Hire Date _____

Job Title & Grade _____  Job Date _____

Problem or incident; rule or policy reviewed and discussed:



Dates of previous counselings or discussion concerning the same rule or policy:


Action required of the employee:


Employee Signature _____  Date _____

Manager Signature _____  Date _____


This record will be maintained in departmental files. If further action is required for the same offense, it will be forwarded to Human Resources for inclusion in the personnel file.

---

## Written Warning

The written warning follows in turn as necessary, with this documentation automatically included in the employee's personnel file. (See Exhibit 13–2 for an example of a written warning form.)

An employee whose improper behavior has not been corrected following counseling, oral warning, and written warning is in a position in which failure to change will lead to loss of income via suspension and perhaps loss of employment. By this stage the supervisor and employee have been together on the subject of the employee's behavior problem at least three and perhaps four, five, or six times. It is time for the supervisor to bring other organizational resources into the process.

## Before Suspension

The supervisor should at this point, before proceeding to the suspension step, refer the employee to one of two available sources of further assistance: the employee health service or the human resources department.

If in any of their numerous contacts the employee has given the supervisor reason to believe he or she may be experiencing health problems of any kind, a referral to employee health is in order. If the problem appears to perhaps lie in employee attitude or in possible difficulties unrelated to health, the referral should be to human resources or perhaps to an employee relations specialist or employee ombudsperson.

**Exhibit 13–2** Written Warning

Employee Name _____ ID No. _____

Department _____ Hire Date _____

Job Title & Grade _____ Job Date _____

Notice of Discharge or Dismissal

Employee Name _____ ID No. _____

Department _____ Hire Date _____

Job Title & Grade _____ Job Date _____

Your employment is being terminated for the following reasons:

Previous Disciplinary Actions:

    Date:                                                      Action Taken:

____ Check here to indicate whether the employee desires an exit interview to discuss benefits status. If this opportunity is declined, continuation-of-benefits information will be mailed to the employee's home address.

Employee Signature _____ Date _____

Manager Signature _____ Date _____

This record puts the employee on notice that additional violations will result in more serious disciplinary action such as suspension without pay or discharge.

This referral puts the employee in contact with someone who can possibly point the way toward resolution of some underlying problem. Also, a knowledgeable person other than the supervisor is brought into the process, and this new participant may be able to get through to the employee where the supervisor could not. Finally, this step gives the employee one more distinct opportunity to correct the problem behavior.

*Suspension and Discharge*

If the referral step is unsuccessful, suspension without pay (in many systems ranging from one to five days) and eventual discharge may follow as necessary. (See Exhibits 13–3 and 13–4 for examples of forms used to document suspension and discharge/dismissal respectively.) However, a well-functioning referral program for employee behavior problems will significantly reduce the use of the clearly punitive steps of suspension and discharge.

**Exhibit 13–3** Suspension without Pay

---

Employee Name _____ ID No. _____

Department _____ Hire Date _____

Job Title & Grade _____ Job Date _____

Problem or incident; rule or policy reviewed and discussed:


Specific problem or incident, and rule or policy reviewed and discussed:


Previous Disciplinary Actions:
Date:                                              Action Taken:


Suspended for ___ days from the above date. Report back on regular shift on ____.
**Or**
Time off waived by manager for the following reason (waiver does not lessen the
severity of the action):

Employee Signature _____ Date _____

Manager Signature _____ Date _____

This is a final warning. Failure to respond appropriately may result in discharge.

---

An important point concerning suspension without pay: Note that in Exhibit 13–3, there is the option for the manager to waive the time-off requirement of a suspension. The manager is permitted to use this option on occasions when the enforced time off of a suspension would leave an important job untended or an area critically understaffed. However, the employee must be strongly advised that waiver of time off does not lessen the severity of the disciplinary action as far as the official record and future actions are concerned.

Should you feel you have cause to discharge an employee, you should take your case to the human resources department for thorough review before taking action. Given the legal environment of the times, most organizations today require human resources or administrative review and concurrence in such cases. This review will attempt to determine whether all bases have been covered from a legal perspective and whether the record clearly demonstrates that the employee was given the opportunity to correct the inappropriate behavior. This review, because of the time required, serves another extremely important function: it assures that no employee is ever fired on the spot or otherwise terminated in the anger of the moment.

Some severe infractions must of course be dealt with as they occur. However, an immediate firing is never the answer. The offending employee should

**Exhibit 13–4**  Notice of Discharge or Dismissal

Employee Name _____  ID No. _____

Department _____  Hire Date _____

Job Title & Grade _____  Job Date _____

Your employment is being terminated for the following reasons:


Previous Disciplinary Actions:
   Date:                                          Action Taken:



____ Check here to indicate whether the employee desires an exit interview to discuss benefits status. If this opportunity is declined, continuation-of-benefits information will be mailed to the employee's home address.

Employee Signature_____  Date _____

Manager Signature _____  Date _____

instead be sent home and immediately placed on indefinite suspension pending investigation and resolution.

Not all kinds of infractions will require the application of all the foregoing steps. A mild infraction, such as tardiness (within a few minutes of starting time) may, if it becomes chronic, eventually require all of the steps described above. A more serious infraction, such as sleeping on duty, may call for a written warning or suspension on the first violation and discharge on the second violation. The organization's human resources department ordinarily provides guidance for determining the severity of disciplinary action for specific infractions.

### Performance Problems: "Warnings" Not Applicable

It is inappropriate to apply a progressive disciplinary process to an employee who is exhibiting substandard work. The substandard performer has not broken the rules; to group this person with the supposed rule breakers is to lend a negative aspect to a process that must be as positively oriented as possible.

Substandard performance can be simply described as the production of unsatisfactory results that prevent an employee from attaining or maintaining job standard. The job standard may be further defined as the acceptable level of output achieved by employees in the same or similar job classification, or the standard level of results, defined in advance by the supervisor and clearly identifying the quantity and quality of output expected.

### For the Newly Identified Substandard Performer

The supervisor's primary objective should not be to get rid of the substandard performer, as is frequently the case, but rather to show the substandard performer how to perform acceptably. The supervisor should

- review the job standard with the employee, ensuring that the standard is known and understood and, ideally, that the employee accepts this as a reasonable expectation
- counsel the employee, developing an action plan specifying what must be done to attain standard performance and a timetable for doing so, documenting this thoroughly, as any counseling session should be documented, with a copy of the complete plan supplied to the employee
- conscientiously monitor the employee's progress against the improvement plan, providing assistance as necessary
- remove apparent obstacles to the employee's success when possible and make reasonable accommodations to enhance employee performance

If this process does not correct the problem within the agreed-upon time period, it should be repeated in essentially identical fashion in terms of the creation of a mutually acceptable plan of correction—with necessary modifications from the earlier plan, based on what was encountered in the process—and an agreed-upon target date.

### Again to the Important "Plus"

The second time the employee is taken through the corrective counseling and instruction, the process should include referral to either the human resource department or the employee health office. The reasons for doing so are essentially the same as for making this referral for an employee exhibiting conduct problems, and the advantages of doing so are likewise the same: a new person who can possibly help is brought into the process, and the employee is given the chance to address a possible underlying problem that may be causing the apparent performance problem.

### How Many Times?

Depending on how much, if any, improvement is noted from one time to the next, the foregoing process might be applied three or four times. When finally every reasonable opportunity to improve has been extended multiple times without lasting change occurring, a last-ditch deadline should be established. When this deadline arrives, employment should end unless all conditions of the plan of improvement have been met.

### Dismissal, Not Discharge

When it is necessary to release an employee for reasons of substandard performance, the action should be identified as a dismissal for failure to meet job standards, and not as a discharge. The distinction is important; a discharge for cause is a "firing," and a person so terminated has lost employment through inappropriate conduct and in most parts of the country is not eligible for unemployment compensation. However, an individual who is dismissed for inability to meet the standards of the job is not considered wholly responsible for the termination, so the action is regarded more as a layoff than a discharge and the person so terminated is usually eligible for unemployment compensation.

## Guidelines for Fair and Effective Discipline

### Be Reasonable

At all times strive to keep the severity of disciplinary action consistent with the infraction. It helps if there are stated guidelines for the severity of discipline, but very often you are on your own. Remember the particular action you associated with a certain infraction and try to avoid any variation in the scale of punishment involved.

### Avoid Making Examples

Every employee deserves fair, consistent treatment relative to all other employees. Resist the occasional temptation to make an example of an individual for the sake of discouraging the same kind of behavior by others. Making examples serves only to create fear and resentment, and it destroys the effectiveness of discipline.

### Follow the Rules

The rules in the employee handbook will not cover every situation, but they will apply to many occasions when disciplinary action is warranted. Use the rules, and use them consistently. What applies to one employee should apply to all others for the same offense. Use written warnings when the system calls for them. Do not simply "slide over" an incident deserving a warning without actually issuing the warning; this omission may return to haunt you later.

### Respect Privacy

Do not meddle in the life of an employee outside of the institution. What an employee does on off hours is ordinarily none of your business. The only time you can be concerned with an employee's private life is when you know that the person is engaged in something that can harm job performance or negatively affect the reputation of the organization. Even then you remain on shaky ground because you are risking violation of someone's privacy.

### Avoid Favoritism

Under no circumstances should you allow yourself to favor any employees over others. Undoubtedly there will be some employees you personally like better than others; people are different and your reactions are natural. However, you must make every effort to ensure that disciplinary actions you dispense are consistent among your employees regardless of your personal feelings toward various people.

### Act Only on Clear Evidence

Take disciplinary action only when absolutely certain you are dealing with a truly guilty party. Hearsay or second-hand evidence is totally inadequate and undeserving of more than your passing attention. It is far better to run the risk of allowing someone who deserves punishment to slip through rather than to discipline an innocent person unjustly.

*Avoid Dwelling on History*

When an incident is over and disciplinary action has been delivered, forget it. Do not bring the incident up again; do not continually remind the employee that you remember what happened. The only extent to which you can justifiably deal with history in disciplinary action is through the necessary accumulation of written warnings. This practice, of course, must be spelled out in the work rules of the organization.

## The Inevitable Documentation

At several points in the processes described in the preceding paragraphs the need to provide documentation was mentioned, even to the extent of calling for documentation of so-called oral warnings. It is often too easy to delay the documentation and perhaps forget about it entirely, mainly because documentation is usually not an immediate concern.

After most employment actions take place, all involved parties go forward to other concerns and never look back. Occasionally, however, an employment action is challenged, either internally through a grievance or appeal process or externally through a civil rights or advocacy agency or a lawsuit. And when an action is challenged, all of the documentation related to it in any way is brought to the foreground.

Documents related to performance or conduct problems are used to reasonably establish whether something did or did not occur, whether an employee was or was not spoken with about a certain problem, whether the employee agreed or disagreed with a certain course of action, and so on. These documents are used to establish whether the employee was given the opportunity to improve or correct. Human memories fade or become selective regarding certain kinds of information, and the documentation is relied upon to either support or refute certain contentions.

The importance of the documentation of employment actions cannot be stressed too strongly. In the words of one investigator for an employee advocacy agency, "If it's not properly documented, signed, and dated, we assume it never happened."

## NONPUNITIVE DISCIPLINE

### A Controversial Approach to Disciplinary Action

No matter how fairly and humanely disciplinary action is accomplished, it is sometimes difficult to avoid seeing it as punitive in nature. Although disciplinary action properly taken may have its obvious positive elements in attempting to correct behavior, the warnings employed are sure to appear to some as punishment or at least the threat of punishment. As a result, some organizations have experimented with the concept of nonpunitive discipline in the belief that punishment simply breeds resistance, fosters resentment, and undermines employee willingness.

The nonpunitive approach, controversial at best, is based in part on the belief that placing more responsibility on the employee makes it more difficult for the person to remain hostile toward the organization. Its advocates claim that nonpunitive discipline reduces grievances and discharges, decreases voluntary terminations, and improves morale. Those opposed are inclined to view it as a giveaway in which an individual is "rewarded" for inappropriate behavior with the principal controversial element of nonpunitive discipline: a one-day suspension with pay, or, as it is sometimes described, a *day of decision.*

Although there are variations in its application, nonpunitive discipline might work somewhat in the following manner.

1. Upon committing an infraction requiring correction, the employee is informally counseled concerning the rule broken or the policy violated. The unacceptable behavior is highlighted and the appropriate behavior is described.

2. Upon a second violation the employee is again counseled, but this time the session is more formal and includes the supervisor's manager or a human resources representative, and documentation is generated.

3. In the event of a third violation the employee is advised that if he or she finds the particular rule or policy inappropriate, perhaps it is time to seek another employer. The employee is given a one-day suspension, and the employee is given options in writing: either choose to leave, or agree—in writing—to the requirement for corrected behavior. If the employee agrees to correction, he or she is returned to work and receives full pay for the day off. If the employee does not agree or does not respond by some predetermined time, termination is automatic. (The day off with full pay is often a sticking point with other employees who must take up the slack created by the absence of one who is being paid to "do nothing" for a day.)

4. Should the employee agree and return to work violates the agreement at some later date, then termination is in order.

So-called "nonpunitive" discipline—"nonpunitive" stressed in quotes because, as some see it, the process simply forestalls the punitive nature of disciplinary action to the very end of unsuccessful correction—is generally more appropriate for professional and technical personnel than for rank-and-file or entry level personnel. In brief, it will likely work only with those employees who fully appreciate the implications of the "day of decision" and will take it seriously.

## COACHING: STOPPING TROUBLE BEFORE IT STARTS

It is unrealistic to believe that all problems of employee conduct and all instances of substandard performance can be corrected before they start; that is, that they can, in all instances, be avoided. No matter how effective the individual manager may be, these kinds of difficulties can be expected to occur. What the manager can control to some extent, however, is how often these kinds of difficulties arise. The supervisor who finds that the employee problems occur constantly may be overlooking his or her essential role in coaching employees.

We may legitimately refer to coaching as an essential ongoing process that has the capacity to minimize the need for the manager to address employee problems through the corrective processes. In other words, the truly effective manager will be effective as a coach of employees, and effective coaching will lessen the need to apply corrective processes. One might be tempted to place coaching before counseling as the first step of any corrective process, but this is not appropriate. Counseling applies at the presence or emergence of a problem; coaching is a continuing process that applies before a problem occurs.

One way to gain an appreciation of the need for coaching is to think back on one or more employment experiences in which you found yourself feeling on the brink of being overwhelmed by a new job. You were taught the steps to perform, you were shown the job as performed by another, and you were turned loose to make your way on your own. Very soon, however, the questions began to arise: That seemed not to work as I was shown. What did I do wrong? This is a little different from what was demonstrated. What do I do now? What do I do when this particular exception occurs? And so on. The frustrations and uncertainties arise until you feel overwhelmed by the job; you fear that you may not succeed at this, or that you may inadvertently do something that will cause you to lose your new-found job. In fact some new employees who find themselves feeling overwhelmed simply eliminate the feeling by removing themselves from the job. Many new employees have resigned under such circumstances, and many such resignations could have been avoided with proper orientation and training followed by effective coaching.

Any manager who supervises the people who perform the hands-on work has a coaching responsibility. Think of this responsibility as an essential extension of orientation and training. Newer employees will of course require more coaching than experienced employees, but at various times it is likely that nearly all employees will benefit from appropriate coaching.

Coaching is simply the provision of ongoing advice, assistance, and encouragement to the extent necessary to enable an employee to perform comfortably and effectively on a continuing basis. As such it is much of the basis for the continuing relationship between manager and employee. The effectively coached employee is far less likely to exhibit behavior that necessitates use of the corrective processes.

## GUTS, TACT, AND JUSTICE

Criticizing employees and parceling out disciplinary action take courage. In most instances it is normal for the supervisor to feel uneasy. We can go so far as to suggest that we should never want to reach the point of becoming completely comfortable with criticism and discipline; this state might suggest a callousness that runs contrary to the character of an effective supervisor.

An employee who has done something deserving of criticism or disciplinary action nevertheless deserves your full consideration as an individual. You must continually be aware of feelings—your own as well as others. However, regardless of individual feelings, what you say and what you do must be said and done out of consideration for the needs of the institution, its patients, and its employees.

---

## REVIEW QUESTIONS

1. In most instances, what is—or should be—the primary purpose of disciplinary action? Why?
2. What is necessary to make *constructive criticism* truly constructive?
3. Why is it advisable to treat *problems of performance* differently from *problems of conduct*?
4. Why are most organizations' disciplinary processes progressive in nature, and why are there usually different numbers of progressive steps for different infractions?
5. If disciplinary action is supposed to be progressive and provide the opportunity for correction of behavior, why are there some infractions for which an employee may be discharged for a single violation?
6. How does *counseling* differ from *oral warning*?

---

## CASE: A GOOD EMPLOYEE, BUT. . .

Housekeeping supervisor Ellie Richards was faced with a situation that left her feeling uncomfortable about the action she would have to consider taking. In discussing the matter with Stan Miller, the other housekeeping supervisor, she began with, "I have no idea how I should deal with Judy Lawrence. I just don't recall ever facing one like this before."

Stan asked, "What's the problem?"

"Excessive absenteeism," Ellie answered. "Judy has rapidly used up all of her sick time, and most of her sick days have been before or after scheduled days off."

"What's unusual about that? Unfortunately, we have several people who use their sick time as fast as it's accrued. And most get 'sick' on very convenient days."

"What's unusual is the fact that it's Judy Lawrence. She's been here 7 years, but this apparent sick-time abuse has all been within the past few months. She's used her whole sick-time bank in 7 months. And most recently she was out for 3 days without even calling in."

Stan said, "You can terminate her for that."

"I know," said Ellie.

"Especially when you take her other absences into account. You've warned her about them?"

After a moment's silence Ellie said, "No, not in writing. Just once, face to face."

"Any record of it? Fill out a disciplinary dialogue form for her to sign?"

"No," said Ellie. "I really hated to. I know I should have taken some kind of action by now, but I can't seem to make myself do it."

Stan asked, "Why not?"

"Because she's always been such a good employee. She's always been pleasant, she's always done what she's told to do, and she's always done quality work. She's still that way, except for her attendance problems of the past 7 months."

Ellie shrugged and continued, "I guess what I'm really hung up on is: How do I discipline someone who is usually a good employee, and do it in such a way that it doesn't destroy any of what is good about her?"

Stan shook his head and said, "Good performer or not, I'd say you ought to be going by the policy book. That's all I can suggest."

## Questions

1. How would you advise Ellie to proceed in the matter of Judy Lawrence?
2. Do you feel that Ellie's failure to take action thus far affects her ability to take action now? Why or why not?

## CHAPTER 14

# The Problem Employee and Employee Problems

*In so complex a thing as human nature, we must consider it
hard to find rules without exception.*
—*George Eliot*

## CHAPTER OBJECTIVES

☛ Qualify the term "problem employee" and review the hazards involved in applying labels to people.

☛ Provide suggestions as to why the problem employee may indeed present problems for the supervisor.

☛ Present general guidelines for handling troublesome employees.

☛ Recognize the "dead-end employee" as a special case, and suggest approaches for dealing with this person.

☛ Offer guidelines for the control of absenteeism.

☛ Provide guidance for relating to employees whose performance is affected by personal problems.

## SITUATION: WHAT DO WE DO ABOUT A FIRST-CLASS GROUCH?

"As your assistant, I'm certainly not trying to tell you what to do," said Marie Stark. "You're the boss, and I'm only pointing out—again—a problem that's leading us into lots of grief."

"I know," laboratory administrator Morris Craig said with more than a trace of annoyance. "I'm trying to take it the way you mean it. I've heard it from several people and I know we've got a problem with Jennifer. I just don't know how to deal with it, that's all."

"It has to be dealt with," Marie said. "As lab receptionist Jennifer is in a position to leave a first and lasting impression on a lot of people, and she's generating an endless trail of complaints. I've heard from patients, staff, and physicians alike—just about anyone you care to name—about her curt, rude treatment of them. It's been going on for months, and it's getting worse. And now she's starting to mix up appointment times as well."

Morris said, "I know. I had hoped that whatever was bugging her would pass. But it hasn't. She's gone from bad to worse. And it's too bad—she's been here a long time, and this is only relatively recent."

"One of us needs to talk with her. Or at least make some attempt to find out what's wrong."

Morris spread his hands, palms up, and said, "I've tried to talk with her. Just a week ago I gave her a chance to talk in private. I even asked if I could help out in any way, but—." He shrugged helplessly.

"But what?"

227

"She told me nothing was wrong, or something like that. I got the impression that she was telling me—kind of roundabout—to mind my own business."

"Well, something is wrong," Marie said, "and we need to do something about it. Our receptionist is coming across as a first-class grouch and the department is suffering."

*Instructions*

As you proceed through this chapter, look for the elements of a tentative approach for dealing with the apparent attitude problem presented by the laboratory receptionist. Make certain you provide for reasonable opportunity for correction of behavior and that you account for

- possible ways of assisting the employee with "the problem"
- the necessarily progressive nature of any disciplinary action considered
- the needs of the department

## IS THERE SUCH A PERSON AS A "PROBLEM EMPLOYEE"?

We might legitimately ask whether there really is such a person we can call the "problem employee." Considering your answer in practical terms—from the viewpoint of a supervisor—you might be tempted to say there is such a person and offer several real-life examples from among the employees in your department. Indeed, sometimes there may seem to be many problem employees.

In actuality, however, who knows how many, or how few, problem employees there really are? A person may be a true problem employee, but you may see only the apparent problem. Also, you, by your leadership style and through your expectations of the individual, may well be part of the problem.

Usually the problem employee will be neither a very good nor a very poor performer. Rarely can outstanding workers, that is, those exceeding management's expectations in terms of quality of work, amount of work, and interpersonal relations, be considered problems. In addition, the worker whose performance has been chronically substandard and generally unacceptable should no longer be there to present a problem, assuming that persons who turn out to be simply unable to do their jobs are properly weeded out after being given every reasonable opportunity to learn. Rather, the problem employee is usually a worker whose performance, both functionally and interpersonally, falls perhaps a bit short of the average. The problem employee is tough to instruct and correct, tough to motivate, and generally troublesome to handle.

Beware, however, of the label "problem employee." One source researched for material applicable to this discussion (a source not identified for reference since none of its information was used) presumed to identify 24 "types of problem employees."

Problem employee "types," perhaps labeled by terms you have used from time to time, such as "know-it-all," "wise guy," "blabbermouth," and "complainer," tend to zero in on one or two narrow behavioral characteristics and magnify them to the extent that they overshadow the whole person. Also, categorizing a person tends to lead to the assumption that the person is in fact that way and thus tends to channel a relationship with the individual along certain narrow lines. We can be led into automatically reacting to certain people in certain given ways. For instance, if you need something from the business office staff but you know that "stubborn so-and-so" is in charge today you may readily adopt a hard-line approach without realizing you are doing so.

People, and thus employees, are all different. The majority of your employees behave in somewhat the same fashion, owing largely to the rules, methods, and procedures they are required to follow as members of the organization. However, this common behavior in no way means that they are alike. Each has a particular personality, and each is a collection of attitudes and feelings that add up to a unique individual.

Some supervisors are unaware of, or perhaps ignore, the differences between employees that mark some as so-called problem employees. They may unconsciously decide that it is easier to stand on the authority of the supervisory position and use orders and ultimatums for handling the problem employee.

The problem employee, however, can be a particularly interesting challenge for the supervisor. Sure, a particular employee may be difficult to get along with, but learn to get along with one problem employee and your skills at relating with people will improve all the way around.

People, whether our employees or others we come into contact with, cannot be pigeonholed or categorized. Even our use of the term problem employee is unfair; although it is a broad category, it still is a category, and we are grouping people together under that single label. Categorizing employees, which we cannot avoid doing to some extent, often leads to a gradual narrowing of the categories and eventually to stereotyping. In addition to being hazardously unreliable, stereotyping is unfair: It almost always constitutes unwarranted generalization, and as G.K. Chesterton said, "All generalizations are dangerous, including this one."

Watch out, then, for labels you would apply to employees, especially labels with negative connotations such as stubborn, grouchy, lazy, undependable, dull, and so on. When we use such labels we are erecting obstacles that may prevent us from seeing more favorable, but perhaps less obvious, characteristics that are also present. Also, as discussed in the chapter on performance appraisal, when we apply such labels we are rendering personality judgments that most of us are unqualified to make.

Often we are unwittingly led into accepting a label generated by someone else. For instance, a new supervisor coming in from the outside may get a rundown on all employees from the departing supervisor: "This one is cooperative, that one is a grouch, this one is headstrong and insists on doing things the wrong way, that one is a crybaby," and so on. It is bad enough that we are inclined to form our own shaky judgments, let alone that we compound the problem by accepting another supervisor's similarly shaky judgments. At the very least we need to form our own impressions of our employees through personal observation and interaction.

When you type or label an employee you are actually setting yourself up to think of the person as actually being that way and expect the person to behave according to that label.

## DEALING WITH THE PROBLEM EMPLOYEE

### Ups and Downs

Recognize that everyone, including you, has good days and bad days. The mood of the day, how things have been going, how you feel physically, and many other factors have a bearing on how you come across to others at any particular time. So it is with your employees. Most of the people who work in your department have their good days and their bad days, and how each of them appears to you on a few occasions may well determine your general regard for them or your view of them as likely problems.

As in your relations with all employees at all times, try to be empathic. Try putting yourself in the employee's position, and try to appreciate fully why that person feels and acts in such a way. When you see the visible suggestions of problems in your employees, make yourself seriously consider reasons why you behave as you do under possibly similar circumstances. What causes your coolness, distance, irritability, or other less-than-desirable behavior?

In dealing with the problem employee, recognize initially that direct, forceful attempts to alter behavior will probably fail. For instance, meeting deep-seated stubbornness head-on with hard-nosed determination is more likely to be destructive than constructive. Recognize that very often we cannot change so-called difficult people but that often we can accept and perhaps even utilize their peculiarities.

### Time to be Troublesome

One of the keys to dealing with the problem employee is to keep the person constructively occupied. The act of doing meaningful work, with energies directed into obviously useful channels, is by far the best cure for many problem employees. Activity is certainly not the cure for everything, but it can remove some problems, such as irritability, boredom, or frustration owing to inactivity, and it can keep the lid on other problems. When we have time on our hands we tend to dwell on ourselves and our troubles, and the things that bother employees are more likely to come to the surface and be magnified when they are idle or underutilized.

Whenever possible, use your employees in the capacities for which they are best suited. Everyone is a collection of numerous qualities; not everyone does everything with the same degree of success or is equally suited to all assignments. While we should recognize that the needs of the institution and its patients come first and it is often necessary to place people in less-than-ideal assignments, there is nevertheless a degree of management responsibility to use employees in the manner to which they are best suited. When employees are utilized such that their talents and preferences are applied to best advantage, problems are less likely to develop.

Many employees find time in which to be troublesome because they are not sufficiently challenged by their work. Some simply do not care for what they are doing—there are numerous tasks in a health care institution that few people would enjoy doing day in and day out. Part of the solution to the problem of keeping employees constructively occupied could include offering increased responsibility to those who are able to assume it and rotation of job duties, where possible, to spread around the least desirable tasks so they have minimum negative impact on any few select persons.

### The Whole Person

In the long run you will find it practically impossible to separate the person off the job from the person on the job. To a greater or lesser extent, people bring their outside problems onto the job and carry their job-related problems off the job. With some employees this crossover is minimal. With others, however, a small crisis in either facet of their existence can affect attitudes and behavior in the other. Thus the employee who becomes sullen and withdrawn may have done so either because of some job-related experience or because of something that happened off the job. If someone has become moody or stubborn or invited the application of some similar label, then that alone should give you cause to wonder what is behind the behavior.

The behavior projected by an employee can be an emotional defense against treatment received on the job. Because people are different, some distinctly so, the same approach will not work with everyone. As a supervisor, do you make it a practice to remain on friendly terms with everyone—friendly, but impersonal and businesslike—conscientiously trying not to play favorites while you avoid getting "too close" to your employees? To some of your employees this will be appropriate behavior; you will be seen as a good supervisor. However, some employees will see this same behavior as artificial and perhaps label you as "cold" or "phony." (It is not just the supervisors who do the labeling.)

Do you make an effort to get to know all your employees, openly expressing interest in them as individuals and inquiring into their personal interests? Again, to part of your employee group this behavior will make you a good supervisor. To others, however, you will seem nosy, inquiring into things that are none of your business. Is it your practice to circulate about the group during the workday to simply show people you are there, available, and interested? If so, this behavior will be accepted by some employees as appropriate supervisory behavior while some others may see you as distrustful because you are constantly checking up on them.

Whatever you do in your efforts to be a good supervisor, a few employees are likely to react negatively. These negative reactors are likely to be your "problem employees."

### SEVEN GUIDELINES

In dealing with problem employees, remember the following seven guidelines:

1. Listen. Make it clear that you are always available to hear what is both-

ering your employees. Display an open attitude, conscientiously avoiding the tendency to shut out possible unpleasantries because you don't want to hear them. Many employees' doubts, fears, and complaints are created or magnified by a closed attitude on the part of the supervisor, so your obvious willingness to listen will go a long way toward putting some troubles to rest.

2. Always be patient, fair, and consistent, but retain sufficient latitude in your behavior to allow for individual differences among people. Use the rules of the organization as they were intended, stressing corrective aspects rather than punishment. Apply disciplinary action when truly deserved, but do not use the threat of such action to attempt to force change by employees.

3. Recognize and respect individual feelings. Further, recognize that a feeling as such is neither right nor wrong—it is simply there. What a person does with a feeling may be right or wrong, but the feeling itself cannot be helped. Do not ever say, "You shouldn't feel that way." Respect people's feelings, and restrict your supervisory interest to what each employee does with those feelings.

4. Avoid arguments. Problem employees are frequently ready and willing to argue in defense of their feelings or beliefs. However, by arguing with an employee you simply solidify that person in a defensive position and reduce the chances of effective communication of any kind.

5. If possible, let your supposedly stubborn or resistant employees try something their own way. As a supervisor you are interested first in results and only secondarily in how those results are achieved (as long as they are achieved by reasonable methods). There is no better way to clear the air with the employee who "knows better" than to provide the flexibility for that person to try it that way and either succeed or fail. In other words, the employee who appears stubborn or resistant may not be so by nature but may rather be reacting to authoritarian leadership. More participative leadership might be the answer.

6. Pay special attention to the chronic complainers, those employees who seem to grouch and grumble all through the day and spread their gloom and doom to anyone who will listen. Chronic complaining is, of course, a sign of several potential problems and also breeds new problems of its own. The chronic complainer can affect departmental morale and drag down the entire work group. You should make every effort to find out what is behind the complaining, and perhaps even consider altering assignments such that a complainer is semi-isolated or at least limited in the opportunity to spread complaints.

7. Give each employee some special attention. The supervisor-employee relationship remains at the heart of the supervisor's job, and each employee deserves to be recognized as an individual as well as a producer of output. Honest recognition as individuals is all that some of our so-called problem employees really need to enable them to stop being problems.

## A SPECIAL CASE: THE DEAD-END EMPLOYEE

The "dead-end employee" is discussed in this chapter because this person is caught up in a set of circumstances that frequently leads to the development of certain problems. The dead-end employee is that employee who can go no further in the organization. Promotion to supervision may not be possible because basic qualifications are lacking; promotion into a higher level is not possible because the employee is already at the top of grade; pay raises are infrequent because the employee has reached the top of the scale and can move only when the scale itself is moved. In short, the dead-end employee is blocked from growth and advancement in all channels. This employee is a special problem in motivation because there are no more material rewards left with which to prevent creeping dissatisfaction from setting in, and other rewards, the true motivators that should be inherent in the job, are limited.

It is unfortunate that many dead-end employees become problems because these employees very often have the most to offer the organization. It falls to the supervisor to deal with the problem by appealing to the individual through true motivating forces that stress job factors rather than environmental factors.

In dealing with the dead-end employee, remember the following:

- Consult the employee on various problems and aspects of the department's work. Ask for advice. It is possible that an employee with years of experience in the same capacity has a great deal to offer and will react favorably to the opportunity to offer it.

- Give the employee a bit of additional responsibility when possible, and let the person earn the opportunity to be more responsible. Some freedom and flexibility may be seen as recognition of a sort for the employee's past experience and contributions.

- Delegate special one-time assignments. Again, years of experience may have prepared the employee to handle special jobs above and beyond ordinary assignments.

- Use the dead-end employee as a teacher. The experienced employee may be quite valuable in one-on-one situations, helping to orient new employees or teaching present employees new and different tasks.

- Point the dead-end employee toward certain prestige assignments such as committee assignments, attendance at an occasional seminar or educational program, or the coordination of a social activity such as a retirement party or other gathering.

Note that all of the foregoing suggestions deal with ways of putting interest, challenge, variety, and responsibility into the work itself. In dealing with the dead-end employee, special attention must be given to true motivating forces because the potential dissatisfiers, that is, the environmental factors such as wages and fringe benefits and working conditions, are present in force. If the employee has come to regard an occasional pay increase as deserved reward for putting up with the same old nonsense, when the top of the scale has been reached and pay raises stop, then dissatisfaction will begin. All the suggestions made relative to the dead-end employee are intended to help the person find sufficient motivation in the work itself and avoid the weight of the dissatisfiers.

There are other potential solutions to the problem of the dead-end employee, conditions permitting. Maybe it is possible to transfer the person to a completely different assignment or perhaps set up a rotational scheme in which several employees trade assignments on a regular basis. Also, the dead-end employee may be cross-trained on several other jobs within the department and thus be given a chance to do a variety of work and become more valuable to the department.

Perhaps it is unfair to discuss the dead-end employee in a chapter on "problem employees," since many such employees may present no problem at all. However, it is to the supervisor's advantage to recognize the dead-end employee as at least a slightly special case that a bit of conscientious supervisory attention can keep from becoming a real problem.

## ABSENTEEISM

As well as being a significant problem in its own right, absenteeism is usually a symptom of other problems. To the supervisor, absenteeism is an immediate problem of sometimes significant dimensions. Even a modest percentage of absenteeism in the department is likely to upset schedules and cause much supervisory time and effort to be devoted to juggling personnel and assignments to cover necessary tasks.

The employee who develops a pattern of chronic absenteeism becomes a problem employee. Chronic absenteeism, in turn, should suggest that this employee may have problems, personal or otherwise, that are being at least partly revealed by their effects on work attendance.

To some extent absenteeism haunts supervisors and managers in every industry and every conceivable organizational setting. Of course a great deal of absenteeism is legitimate; people get sick and have other difficulties that sometimes keep them away from work. A considerable amount of absenteeism, however, is not legitimate—at least not to the extent to which we define legitimate in terms of organizationally recognized reasons for employee absence. In addition, there is no sure way of determining how much absence is legitimate and how much is not.

It has been estimated that absenteeism costs the country in excess of $10 billion per year in lost output and other costs. When someone fails to show up for work, usually one of two things happens: (1) the employee's work goes undone that day or (2) someone else must be assigned to do the absent employee's work. In both cases significant cost can be involved. Perhaps sick leave benefits are paid to the absentee, wages are paid to a replacement employee, or revenue is lost because the employee was not there to perform, and numerous rippling inefficiencies occur that ultimately have a dollar impact on the organization.

To a degree, absenteeism is governed by employee attitude. Employee attitude is in turn influenced by numerous factors. An employee experiencing a negative turn in attitude is likely to discover that unwarranted absence, once indulged in, is just that much easier the next time around. This can be especially true if absenteeism is in effect aided by silent or tolerant supervision.

Since there are legitimate reasons for employees to be absent, absenteeism is a problem that can never be completely cured. However, absenteeism can be reduced and controlled through conscientious supervisory attention.

## Guidelines for Reduced Absenteeism

For control of absenteeism in your department, consider the following eight guidelines:

1. In dealing with employees, stress that employment is a two-way street. Sick leave is an employee benefit with an associated cost, provided for use when needed. It is more privilege than right and as such should not be abused. Let your employees know that absence should not be taken for granted, and let them know what it does to your department in terms of added cost and lost output.

2. Let your employees know that their attendance is important to the operation of the department. Openly publicize your concern for absenteeism and its effects on department performance.

3. Start new employees the right way, including in their orientation your expectation of regular attendance. Make sure they clearly understand all the rules governing absenteeism and the use of sick leave benefits.

4. Keep accurate attendance records, and do so with the knowledge of each employee. Do not put yourself in the position of having to have another department (for instance, personnel or payroll) research an employee's attendance record when a question arises.

5. Have absentees report to you when returning to work. This generally will not bother legitimate absentees, but it puts a certain amount of pressure on the healthy "stay-aways." In any case, even assuming that a particular absence may indeed be legitimate, you should be sufficiently interested in your employees' well-being to briefly check with someone returning from a day or two of absence.

6. Do not allow your system to reward for absenteeism. For instance, in some departments in which employees rotate to provide weekend coverage there may be people who seem to experience "illness" only when scheduled to work on Saturday or Sunday. Arrange your scheduling so that a person who calls in sick on a scheduled Saturday or Sunday will be rescheduled to work that day on the following weekend so the employee cannot avoid working a fair share of weekends through the use of sick leave.

7. Discuss unusual patterns of absence with the employees involved. If someone's supposed illness or personal problem always creates a long weekend or stretches a holiday into two days, at least make it known that you are aware of the pattern and feel perhaps it would be more than coincidence should this pattern continue.

8. Use incentives available to you as a supervisor to discourage absenteeism. For instance, it would make sense to delegate a special assignment or a particularly interesting or appealing task to someone you can reasonably count on to show up regularly for work and to make it known that this measure of dependability is one of your reasons for selecting the person you chose. Also, make appropriate use of employee's attendance records at performance appraisal time. While attendance is not likely to weigh heaviest in a performance appraisal, unless, of course, it is exceptionally poor, you can certainly apply attendance in its proper relationship with other appraisal factors in either extending or withholding praise and reward.

### Morale and Motivation

Employee morale and individual motivation to perform are key factors in a department's rate of absenteeism. Generally, low morale and lack of individual motivation will encourage increased absenteeism. Some people stay away from work because they are ill and would do so in any case. However, many absences happen when employees are feeling "on the fence"—neither especially sick nor particularly well. If this "blah" feeling happens to coincide with a "blah" attitude toward the job, the employee will stay home as long as sick-time benefits remain available.

All the factors having a bearing on the employee's attitude toward the organization, the job, and the work—the motivators and dissatisfiers discussed in Chapter 11—can influence attendance. Some of the most frequent causes of unwarranted absences are boredom, repetition, lack of interest, lack of challenge, and the inability to see positive results from one's efforts. Anything the supervisor can do to improve the chances of employee self-motivation will also be positive steps toward reducing and controlling absenteeism.

### ABUSE OF SICK TIME

For many years, health care organizations, not generally known as high-paying employers, compensated in part for unattractive salary levels by providing relatively generous benefits. One such benefit was paid sick time. In most instances sick time was provided as a *welfare benefit*, one that is there to be used when needed but if not needed it disappears after some specified time. However, many employees came to regard their sick time as an *entitlement,* and since sick time was subject to a use-it-or-lose-it requirement they felt justified in using sick days as they would vacation or personal days.

The entitlement view of paid sick time led to its abuse, contributing to absenteeism and prompting some organizations to drastically alter their sick-time benefits. In recognition of rising costs of doing business, and in what has perhaps been a long overdue reaction to chronic abuse of sick time in some quarters, employers began seeking ways to reduce the number of sick days utilized and generally curb the abuse of sick time.

Organizations that offer a paid sick-time benefit have found that employees average 5 to 6 sick days per year, for a cost of about 2% of total payroll.[1] Some organizations have also learned that the amount of sick time used is related to the amount of the benefit. Consider, for example, the experiences of two hospitals located in the same community. At one where the sick-time benefit was a generous 12 days per year, usage averaged 7 days per employee per year. At the other, where just 5 days per year were provided, usage averaged 3.5 days per employee per year.

### The Emergence of Paid-Time-Off (PTO) Plans

In an effort to reduce the payroll impact of sick time, many employers have been combining various forms of paid leave—primarily sick time, vacation, and personal time—into a single bank. These paid-time-off arrangements, referred to simply as PTO plans, encourage employees to use leave only when necessary because time used for one purpose reduces the time available for other purposes. Such a plan is replenished regularly, usually per pay period or per month, as employees earn additional paid-time-off determined by some factor based on worked hours or paid hours. This kind of plan can be effective for both hourly and salaried employees, as it places greater responsibility in the hands of employees who are for the most part willing to decide how this benefit is used. A PTO plan generally reduces the company's potential exposure. When a plan is conceived, for example, what might once have been a 12-day-per-year benefit is reduced to, say, 4 or 5 days to be combined with other paid time off. But these 4 or 5 days belong to the employees to use as they see fit. In other words, these days become an entitlement. Some plans even allow employees to cash in a certain amount of unused time, providing an additional incentive to avoid unnecessary absences.

Although the use of paid sick leave is decreasing, absenteeism will continue to be a problem if it is allowed to exist unchecked. As suggested in the foregoing sections, the best control over absenteeism and thus over sick time abuse is the immediate supervisor's visible attention to attendance. As far as employee absenteeism is concerned, we usually get what we expect or what we seem willing to tolerate. Making it clear that abuse of time off will not be tolerated will go a long way toward keeping such abuse to a minimum.

## THE TROUBLED EMPLOYEE

Employees with personal problems—those that people cannot help but bring to work with them—are rarely able to do their best work. As a supervisor you may be in a difficult position relative to the troubled employee. Getting the work of the department done, and done well, is your responsibility. How your employees perform their duties in completing the department's tasks is also your business. As an appropriately people-oriented supervisor you should be interested in the employee as a whole person, but the employee's private life and personal problems are none of your business; they represent an area you cannot enter without specific invitation.

In dealing with the apparently troubled employee, do not prod, and do not push. Make yourself available to the employee, and make known your willingness to listen. You may have to go as far as to provide the time, the place, and the opportunity for the employee to talk with you, without specifically asking the employee to "open up." Quite often, if your openness is evident the troubled employee will turn to you.

In relating to the troubled employee, remember the following:

- Listen—but be aware at all times of the temptation to give advice. Some of the most useless statements you can make begin with, "If I were you. . ." Also, although many troubled employees could use advice, it is usually advice that you are unqualified to deliver. The best you can do under most circumstances is gently to suggest that the employee seek help from qualified professionals.

- Be patient—and show your concern for the employee as an individual. Although you should naturally be concerned with an individual's impairment as a productive employee, do not parade this before the troubled person. Rather, be patient and understanding. Perhaps, when possible, you can even be patient to the extent of easing off on tight deadlines and extra work requirements until the person is able to work through a problem.

- Do not argue—and do not criticize an employee for holding certain feelings or reflecting certain attitudes. Avoid passing judgment on the employee based on what you are seeing and hearing.

- Be discreet—let nothing a troubled employee tells you go beyond you. Be extra cautious if an employee tends toward opening up to the extent of revealing much that is extremely personal and private. While it often does good for someone to be able to simply talk to someone else about a problem, a person runs the risk of saying too much and might afterward feel extremely uncomfortable about having done so. If you can, try to demonstrate that you sympathize and understand without allowing the employee to go too far. Always provide assurance that what you have heard in such an exchange is safe with you.

- Reassure—when you are honestly able to do so, provide the employee with reasonable assurance of things of importance such as the security of the employee's job, the absence of undue pressure while problems get worked out, and the presence of a friendly and sympathetic ear when needed. You need not even know the nature of the employee's outside problem to supply very real assistance by reducing the job-related pressures on the individual.

In dealing with the troubled employee in general, the good supervisor will listen honestly and sympathetically and do what can be done to reduce pressure on the employee but will leave the giving of specific advice related to the problem to persons qualified to deal with such matters.

### Employee Assistance Programs

An employee assistance program (EAP) is a program designed to operate in a work setting to help employees cope with personal problems that impair their job performance.[2] Originating during the 1970s, EAPs continue to proliferate steadily throughout health care as well as in other industries. Should your organization have an active, reasonably publicized EAP in place, your troubled employees may find that they have sources of appropriate help at hand.

A well-functioning EAP can help increase work quality, reduce productivity losses, and control tardiness, absenteeism, and other undesirable conditions that affect job performance when employees' personal problems carry over into the work environment. A great many kinds of personal problems—drug abuse, alcoholism, and compulsive gambling, as well as marital, legal, financial, and emotional difficulties—can harm an employee's performance. The EAP is intended to provide employees who are troubled by such problems with personal, confidential assistance.

Assembled and funded in a manner similar to many of the institution's other employee benefits, the EAP consists of a network of service providers available to employees in need of specific kinds of assistance. For the sake of complete confidentiality, few if any of the services are ever provided by a department or division of the institution whose employees the program serves. All employees will know about the EAP, but the institution's only direct involvement will be through the services provided by an EAP coordinator who, more often than not, will be an employee of the EAP provider.

As a supervisor in an organization that operates an EAP, you will have received special training that enhances your ability to recognize job-performance problems that might result from personal difficulties. When you encounter such circumstances with a particular employee, you may be able to suggest, perhaps as an alternative to normal disciplinary processes, that the employee consider visiting the EAP coordinator.

An employee might enter the program independently, directly approaching the EAP coordinator without referral. Most EAPs encourage self-referrals from employees who believe they are heading for trouble, if not already in trouble. Beyond management referral and self-referral, third-party referral is also possible—perhaps from a family member, clergyman, personal physician, or other concerned party.

Although employees' lives outside of the workplace are truly none of your legitimate concern, employees' work performance indeed is. Having learned the more common signs that indicate the likely presence of serious personal problems—serious at least to the extent of affecting job performance—you are then able to tell employees how to gain access to the EAP should they desire help. The supervisor neither commands nor directs; the supervisor simply recognizes the signs and reminds employees of the availability of the EAP.

Over a period of time, as an EAP matures and employee acceptance grows, self-referrals tend to increase relative to other kinds of referrals, and the focus of the program gradually moves from crisis intervention to preventive care. A mature, well-functioning EAP can be the most comprehensive resource available for dealing with the troubled employee.

## ONE AND THE SAME?

Having read the "Situation" that opened this chapter and having gone through the pages that follow it, it should be evident that the problem employee and the employee with problems are often one and the same. As also stated elsewhere, it is virtually impossible to separate completely the person on the job from the person off the job, and often an individual's personal problems have a decided effect on that person's performance and behavior at work.

Morris Craig has in effect been challenged to determine what to do about Jennifer's performance. Trying to meet individual and departmental needs, having no rationale for understanding the change, and apparently trying to avoid confrontation, he is relying on Jennifer to solve her own problems. Unfortunately, she seems unwilling to solve them and unwilling to discuss them, and Craig's delaying tactics are only compounding the problem.

As always, Craig must deal with the results of behavior, with specific instances to cite, but if something can be learned about the cause he can help point Jennifer in the direction of a solution. If the trouble is work related, such as burnout, job satisfaction might be improved through rearranging duties, cross-training with others, providing new responsibilities, or other job-enriching actions. If the causes appear to be external and personal, a leave of absence or EAP referral might be appropriate.

Stark's recommendation is an excellent first step, especially with an employee whose past behavior has been acceptable. Jennifer may avoid discussing specific concerns with her male boss, but she might talk with a female colleague. Furthermore, staff might help resolve the problem without Craig's involvement. This approach emphasizes commitment of the work group to its members and departmental goals, a functional aspect the department seems to lack.

At this time Craig also could complete a special performance appraisal. Open, honest dialogue is required. Jennifer knows her responsibilities and is probably aware of her behavior, her perception of the job, her role within the department, and adverse influences on her work, so her recommendations are important in a mutually satisfactory resolution.

As a last resort, disciplinary action may be required to prevent further disruption. Craig must clearly indicate to Jennifer why such action is required and must describe organizational policy, identify expected behaviors, and provide regular monitoring and follow-up. Her behavior could be owing to dire external circumstances completely beyond her control. Craig and others might feel considerable sympathy toward her, but nevertheless this behavior cannot be allowed to continue because of the damage it does to the department. The responsibility rests with Jennifer. Regardless of cause, she either must change her behavior and improve her performance or ultimately lose her employment.

## SPECIAL CASES: SOME SIGNS OF THE TIMES

In addition to providing more useful information and advice to its users, another reason for issuing a new edition of a book is to address changes that have been occurring in the field of concentration. In our concern with problem employees and employee problems, in recent years—say within the past decade or so—we have been experiencing some discernible patterns of employee behavior that were not especially evident when the initial edition of *The Effective Health Care Supervisor* was published in 1982.

From numerous situations ranging from the nearly insignificant to the potentially deadly serious, two patterns of employee thought and behavior appear to be growing in significance. The first pattern has been with us increasingly in many areas of life for quite some time but seems to be growing more pronounced in the workplace; it is the increasing inability of people to take responsibility for their own circumstances and behavior. This growing tendency has been strongly aided and abetted by government. In passing an accumulation of laws regulating essentially every dimension of employment, our government has fostered for many people the impression that if one does not like or agree with a particular act or decision, then one is being damaged by external forces. This attitude seems to be supported by the modern popular psychology movement that strongly suggests that almost anything "wrong" stems from environment, background, or past experience. (A thorough exploration of cause lies well beyond the scope of this discussion.)

Regardless of cause, the trend toward the inability to accept responsibility for one's own circumstances is present and must be addressed in employee relations. It makes the task of supervision more difficult because one who does not—in many instances, actually cannot—accept responsibility generally does not accept correction as legitimate. Surely anyone who has supervised for a few years has encountered the occasional employee who can do no wrong—whatever happens is always the fault of other persons or external circumstances.

The other troublesome, growing tendency is evidenced in the behavior of an increasing number of employees who seem to be acting out the belief that the work organization exists primarily for their benefit. Once again the government and its efforts to regulate essentially all aspects of employment have helped create this condition, and labor unions and some social action organizations have behaved as though employment, rather than service to patients, clients, or customers, should be the work organization's first concern. Again, however, the problem's causes are far broader and more complex than a pair of simply stated possibilities.

Today we have an increasing number of employees who want to work just the hours they want to work, arrive and leave at times that best suit their own needs, do their jobs the way they would like to do them regardless of what the organization's customers need, leave the job for prolonged periods when their circumstances suggest doing so, and be guaranteed return to a secure position on their own terms when they wish. In short, they consider the organization's primary responsibility as ensuring their livelihood.

It would be great if today's work organizations could do for everyone what some of their employees want. The essential difficulty with this posture, however, is that it places the concerns of the employee above the concerns of the customer. This suggests that there is an extremely important message that today's managers at all levels must continually communicate to their employees: If our primary external customers—or, specific to health care, our patients—are not always our first concern, they will eventually become someone else's customers. Then we will have no employees to be concerned about.

Neither of these trends shows signs of abating at the present time, so their effects will cause employee relations concerns for the foreseeable future.

However, we can also be assured that conditions will eventually change to the extent that we will be faced with trends in employee relations not yet imagined.

## THE REAL "PROBLEM"

The true people-problem of the supervisor is not the problem employee as such, but rather it is the basic challenge presented by the vast differences to be encountered among people. Everybody is different, so there is no single "right way" of dealing with all employees. Should you have 12 employees reporting to you it is conceivable that for you there may be 12 different "right ways" of dealing with these employees.

A good general rule for supervision is to give as much—or more—time to a new employee as you would devote to a new major assignment. Get to know your people even better than you know your work. Regardless of the function you supervise, your employees are your greatest resource. It is ultimately your humane and understanding use of the human resource that will determine your success as a manager.

---

## REVIEW QUESTIONS

1. What are the implications of a supervisor regularly referring to three specific employees as *the grouch, the whiner* and *the pain*?
2. What is your responsibility if you believe a certain employee has personal problems that are affecting work performance but does not acknowledge problems or is unwilling to talk about them?
3. What is referred to in saying an employee has "time to be troublesome?"
4. What are the major characteristics of the *dead-end employee*?
5. What is the most important aspect of a supervisor's approach in dealing with absenteeism in the work group?
6. What are the key factors contributing to increased absenteeism?
7. Why is there no single correct way of dealing with employees?
8. Accepting the admonition that you cannot give a troubled employee advice (as in "If I were you," etc.), what *can* you do for the troubled employee?

---

## CASE: THE GREAT STONE FACE

Six months ago you were hired from outside of the hospital as a supervisor. You supervise a group of 20 people, most of whom have been there several years.

One of your employees, Alicia Benson, is assigned an extremely intricate job that requires considerable extra training. None of your other employees is able to do Alicia's job because your predecessor never trained anyone else in the job.

Alicia strikes you as good at what she does. However, she has days—at least one a week—on which she refuses to speak with her coworkers. Her silences are well known; the other employees refer to her as "the great stone face." Since her regular duties require contact with other employees, when one of her silent moods strikes, the department's work flow is impaired and people begin to complain.

On several occasions you have given Alicia the opportunity to talk with you, but so far she has given you no clue as to any difficulty that might be behind her moods. All of your indirect offers of help have been ignored and when directly asked if anything is bothering her she ducks the question.

## Instructions

Develop a tentative approach to the overall problem presented by Alicia's behavior, considering not only the "problem employee" specifically, but also the effects of her mood changes on the department. (An "if-then" approach is suggested. For instance, "If I try this particular direction and such a response is forthcoming, then I'll go on to try. . .")

As circumstances permit, share your thoughts on the problem in a discussion group.

---

**NOTES**

1. Asbury Park Press, "Company Sick-Day Policies Vary," *Democrat & Chronicle,* Rochester, NY, 5 January 2004.
2. Hospital Education and Research Fund, *On Instituting a Hospital-Based Employee Assistance Program: A Compendium* (Albany, N.Y: 1987).

## CHAPTER 15

# The Supervisor and the Human Resource Department

*I use not only all the brains I have, but all I can borrow.*
—*Anonymous*

## CHAPTER OBJECTIVES

☛ Introduce the human resource department as a vital staff function that exists to support operating management and the employees.

☛ Outline the functions of human resources and indicate how these functions relate to the role of the supervisor.

☛ Describe a number of action steps the supervisor can take to ensure that he or she will obtain appropriate service from human resources when needed.

☛ Suggest what the supervisor can do to establish a working relationship with human resources that will lead to improved human resource service to the organization.

## SITUATION: A FAVOR OR A TRAP?

One morning, well before the start of your department's normal working hours, you were enjoying a cup of coffee in the cafeteria, sorting out some notes concerning your intentions for the day, when you were approached by one of your employees. The employee, Marge Nelson, who is one of your two or three most senior employees in terms of service, seated herself across from you and said, "There's something going on in the department that you need to know about, and I've waited far too long to tell you." Marge proceeded to tell you ("In strictest confidence, please, I know you'll understand why") that another long-term employee, Carrie James, had been making a great many derogatory comments about you throughout the department and generally questioning your competence.

For nearly 10 minutes Marge showered you with criticism of you, your management style, and your approach to individual employees, all attributed to Carrie James. On exhausting her litany Marge proclaimed that she did not ordinarily "carry tales" but that she felt you "had a right to know, for the good of the department—but please don't tell her I said anything."

Although Marge's comments were filled with "she saids" and "she dids," she being Carrie, and generally twice-told tales without connection to specific incidents, something extremely disturbing clicked in your mind while you were listening: Recently your posted departmental schedule had been altered, without your knowledge, in a way indicating that someone had tried to copy your handwriting and forge your initials. Two separate, seemingly unconnected comments by Marge together revealed that one of only two people could have

244

altered your schedule. Those two people were Carrie James—and Marge Nelson herself.

As Marge finally fell silent you were left with an intense feeling of disappointment. You wondered if you could ever again fully trust two of your key employees.

*Instructions*

As you proceed through the chapter, consider how you will address the following three questions:

1. What should be your immediate response to Marge Nelson? Why?
2. Do you believe you have the basis on which to proceed with disciplinary action?
3. How can the human resource department help you in these circumstances?

## "PERSONNEL" EQUALS PEOPLE

As a supervisor or first-line manager of any other title you are charged with the task of facilitating the work performance of a number of people. In this role you are expected to ensure that the efforts of your group are applied toward attainment of the organization's objectives. This must be done in such a way that the group functions more effectively with you than it would without you. And, as a first-line manager by any title, there are some days when you can use all the help you can get.

Help is where you find it in your organization, and one place where the supervisor can find help in abundance is the human resource (HR) department.

Human resources is today's more all-encompassing title for what most organizations once called personnel. Whatever the label, however, the true operative word is *people*. Management is frequently described as getting things done through people. People do the hands-on work and other people supervise them, and still other people oversee the supervisors and managers.

As surely as even the most sophisticated piece of medical equipment requires periodic maintenance to ensure its continued functioning, so, too, do the human beings who supply patient care require regular maintenance. And given that the "human machine" is generally unpredictable and varies considerably from person to person in numerous dimensions, the supervisor's "maintenance" will encompass many activities.

There are many places in the organization where the supervisor can go for help with various tasks and problems. For people problems, however, and for some straightforward people-related tasks that cannot yet be described as problems, the supervisor's greatest source of assistance is the human resource department. It remains only for the supervisor to take steps to access that assistance. It is to the individual supervisor's distinct advantage to know exactly what should be expected from human resources and how to get it when needed.

## A VITAL STAFF FUNCTION

As a service department, human resources should be prepared to offer a variety of employee-related services in a number of ways. Human resources should anticipate numerous kinds of difficulties and needs and should communicate the availability of assistance throughout the organization. For example, a personnel policy manual dispenses advice and guidance in employee matters, and top management's instructions to supervisors to seek one-to-one guidance from human resources in matters of disciplinary action are essentially "advertising" for human resource services.

But even though human resources should be prepared to help in a variety of ways and should have so advised all of management's ranks, the human resource department cannot anticipate every specific need of each individual supervisor or manager. To truly put the human resource department to work, the supervisor must be prepared to take his or her needs to the HR department and expect answers or assistance.

The names human resources and personnel are still often used interchangeably and are presently used about equally as the designation for this particular service. Most common among a few other designations encountered are employee relations and labor relations. These latter two labels have also found use as descriptors of subfunctions of modern HR, with employee relations used relative to dealing with employee problems and problem employees, and labor relations referring to dealing with unions. Regardless of label, however, the mission of this particular service department should remain the same—to engage in acquiring, maintaining, and retaining employees so that the objectives of the organization may be fulfilled. As a critical staff function, HR does none of the actual work of the health care organization; rather, human resources facilitates the work of the organization by concerning itself with the organization's most importance resource.

## A SERVICE OF INCREASING VALUE

The human resource department has long been a resource of increasing value to the organization at large and the individual supervisor in particular. Its value has increased because of rational responses to a number of forces, both external and internal to the organization, that have resulted in additional tasks for someone. Two major forces have been the expansion in the number and kinds of tasks that have fallen to HR, and the proliferation of laws affecting aspects of employment. A third notable force is the tendency toward organizational "flattening" evident in present-day health care organizations.

### Increase in Employee-Related Tasks

Like the majority of departments in a modern organization, there was a time when HR did not exist. And also like other departments, HR arose to fill a need.

The earliest human resource departments were commonly known as employment offices, which were created as businesses grew large enough to see the advantages of centralizing much of the process of acquiring employees. Employment and employment-related record keeping made up all the work of the employment office.

When wage and hour laws came into being, the "employment office" absorbed much of the concern for establishing standard rates of pay and monitoring their application relative to hours worked. This began the compensation function.

As organizations began to provide compensation in forms other than wages in response to new laws and other pressures both internal and external, the employment office took over the administration of what became known as "fringe benefits." And as organizations responded to labor legislation and to labor unions themselves, labor relations functions were added to the growing list of activities that shared a common theme: all had something to do with acquiring, maintaining, or retaining employees.

Other people activities were added as needed, and what had once been the employment office became personnel, literally, "the body of people employed by (the organization)." During the last two decades the term personnel began to be replaced by the term human resources, but the essential meaning remains the same. All the while, the HR function grew in value as it took on an increasing number of employee-related functions.

## Proliferation of Laws Pertaining to Employment

A number of laws were of course primary in causing much of the increase in employee-related tasks described in the foregoing section. For example, the establishment of Social Security, workers' compensation, and unemployment all created benefits tasks for HR, and much labor relations activity was brought about by laws. In addition, various antidiscrimination laws, including the Civil Rights Act of 1964, the Age Discrimination in Employment Act, and the Equal Pay Act, brought with them much new work for HR.

The antidiscrimination laws have forever changed the way many organizations do business. They have created a strongly law-oriented environment in which lawsuits and other formal discrimination complaints have become routine HR business. They have also turned employee recruitment in general, and specific processes such as performance evaluation and disciplinary action, into legal minefields filled with traps and pitfalls for the unwary. And in the process, they have created more work for HR and have created myriad reasons for the individual supervisor to turn to HR on more occasions.

## Tendency toward Flattening

The tendency toward organizational flattening—the elimination of entire layers of management—has not appreciably added tasks to HR or increased the inherent importance of the HR function in and of itself. However, this force has markedly increased the importance of human resources to the individual supervisor.

Recent years have seen financially troubling times overtake many of the nation's hospitals. As hospital reimbursement is tightened and income grows at a lesser rate than costs, the resulting financial pinch is often felt in staffing, including numbers of management personnel. The first managers to suffer— as also has been the case in many other kinds of organizations—are middle managers.

Financial problems have caused significant reductions in middle management positions, but all such reductions have not been owing to money troubles alone. Increasing reliance on certain modern approaches to management, those approaches calling for increased employee participation and the making of decisions as close as possible to the bottom of the hierarchy and thus closest to where the action is, also have resulted in the necessity for fewer middle managers.

Regardless of how it occurs, a reduction in the number of middle managers means that more decisions must be made closer to the bottom of the organization. This means that certain decisions that might once have been made by a middle manager—like, for instance, sanctioning an employment offer at a rate above the normal entry rate, deciding how far to proceed in a particular disciplinary action, or determining how to proceed in a situation that includes a high degree of legal risk—are forced down to the level of the supervisor.

The more employee-related decisions are forced to the first line of management, the more the first-line manager—the individual supervisor—has to depend on the guidance and support of the human resource department. Thus the tendency toward flattening has increased the value of HR to the supervisor.

## LEARNING ABOUT YOUR HR DEPARTMENT

To be able to get the most out of the organization's human resource department it is first necessary to understand the nature of the HR function, to know how HR relates organizationally, and to be familiar with the functions performed by your particular HR department.

### The Nature of the Function: Staff Versus Line

Human resources has already been described in these pages as a staff function. As opposed to a line activity, which is a function in which people actually perform the work of the organization (for example, nursing or clinical laboratories), a staff function enhances and supports the performance of the organization's work. The presence of a staff function should make a difference to the extent that the organization's work is more effectively accomplished with the staff function than without it.

The distinction between line and staff is critical to appreciate because a staff function cannot legitimately make decisions that are the province of line management. Operating decisions belong to operating management; they must be made within the chains of command of the line departments. The primary purpose of human resources in enhancing and supporting work performance is to recommend courses of action that are (1) consistent with legislation, regulation, and principles of fairness, and (2) in the best interests of the organization as a whole.

It is not unusual for some managers to blame human resources for decisions other than those they would have made by themselves. Complaints such as "Personnel made me do it," or "This is the HR department's decision," are not uncommon from managers whose preferred decisions are altered because of HR's recommendations. However, human resources generally does not—and should never—have the authority to overrule line management in any matter, personnel or otherwise. If, as occasionally is the case, a personnel decision of line management must be reversed for the good of the organization, the over-ruling is done by higher line management. Human resources may have to reach out and bring higher management into the process when a supervisor insists on pursuing a decision that HR has recommended against, but it must remain line management that actually decides.

As to whether line management readily listens to its advisors in human resources depends largely on the apparent professionalism of the HR function and HR's track record in making solid recommendations.

## The Human Resource Reporting Relationship

The modern HR department will report to one of the two top managers in the organization. Depending on the particular organizational scheme employed, the human resource manager might report to the president or chief executive officer (CEO) or perhaps to the executive vice president or chief operating officer (COO). Generally, human resources should report to a level no lower than the level that has authority over all of the organization's line or operating functions.

Human resources must be in a position to serve all of the organization's operating units equally and impartially. This cannot be done if HR reports to one particular operating division that stands as the organizational equal of other divisions. If, for example, HR reports to a vice president for general services who is the organizational equal of three other vice presidents, HR cannot equally serve all divisions because of being ultimately responsible to just one of those divisions.

Be wary if your HR department reports in the undesirable manner just described. Regardless of how well the HR function might be managed, at times of conflict, when inevitable differences arise concerning personnel decisions, you may conclude that the division that "owns" HR is usually the division that wins. Independence and impartiality are essential for human resources to function effectively for the whole organization, and independence and impartiality are impossible in perception and unlikely in actuality if HR is assigned to one of several operating divisions.

Be wary also of the occasionally encountered practice of duplicating HR functions within the same facility. For example, one will encounter the occasional hospital in which the department of nursing has its own HR function while another HR office serves all other departments. Although there are occasional advantages to be gained from basing some recruiting activity in the nursing department, splitting or subdividing other HR activities tends to create duplication of effort while increasing the organization's exposure to legal risks.

## The Human Resource Functions

There are almost as many possible combinations of human resource functions as there are HR departments. A great many activities that may be generally described as "administrative" can find their way into the human resource department. However, we will here be concerned with the significant activities or groups of functions that are often identified as the tasks of human resources.

The basic HR functions are as follows:

- *Employment*, often referred to as recruiting. This is the overall process of acquiring employees—advertising and otherwise soliciting applicants, screening applicants, referring candidates to managers, checking references, extending offers of employment, and bringing employees into the organization.

- *Compensation, or wage and salary administration*. This is the process of creating and maintaining a wage structure and ensuring that this structure is administered fairly and consistently. Related to compensation, as well as to other HR task groupings, are job evaluation, the creation of job descriptions, and maintenance of a system of employee performance evaluation.

- *Benefits administration*. This activity is a natural offshoot of wage and salary administration, since benefits are actually a part of an employee's total compensation. Benefits administration consists of maintaining the organization's benefit structure and assisting employees in understanding and accessing their benefits.

- *Employee relations*. This activity may be generally described as dealing with problem employees and employees who have problems. It may range from handling employee complaints or appeals through processing disciplinary actions to arranging employee recognition and recreation activities.

One can see the foregoing four general activities at work in essentially every human resource function regardless of size and overall scope. In a very large organization these will be separate departments within HR, each with its own head and its own staff and perhaps including multiple subdivisions. In a very small organization these are likely to be the tasks of a single person who has other duties as well.

One additional basic function that may be encountered is *labor relations*. Although labor relations may be a functional title that identifies a whole department or simply a human resource department activity, it is also a relatively generic label that applies to the maintenance of a continuing relationship with a bargaining unit, that is, a labor union. Again, depending on size, labor relations may be a subdivision of HR in its own right or simply one of several responsibilities assigned to one person.

Other activities that might be found within human resources include the following:

- *Employee health*. Often part of HR, in health care organizations it sometimes will be a part of one of the medical divisions.
- *Training* (for both managers and rank-and-file employees). With the exception of nursing in-service education, traditionally a part of the nursing department, if a formal training function exists it is most often part of human resources.
- *Payroll*. In the past, it was often part of "personnel," but in recent years payroll has usually resided in the finance division. However, a working interrelationship of personnel and payroll has always been essential, and recent years, bringing integrated personnel/payroll systems, have seen the beginnings of payroll's organizational shift back toward HR.
- *Security and parking*. With increasing frequency, security and parking, because of their strong employee relationships, are becoming attached to HR. However, they are presently more likely to be found attached to an environmental or facilities division.
- *Safety*. As with security, safety is becoming increasingly attached to HR, but is just as likely to be found in the facilities division.
- *Child care*. As an activity that is presented largely as an employee service, an organization's child care function is most likely assigned to human resources.

### Rounding Out Your Knowledge

Using the foregoing paragraphs as a guide, determine exactly which functions are performed by your organization's human resource department. Furthermore, take steps to attach a person's name to each function. You should strive to be in a position in which you understand how the HR department is organized, so you know generally who does what, who reports to whom, and who bears overall responsibility. Moreover, you should also make certain that you know the organizational relationships of sometimes-HR functions (e.g., security) that belong elsewhere in your particular organization, so you can ensure that you always take certain matters to the correct department.

Next, take the time to make a list of the supervisory functions or activities you encounter that can lead you to seek information or assistance from human resources. The lists of most supervisors may have a great deal in common in that they might include the following:

- Employment: Finding sufficient qualified candidates from whom to fill an open position
- Benefits: Providing information with which to answer employees' benefits questions
- Compensation: Providing information with which to answer employees' questions related to pay
- Employee problems: Determining where to send a particular employee who is having difficulty with (whatever the problem area)

- Job descriptions/job evaluations: Determining how to proceed in questioning the salary grade of any particular position
- Policy interpretations: Determining the appropriate interpretation of personnel policy for any particular instance
- Disciplinary actions: Determining how to proceed in dealing with what appear to be violations of work rules
- Performance problems: Determining how to proceed in dealing with employees whose work performance is consistently below the department's standard
- Performance appraisals: Securing guidance in doing appropriate performance appraisals, and finding out how much one can depend on human resources to coordinate the overall appraisal process

The foregoing list can doubtless be expanded by each supervisor who may refer to it. One helpful method of expanding your list includes leafing through your organization's personnel policy manual and employee handbook; this process will bring to mind additional areas of concern that you encounter in your work.

## PUTTING THE HR DEPARTMENT TO WORK

### A Universal Approach

The first, simplest, and most valuable advice to be offered for getting the most out of your human resource department involves the age-old two-step process of initiation and follow-up. It is but a slight variation on a practice followed by most successful supervisors.

The successful supervisor knows that any task worth assigning is worth a specific deadline. The "do-it-when-you-have-a-chance" or "when-you-think-about-it" approach breeds procrastination, delay, and inaction. An assignment—necessarily a well-thought-out, specific assignment—must be accompanied by a target for completion, a deadline which, though it may be generous or even loose, leaves no doubt as to expected completion. And when that deadline arrives and no results have been forthcoming, the supervisor then exercises the most important part of the total process—faithful follow-up. Faithful follow-up is the key; the supervisor who always waits a week beyond the deadline is behaviorally telling the employees that they always have at least an extra week.

Anything needed from the human resource department should be addressed in a similar manner. Relative to the HR department, the process might be summarized as follows:

- Make certain that the function of interest is part of HR's responsibilities, and determine, if possible, who in HR would be the best person to approach on the topic.
- Refine your question or need such that your inquiry is sufficiently specific to permit a specific response.
- When you make contact and convey your need to the appropriate person,

if the answer is not immediately available ask when an answer will be supplied.

- If the promised reply date occurs later than your legitimate need date, negotiate a deadline agreeable to both you and HR.
- If your agreed-upon deadline arrives and you have not received your answer, follow up with the HR department. Follow up politely, follow up diplomatically, but follow up faithfully. Never let an unanswered deadline pass without following up.

This process should be applied to problems, issues, and concerns that you as a supervisor would consider taking to human resources. It should also—and especially—be applied to questions and concerns that your employees bring to you. If an employee's question in any way involves human resource concerns, and if you are unable to respond appropriately, then you need to take the question to HR as though it were your own.

## Some Specific Action Steps

Any number of supervisory needs present opportunities to put the human resource department to work. The more frequently encountered of these include the following.

### Finding New Employees

There are any number of points in the employment process at which the supervisor and HR must work together. Fulfill your end of the working relationship, and expect HR staff to fulfill theirs. For example, if none of the five candidates HR has supplied for a particular position is truly appropriate, ask for more; do not settle for only what you are given if what you are given is not enough. (For your part of the arrangement, do not continue to call for more applicants in your search for the "perfect" candidate if you have already seen two or three who meet the posted requirements of the job.) Also, stay in touch with HR concerning the extending of offers, the checking of references, and the scheduling of preemployment physical examinations and starting dates. Do not be unreasonable: recognize that these activities take time. By making your interest and attention known, however, you will encourage completion of the process.

### Bringing Job Descriptions Up-to-Date

The supervisor ordinarily has a significant responsibility in maintaining current job descriptions for the department. The HR department usually also has the responsibility for associating a pay level with each job and for maintaining central files of up-to-date job descriptions. Your part is best done within your department; job descriptions should be written in large part by those who do the work and those who supervise the doing of the work. However, you need to deliberately involve HR in contributing consistency to every necessary job description and in ensuring that each job is properly placed on a pay scale. Once again, your visible interest in the process will encourage timely completion of HR's activities.

## Disciplining Employees

Regardless of the extent of human resource involvement in the disciplinary process, it is not the HR department that decides upon disciplinary action. The HR department disciplines nobody (except employees of the HR department, as necessary). Any employee deserving of disciplinary action must be disciplined through his or her immediate chain of command. In most organizations it is a requirement for the supervisor to take proposed disciplinary actions through human resources before implementation. Whether or not this is so for your organization, you need to take your best assessment to HR and ask for advice. And you need to expect sound advice, whether in the form of a single recommendation, complete with rationale for doing so, or as two or more alternatives, each with its own possible consequences fully explained. The decision is theoretically all yours, and if it is a poor decision you will bear much of the blame. Do not let HR avoid responsibility by failing to provide specific direction; insist on complete HR participation in deciding upon disciplinary action.

## Evaluating Employees

One of the most important tasks of the supervisor is the appraisal of employee performance. No formal system of performance appraisal can function consistently throughout the organization without the central guidance usually provided by human resources. Although you can certainly evaluate your employees' performance without the assistance of HR, you can do a much more consistently acceptable job of evaluation with HR involvement. Most of human resource's involvement in evaluation should occur automatically as far as the supervisor is concerned. The HR department should provide forms, instructions, schedules, and reminders throughout the process. However, if the HR department is not always on top of the supervisor's employee appraisal needs, according to the needs of the moment the supervisor should do the following:

- Keep track of scheduled review dates and ask HR for forms and timetables if they are not supplied automatically.
- Ask for periodic instruction in how to apply rating criteria, especially if criteria have changed and refresher instruction is not supplied.
- Keep HR advised of how changing job requirements may be affecting the application of criteria based on previous requirements.
- Ask HR for rating profile information, that is, statistical information that reveals patterns in the supervisor's rating practices and shows whether those patterns are changing with time, and perhaps also shows how this specific supervisor's rating patterns compare with those of other supervisors.

## Dealing with Training Needs

If the human resource department has responsibility for any kind of employee training—and in most health care organizations there is a better-than-even chance that this is so—do not wait for needed training to come to you. If there are training needs in your work group, take them to HR. If, for example, you feel several of your employees require training in basic telephone techniques, take your well-defined need to human resources, negotiate a timetable for providing the training, and offer to become personally involved in the training. (With appropriate HR involvement, every supervisor is a potentially valuable instructor in some topic.)

The foregoing are presented as a few specific suggestions but are offered primarily to convey a general idea to the supervisor: The human resource department exists as a service function for all employees; it remains for the supervisor to take each legitimate personnel-related need to HR and to ask for—and expect—an honest response.

## WANTED: WELL-CONSIDERED INPUT

The most effective human resource departments are not one-way dispensers of information and assistance. The most effective human resource departments are those that are responsive to the needs of the organization's work force. However, the HR department can go only so far in anticipating needs and meeting them within the limits of available resources. To be fully effective, the HR department must learn of employee needs from employees and supervisors and must in turn go to top management with solid proposals for meeting the most pressing needs.

Some employees, although usually a minority, take their own questions, concerns, and suggestions to the human resource department. However, many employees will never do so for themselves; their needs, whether conveyed through words, actions, or attitudes, must find their way to human resources and eventually to top management through their supervisors.

Among the kinds of information that the supervisor should pass to human resources are

- reactions to various personnel policies, especially when policies seem to have become less appropriate under changing conditions
- employee attitudes concerning pay and benefits, especially perceptions of inequities and alleged instances of unfair treatment
- complaints—and compliments as well—about employee services such as cafeteria and parking
- comments on the appropriateness of various employee benefits, and perceptions of benefits needed or desired as opposed to those presently given
- potential changes in any or all means of acquiring, maintaining, or retaining employees that might afford the organization a competitive edge in its community

## UNDERSTANDING WHY AS WELL AS WHAT

It is relatively easy to determine what human resources as a department does within the organization. However, it is necessary to go beyond what and develop an appreciation of why this department does what it does and why HR sometimes must espouse a position in opposition to a line department's position.

Consider the case of the supervisor who appeals to the HR department to help resolve a seemingly unending series of difficulties by agreeing to the termination of a particular employee. As the supervisor says, "I simply can't do any more with this person. She's chronically late in spite of all my warnings. Her absenteeism disrupts staffing; she uses up her sick time as fast as she earns it. Her attitude is absolutely terrible; she's been rude to patients and families; and the way she talks to me borders on insubordination most of the time. Her clinical skills are just average at best, and she's a disruptive influence on the unit. I've been patient longer than anyone has the right to expect of me, but nothing has changed. I want to discharge her."

As often occurs in such circumstances, the human resource practitioner hearing the supervisor's request briefly reviews the employee's background and immediately recommends against termination. This may understandably disappoint and upset the supervisor and leave her displeased with the HR department. She may complain, with some justification, that she ought to be supported in her efforts to get rid of an unsatisfactory employee. She may well view HR as obstructive and adopt an adversarial position, perhaps even attempting to solicit the assistance of her own higher management in opposing the human resource position.

Why would human resources be automatically protective of an employee whose relationship with work is as bad as described above? The differences lie in (1) the supervisor's perspective versus the human resource department's perspective and (2) the frequently cited employee personnel file—"the record."

The supervisor's perspective is unit or departmental. The supervisor is legitimately focused on the good of the patients and the good of the unit, and the employee in question threatens both. However, human resources must view the issues in two ways that conflict with the supervisor's perspective. In micro terms, HR must be concerned with the rights of the individual employee; in macro terms, HR must be concerned with the good of the total organization. The organization is of course no more than the sum total of a number of individuals, but in focusing on the one and the all the HR perspective fails to match that of the supervisor, which is necessarily a focus on more than one but much less than all.

Then there is "the record" to consider. In the foregoing case it turns out that all of the supervisor's warnings concerning tardiness were oral warnings of which no record exists. The same was true for warnings of absenteeism, except for a single written warning that is too old to give weight to present disciplinary action. No other warnings appear in the personnel file, and although in the mind of the supervisor this employee has always been less than satisfactory, the personnel file includes several performance evaluations which, although not glowing with praise, suggest at least minimally acceptable performance. In short, there is no basis for termination except in the supervisor's mind.

In regard to problems such as that just described, the HR department is

- defending the rights of the individual, not only because doing so arises from a sense of fairness but also because there are many laws requiring the organization to do so
- protecting the total organization from a multitude of legal risks

Whenever there is a risk that an employee problem or complaint will be taken outside of the organization, it is best to think of any criticism of employee conduct or performance in a single light: If it is not in the record, it never happened. Except in instances of termination for major infractions calling for immediate discharge (and these days even many of these actions are successfully challenged), a discharge must be backed up with a written trail describing all that occurred. It is legally necessary to be able to demonstrate that the employee was given every reasonable opportunity to correct the offending behavior or improve the unsatisfactory performance.

## WITH FRIENDS LIKE THIS. . .

Referring to the "Situation" presented at the beginning of the chapter, clearly this places before you something that could conceivably be a trap but in no way constitutes a favor. Regardless of all the "information" Marge claims to be giving you, all she has in fact done for you is to give you cause to worry. With "friends" like Marge Nelson, who needs enemies?

Your immediate response, while Marge is there in front of you, should include an effort to solicit specific information, to give you something you can verify and use. You will probably not receive specifics but you should make the effort, attempting to learn anything that can be verified. You also should let Marge know that second-hand information is often more troublesome than no information at all; it helps you not at all, but you cannot help worrying because of it. You also might consider asking Marge what her object is in talking with you about such matters, and perhaps suggest that she bring you nothing else unless it is information you can corroborate and act on.

There is no basis on which to proceed with disciplinary action. Disciplinary action should never be based on hearsay.

The human resource department, specifically an employee relations manager or someone with a similar title and duties, can help you sort out the possibilities and better prepare you to deal with both Carrie James and Marge Nelson. Discuss the Marge Nelson conversation in detail with human resources, and especially seek out human resources if you should be similarly approached by Carrie James. Human resources can suggest how you can go about monitoring conditions in your department and can help you avoid being used by one party against another in the event of a James-versus-Nelson struggle in the department. It is highly likely that Marge Nelson's reasons for coming to you with her tales about others fall a bit shy of caring for the "good of the department" and come closer to a personal agenda that includes undermining Carrie James and possibly you as well.

**EMPHASIS ON SERVICE**

As a staff function, human resources is organized as a service activity. Service activities render no patient care; they do not advance the work of the organization. However, they support the performance of the organization's work and in a practical sense become necessary. For example, if a pure service such as building maintenance did not exist, the facility's physical plant would gradually self-destruct. Similarly, without human resources to see to the maintenance of the work force, the overall suitability and capability of that work force would steadily erode.

Recognize human resources for what it is: an essential service function required to help the organization run as efficiently as possible.

Learn what the HR department does, and especially learn why the department does what it does. Provide input to the human resource department. Forge a continuing working relationship with the HR department, making it clear that you expect service from this essential service department. Challenge the HR department to do more, to do better, and to continually improve service—and put the human resource department to work for you and your employees.

---

## REVIEW QUESTIONS

1. What characteristics of the human resource department make it a staff activity rather than a line activity?
2. What were the primary factors causing expansion of human resource activities from this department's original "employment office" function?
3. Why must the individual supervisor be at least nominally conversant with the structure and details of the organization's benefit package?
4. Why might human resources often appear to be opposing a supervisor who desires to take a drastic action such as discharging an employee? What is the purpose of such resistance?
5. Identify the four Basic Human Resource Functions and provide one example of each related to your most recent employment.

---

## EXERCISE: WHERE CAN HUMAN RESOURCES HELP?

Review the human resource functions as outlined in this chapter. Within each major function, identify the subfunctions that involve you as a supervisor. (For example, under the employment or recruiting function you will probably have no role in locating or screening applicants, but you will be actively involved in interviewing job candidates. As another example, you will have no active responsibility for administering benefits, but you will often be expected to come up with answers to your employees' questions about benefits.)

When you have generated a complete list of human resource subfunctions that require your active involvement, determine who in your human resource department is most involved with each and associate one or two names with each subfunction. Most supervisors' lists will be likely to include selection interviewing, answering benefit questions, doing performance evaluations, and taking disciplinary action. This can become the basis of a reference list to help familiarize you with the individual specialties and strengths of the organization's human resource practitioners.

As an additional activity, review your list of pertinent human resource subfunctions against Chapter 27, "The Supervisor and the Law." For each human resource subfunction with which you are involved, indicate the major areas of legislation (e.g., "antidiscrimination laws") and the specific laws (e.g., "Immigration Reform and Control Act") that are of concern to your performance of the subfunction.

# PART IV

# The Supervisor and the Task

## CHAPTER 16

# Ethics and Ethical Standards

*I look upon the simple and childish virtues of veracity and*
*honesty as the root of all that is sublime in character.*
*— Ralph Waldo Emerson*

## CHAPTER OBJECTIVES

☛ Define ethics within the context of the modern health care organization.

☛ Introduce the major areas of concern in the area of medical ethics.

☛ Introduce business ethics within the specific context of the health care manager's work environment.

☛ Describe the areas of ethical concern having the greatest impact on the role of the manager in health care, specifically conflict of interest and regulatory compliance.

☛ Outline possible ethical standards of conduct for the health care organization.

☛ Review the manager's responsibility for modeling ethical behavior for his or her employees.

## SITUATION: IS THE BOSS ALWAYS THE BOSS?

Carl Mason is controller of Morgan General Hospital. He reports to Robert Green, vice president for finance. Green, formerly controller, has been with the hospital for more than 20 years and has been in his present position for 5 years. Mason is the third controller reporting to Green in less than 5 years. He has never heard a predecessor's opinion of Green, but his own is that Green tends to micromanage, hanging on to as much control as possible within the departments of the finance division.

As a result of some recent dramatic systems changes, Mason's information services department expanded, but general accounting and patient accounting were both found to be overstaffed relative to current needs. Mason accepted the eventual necessity of reducing staff in both accounting groups; however, the budget year was coming up and he had not been able to achieve the needed reduction through attrition. It looked as though he might have to lay off two people unless he was lucky enough to have someone resign or retire. The only person anywhere near retirement was Ned Kline, who often expressed his intention to work until age 65. Kline was 9 months shy of turning 62 years old.

Along with Mason's personnel budget projections, Green requested a plan for bringing staff down to the required level. Mason submitted two names for layoff: Brown of general accounting and Miller of patient accounting. Green responded by suggesting that Mason instead get rid of Jerry Victor and Ned Kline, both of patient accounting. Mason did not agree, and he asked for Green's reasons. Green responded that he believed Victor and Kline to be the two least productive people in accounting and that Kline had a chronic attitude problem. Mason disputed both of these suggestions, pointing out that he had gone by straight seniority in his recommendations although he had been given no criteria for designating employees for layoff. Mason considered Victor capable, and Victor was third from the bottom in seniority. Brown and Miller were the logical ones to go on a last-in, first-out basis. He generally agreed with Green about Kline's productivity and attitude, but he felt he had to point out that Kline was always known as a complainer but the issue was never addressed. In fact, Kline's personnel file held more than 20 years' worth of "satisfactory" performance evaluations and not a single criticism or complaint. If keeping Kline this long had been a management mistake, Mason reasoned, it was unfair as well as risky to get rid of him at his present age.

Green told Mason to do what he thought was right; he was only offering suggestions.

Mason knew there was no love lost between Green and Victor; they had occasional differences on business matters, and when they communicated at all it was curtly. Mason felt that Green was using the layoff to get rid of people he did not particularly like.

One week later Green asked Mason if he had revised his recommendations. The layoffs were to take place in stages, with a pay period between individual layoffs. One had to go at the end of the current week; Mason indicated that his first choice to go was Brown. Green repeated his earlier recommendation to lay off Kline and Victor. He felt that Kline would not be hurt because he was vested in the retirement plan and was known to own some rental property on the side.

On Wednesday, two days before the target for the first layoff, Mason prepared a termination notice for Brown. He went to Green for the required signature, but Green refused to sign. He said to Mason, "What would you do if I gave you a direct order to lay off Kline and Victor?"

Mason answered, "I don't know."

Green said he was going to keep the notice until the following day and do some thinking. When Mason went to see Green the next day he found that Green had not signed the layoff notice for Brown, but had rather prepared— and already signed as higher management—termination notices for Kline and Victor. He showed them to Mason and said, "I feel that it's in the best interests of this hospital if these two are the people who leave. They're the least capable employees in the finance division, and when push comes to shove, the finance division is me. I'm sorry you chose to ignore my suggestions, so I'm giving you a direct order: Sign these two layoff notices and get Victor out of here this week and Kline at the end of the next pay period."

*Instructions*

As you proceed through this chapter, imagine yourself in the position of Carl Mason and consider what ethical dilemmas are presented, what courses of action might be open to you, and what you believe you would have to do if you were placed in this position.

## ETHICS AND THE HEALTH CARE MANAGER

The primary definition of ethics for the purposes of this chapter is: the system or code of morals of a particular group, profession, religion, etc. A somewhat broader definition is that of ethics as a field of study in its own right: the study of standards of conduct and moral judgment; moral philosophy.[1] The former definition is of course the one placing ethics in the context of the work organization, but whether we ascribe to this definition or another we will find that in all definitions of ethics there is mention of morals or morality. Indeed, one of the briefest but most useful descriptions of ethics is moral code.

Whether written or unwritten, every organization has a system or code of morals based on how its leaders want to relate to customers and others and thus directing how the organization's employees should behave as well. An increasing number of organizations, within health care and otherwise, are issuing formal ethical standards of conduct for their employees.

Individual occupations, notably the health care professions, likewise have published ethical standards proscribing the conduct of their members. In most instances, people admitted to membership in a profession agree to ascribe to these ethical standards of conduct as a condition of entry.

Individuals also have standards of conduct, although for most people these standards must be inferred from their behavior. (And as far as individual standards are concerned, one's observable behavior is usually a far more accurate indication of true ethical standards than one's own words might be in attempting to articulate these standards.)

Whether exhibited by an individual or by an organization, behavior is generally governed by these ethical standards of conduct plus legal requirements in the form of applicable laws and regulations. Within the health care organization we might find it convenient to consider medical ethics and business ethics as worthy of separate consideration. The medical ethics arena is complicated and growing more complex each year, presenting much more thorny and emotionally charged issues than business ethics. Fortunately many medical ethics issues are addressed at administrative and board levels and are embodied in policies governing behavior; it also is fortunate that medical ethics concerns do not impact all employees. Issues of business ethics, on the other hand, although less complex and less emotionally charged than medical ethics issues, are of concern—or should be of concern—to all employees at all organizational levels.

## MEDICAL ETHICS: SOME OF THE ISSUES

The complex and generally emotionally charged medical ethics issues include the following:

- Genetic testing and its uses, including the attendant issues of patient confidentiality. A primary concern is that information acquired through genetic testing could be used to discriminate in hiring and insuring, which would allow employers and insurers to weed out prospects that exhibit a genetic predisposition toward potentially serious or chronic conditions. Could we indeed see the day when a genetic predisposition toward a certain disease could be considered a preexisting condition?

- Genetic manipulation, with supporting arguments citing the ability to eventually correct or prevent potentially serious conditions and opposing arguments citing the dangers in attempting to do so and questioning the morality of such manipulation.
- Cloning, with present claims of human cloning soon becoming practical, countered with arguments concerning the perceived dangers in this newly evolving technology and, again, the morality of the process.
- Reproductive freedom, which includes all facets of the abortion issue fraught with moral and religious arguments and pitting concepts of individual rights against the rights of the unborn, plus consideration of sterilization and artificial methods of birth control, as well as prenatal diagnosis of fetal disorders.
- Patient self-determination, addressing the right of an individual to designate the extent to which he or she will be cared for under certain extreme circumstances and generally to accept or refuse treatment, and the right to complete an advance directive as permitted by state law. The Patient Self-Determination Act (PSDA), passed as part of the Omnibus Budget Reconciliation Act (OBRA) in 1990, included the requirement for providers to furnish information to patients on admission concerning their rights under law to make health care decisions. It also required states that did not already have some legal form of advance directive to put one in place. An advance directive can be instructional, in which one specifies certain treatment in advance of a terminal illness or certain condition (e.g., a "living will"), or proxy, in which a competent adult chooses another person to make health care decisions for him or her (a "durable power of attorney" for health care). Advance directives themselves give rise to many ethical controversies as it is argued whether they primarily protect patient autonomy or simply allow providers to avoid responsibility for life-or-death decisions. And, of course, there is within the broader concept of patient self-determination the issue of physician-assisted suicide for the hopelessly ill, a virtual battleground of moral, ethical, and religious issues.
- Since acquired immunodeficiency syndrome (AIDS) first emerged, disclosure of one's positive status for human immunodeficiency virus (HIV) infection has been a significant ethical issue. On one side is the public nature of AIDS and the desire to protect the general population; on the other are the rights of the individual to privacy and confidentiality and the fears—frequently justified—that one's HIV-positive status will become the basis for discrimination in areas such as employment and the provision of health care.

Fortunately for the health care department manager, the known and anticipated medical ethics issues will, in many instances, be addressed by policies established by the institution's board of directors. For example, a hospital in which abortions are performed will ordinarily have a policy exempting nurses who are opposed to abortion from participation in such procedures.

To address medical ethics issues that may not be clearly covered by policy and those that would appear to involve exceptions or extraordinary circumstances, larger health care organizations, specifically hospitals, health systems, and medical centers, ordinarily have ethics committees.

## When Medicine and Business Meet

Beginning in the 1960s when concern over escalating health care costs first emerged and health care organizations were urged to adopt cost-control practices, managers frequently heard statements such as: "A hospital should be run like a business."

Think about that statement. Should a hospital definitely be run like a business? There is surely no doubt that a great many sound business practices belong in a health care organization as well as any other enterprise. Consider, however, that running a health care entity of any size, from a solo medical practice to a major medical center, as a business has raised—or at least made more prominent—a number of ethical issues as follows:

- There is always the issue of who gets service and who does not. Many will say that all deserve service according to their needs, but when there are more apparent needs than there is service capacity, who will determine who is served and how will this be determined? Since a business must remain solvent in order to continue in business, who gets service may at times be determined by ability to pay. The ethical and moral issues involved in the apportionment of services have long been with the industry and remain so whenever a decision to provide service is based on ability to pay via either one's personal economic status or particular insurance plan.

- As the incomes of some providers, specifically physicians, have risen over the recent four decades, questions concerning compensation have arisen. How much compensation is legitimate? In defense of high fees and high earnings some will point out the long, difficult, and costly education involved in becoming a physician. Those who defend high physician incomes will frown on those who question high medical fees, suggesting these people are "putting a price on their health." Yet others will claim that one's health, precious indeed, is being held hostage by the ability to pay.

- Not too many decades ago it was generally considered unethical for professionals, especially physicians, dentists, and attorneys, to advertise. We hardly need to point out that today health care organizations from individual practitioners to multihospital systems advertise regularly. Few people find this practice unethical, any more than they find competition among providers to be unethical. Occurring gradually over a few decades, this change in practice illustrates perfectly how a set of ethical standards, or a moral code, can change with the times.

Considerably more pertinent to the individual health care manager, however, are the business ethics governing the situations that the manager encounters on virtually a daily basis.

## BUSINESS ETHICS AND THE HEALTH CARE ORGANIZATION

### Regulatory Compliance

An organizational commitment to integrity is often expressed in the form of a regulatory compliance program. As the name implies, the purpose of such a program is to ensure compliance with all applicable laws and regulations. Program emphasis, however, usually concerns compliance in billing and reimbursement from Medicare, Medicaid, other government programs, and private insurers. Many such programs are directed toward achieving thorough and accurate compliance with areas of concern that the Office of Inspector General of the Department of Health and Human Services (DHHS) has identified as receiving insufficient care and attention; that is, areas that are susceptible to fraud and abuse as well as error.

Among the areas of concern identified by HHS are the following:

- duplicate billing, or billing for services not actually rendered
- "unbundling," the practice of submitting bills piecemeal to maximize payment for services or tests that would ordinarily be billed together
- "upcoding" to provide a higher rate than the code that reflects the actual service
- using a diagnosis-related group (DRG) code that provides a higher rate than the code that most accurately describes the service rendered (known as "DRG creep")
- rendering outpatient services in conjunction with inpatient stays
- filing false or erroneous cost reports
- billing for discharge in lieu of transfer
- limiting a patient's freedom of choice
- failing to refund credit balances
- utilizing incentives that violate anti-kickback regulations or other similar statutes
- engaging in questionable financial arrangements between hospital and hospital-based physicians
- participating in violations of the Stark physician self-referral law (more detail will be provided later)
- violating patient anti-dumping regulations
- knowingly failing to provide covered services or necessary care to health maintenance organization (HMO) members

The elimination and continuing prevention of fraud, abuse, and waste in all aspects of health care billing and accounting are the goals of any sound regulatory compliance program, and the health care department manager is ethically obligated to support all personally applicable aspects of the program to the best of his or her ability. All employees are responsible for understanding and complying with all laws and regulations applicable to their jobs, and the manager is responsible for ensuring that employees have all the information they need to enable them to do so.

## Conflict of Interest

An organization's employees most certainly have the right to engage in outside financial, business, or other activities as long as these activities do not interfere with the conscientious performance of their duties. It is necessary to avoid both actual conflict of interest and any behavior that creates the appearance of conflict of interest; a merely perceived conflict of interest is genuine to the perceiver.

Conflicts of interest exist when employee loyalty is divided between an individual's organizational responsibilities and any outside interest. A potential conflict of interest is present whenever an objective observer of one's actions would have cause to wonder whether the observed actions are motivated solely by organizational concerns or external concerns.

Conflict of interest is the area of ethical concern likely to emerge most frequently in the health care manager's management of a department or group. Some of the following guidelines or principles apply to all employees at all levels. Some are most pertinent to specific employees, such as those responsible for purchasing. A great many of them are of concern to every department manager as they affect employee behavior.

- Avoid placing business with any firm in which you or your family or close business or personal associates have a direct or indirect interest (usually financial).
- Derive no personal financial gain from transactions involving the organization unless the organization is advised of—and approves of—your potential benefit.
- Conduct all aspects of a personal business venture outside of the organizational environment and on non-work time. This is an area of significant concern as it is an ethical principle regularly violated and often implicitly condoned by department management through failure to address the offending behavior. For example, the employee who, while at work, solicits orders for cosmetics, food containers, or jewelry is in active violation of ethical standards; the person who makes photocopies for a part-time activity while on work time and using the organization's equipment is similarly in violation technically.
- Do not employ a relative in any situation where you have hiring authority or supervisory responsibility.
- Avoid soliciting, offering, accepting, or providing any consideration that could be construed as conflicting with the organization's business interests, such as meals, gifts, loans, entertainment, or transportation.
- Do not accept gifts exceeding the maximum value established by the organization (limits may exist in amounts up to perhaps $50 but are commonly lower); never accept gifts of cash in any amount.
- Safeguard patient and provider information against improper access or use for financial gain by unauthorized interests.
- Never charge, solicit, or accept any gift, donation, or other consideration as a precondition of admission, expedited admission, or continued stay.

- Require vendors and contractors to abide by your organization's ethical standards in their business relationships with the organization, and maintain impartial relationships with all actual and potential vendors and contractors.
- Do not endorse any product or outside service on behalf of the organization.
- Abstain from any discussion or decision affecting your employing organization and make clear your reasons for abstaining when serving as a member of an external organization or board of directors or in a public office.

If in doubt, always disclose the situation and seek resolution of an actual or potential conflict of interest before taking what might later be deemed an improper action. Questions concerning a potential conflict of interest can usually be addressed with the organization's human resource department.

Finally, in many organizations all department managers are asked to sign a conflict-of-interest statement either indicating the presence of potential conflicts or the absence of such. This statement is usually renewed annually; ordinarily it is the same conflict-of-interest statement executed by members of the board of directors.

## Use of Organizational Assets and Information

It is considered the responsibility of all employees to protect the assets of the organization against loss, theft, and misuse. The organization's property may neither be used for personal benefit, nor may it be loaned, sold, given away, or disposed of in any manner without appropriate authorization. Material that is declared surplus, obsolete, or scrap must ordinarily be disposed of according to specific organizational policies.

An organization's assets are intended for use for business purposes only during legitimate employment. Improper use ordinarily includes unauthorized personal appropriation or use of tangible assets such as computers and copiers and other office equipment, medical equipment, vehicles, supplies, reports and records, computer software and data, and facilities. Intangible assets such as intellectual property, trademarks and copyrights, proprietary information including computer programs, confidential data, business plans and such must be protected as vigorously as tangible property.

It also is necessary to protect patient property and information in accordance with established policies requiring that patient information is to be shared only with those who are authorized to receive such information and have a legitimate need for it.

The responsibility for protection also extends to proprietary information entrusted to the organization by vendors, both actual and potential, referral sources, contractors, service providers and others. This standard invariably includes the requirement to use only legally licensed computer software, with the use of bootleg or pirated software considered unethical—not to mention illegal.

Concerning information, an organization's ethical standards of conduct may set forth the following principles:

- It is prohibited to disclose business secrets or proprietary information to anyone external to the organization, whether during or after employment, except as specifically authorized.
- All organizational property and information in one's possession must be surrendered upon termination of employment.
- It is prohibited to use, either directly or indirectly, inside information (i.e., information acquired through employment with the organization) for personal gain or the gain of others.

### Referral Practices

The laws governing Medicare, Medicaid, and other federally sponsored programs prohibit the payment of any form of remuneration in return for the referral of patients. It also is illegal to induce the purchase of goods or services by Medicare or Medicaid for such referrals. The federal anti-kickback statute imposes criminal penalties on individuals and organizations that knowingly and willfully seek or receive compensation in return for referring patients or arranging for the provision of services for which payment may be made under a federal health care program. The kinds of payments prohibited by the statute include kickbacks, bribes, and rebates.

The Self-Referral Law (the Stark law) prohibits a physician with a financial relationship with an entity providing any designated health service from referring Medicare and Medicaid patients to that entity unless the service or relationship falls within the Stark law's statutory exemption. The law also prohibits an entity from billing federal health care programs for items or services ordered by a physician who has a financial relationship with that entity. The Stark law, in other words, sought to eradicate the practice of some physicians of referring or sending patients to other provider organizations (e.g., clinical laboratories, radiological services, pharmacies, medical supply firms, etc.) of which they were owners in whole or in part.

The foregoing may be incorporated in an organization's ethical standards of conduct in the following manner:

- No employee shall solicit, receive, offer to pay, or pay remuneration of any kind in exchange for referring or recommending referral of any individual to another person, department, or division of the organization for services or in return for the purchase of goods or services to be paid for by a federal program.
- No employee shall offer or grant any benefits to a referring physician or other referral source to secure the referral of patients or patient business.
- No physician shall make referrals for designated health services to entities in which the physician has a financial interest through either ownership or a compensation arrangement.
- No physician shall bill for services rendered as a result of an illegal referral.

## Political Activity

It is common to find in an organization's code of conduct an expectation that employees who participate in government through political activity will ensure that they are not seen as representing the organization in doing so. There is, in fact, a legal prohibition against political activity by not-for-profit hospitals and nursing homes and such; participating in political activity can jeopardize the employer's tax-exempt status. Specifics in the code of conduct may include the following:

- An employee speaking out on public issues must avoid the impression or appearance of speaking for the organization.
- Employees who hold public office must do so as individuals, not as representatives of the organization; they must pursue the duties of such office in a manner that does not conflict with organizational responsibilities.
- No organizational funds may be used to support any political activity, and no one may make political contributions on behalf of the organization.
- No employee may be reimbursed in any manner for political activity.
- No organizational facilities may be used for political activity.

## Privacy and Confidentiality

### Employee Privacy

Although personnel files will ordinarily remain the property of the employer, the organization having a privacy policy in place will strictly limit access to personnel files to those having a legitimate need for the information. Such a policy will usually state that personnel information will be released externally only upon employee authorization or to satisfy legitimate legal requirements (court orders, subpoenas, etc.).

### Patient Confidentiality

Patient records, results of tests, diagnoses, and any other information relating to or concerning individuals to whom the organization is providing or has provided service should be held in the strictest confidence. It is considered a violation of the ethical code of conduct to reveal patient information to anyone outside of the organization without the express written authorization of the patient (or the patient's guardian, administrator, or executor), or a court order or other appropriate legal instrument.

Internal to the organization, patient information is to be retained in confidence. It is to be revealed on a need-to-know basis only.

## Admission and Care of Patients

A health facility's ethical code of conduct will customarily require the organization and its employees to do the following:

- Admit and care for persons without regard to their race, color, creed, national origin, or economic status, accepting and treating all with a caring response to their needs.

- Provide each patient (for hospitals) or resident (for nursing homes or other long-term setting) with a patient's bill of rights.
- Treat all patients or residents in a manner that fosters trust, extending every reasonable consideration to diversity of background, culture, religion, and heritage.
- Involve patients, whenever possible, in decisions regarding their treatment, and assist them in understanding proposed treatments and potential risks and outcomes.
- Respect the privacy and individuality of all who come to the organization for service.

## Employee Relationships

The following is a suggested model for the section of an organization's ethical standards of conduct that addresses relationships with employees:

(The organization) recognizes people as valued resources. Employee relationships built on mutual respect are essential to maintaining a high level of integrity in our work.

Every employee will be treated and judged as an individual on the basis of individual qualifications without regard to race, sex, sexual orientation, religion, national origin, age, disability, veteran status, or other characteristic protected by law. This pledge extends to all areas of the employment relationship including hiring, promotion, benefits, training, and discipline.

(The organization) will conscientiously observe all federal, state, and local laws and regulations applicable in any way to the employment relationship.

(The organization) is committed to providing a work environment in which employees are free from harassment, sexual or otherwise. No employee will be made to feel uncomfortable in the work environment through exposure to coarse, profane, or derogatory comments or sexual language.

Employees are encouraged to express themselves freely and responsibly through established channels and procedures. Complaints will be treated as confidential information and will be revealed only to those who need to know as part of a process of investigation or resolution. (The organization) will not tolerate any interference, retaliation, or coercion by any employee against an employee who registers a concern or complaint.

We will observe the standards of our profession and exercise judgment and objectivity at all times. Significant difference of professional opinion should be referred to the appropriate management for prompt resolution.

We shall show respect and consideration for one another regardless of position, status, or relationship.

(The organization) will promote its ethical standards of conduct among all physicians who practice in our facilities and encourage their observance and support of these standards.

## WHEN CODES CLASH: MASON VERSUS GREEN

It was noted early in the chapter that individuals have ethical standards of conduct, although any person's "code" is unwritten. Unwritten or not, however, personal ethical standards, part and parcel of an individual's moral code, can be extremely strong determinants of behavior and can be capable of creating considerable frustration and dissonance when colliding with conflicting standards.

The lesson that should initially jump out of the "Situation" introduced at the beginning of the chapter is that every organization of any appreciable size should have a written policy for determining how employees are identified for layoff when reduction in force is necessary. If Morgan General Hospital had such a policy, chances are that policy would dictate how the layoff would proceed and neither Mason nor Green would have any real decision to make. Apparently, however, there is no such policy, not an uncommon situation in an organization that has never had a layoff in the past so that no one has thought to create such a policy.

An age-old exchange of remarks goes something like: Person 1 says, "Well, the boss ain't always right," and Person 2 responds by saying, "Yes, but the boss is always the boss." Unfortunately, the boss usually is always the boss in the sense of being the party who by virtue of positional authority can willfully prevail when there is a difference of opinion with a subordinate. It is clear that Robert Green is accustomed to getting his own way with subordinates, micromanaging to an extent that might make subordinate managers wonder why they are needed at all.

Carl Mason understandably would like to use normal attrition to reduce staff the painless way, but since attrition did not occur he fell back on what to him was probably the fairest approach to take: last in, first out. In the absence of written rules for selecting who must go, one is least likely to be challenged, legally or otherwise, for using seniority. However, even the absence of written rules does not mean that management can do anything without sparking a negative reaction of some kind. If management is inconsistent in designating people for layoff—say Green lays off those whom he likes least, while in another department straight seniority is used—the inconsistency may be sufficient to prompt complaints to some external advocacy agency.

Because Carl Mason's moral code appears to be in direct conflict with that of his superior, his alternatives are few and are not especially encouraging. He can

- capitulate and do as ordered, which may leave him feeling he has compromised his principles by "selling out"
- refuse the direct order and take his chances with what follows, perhaps loss of employment or loss of management position
- go around Green to either the next highest level of management (a move often akin to organizational suicide) or human resources (not as risky as going to the boss, but still potentially hazardous)
- tender his resignation and seek employment elsewhere

Ultimately what Carl Mason does may depend on a wide variety of factors including his family situation, his financial situation, his age and career stage, the job market for people with his skills, his integrity, and the strength of his personal beliefs.

## ADDRESSING ETHICAL ISSUES

Ideally, an organization should publish its ethical standards of conduct and disseminate them to all employees. These standards also should be distributed externally as appropriate to vendors, contractors, third-party agents, and others as necessary to advise these entities of what to expect in business dealings with the organization.

It also is advisable to put in place a system for reporting alleged or potential violations of the organization's ethical standards. Each employee is urged to report what he or she believes may be a violation of these ethical standards. Reports should be immediate, thorough, and directed to either the individual's immediate supervisor or the chief human resource officer. For potential violations that might appear especially sensitive and for those of such a nature that direct reporting might compromise the reporting employee, it would be advisable for the organization to establish an "employee ethics hotline" number. An employee may use this number to make an anonymous report or to request guidance in describing or addressing a potential violation.

As mentioned earlier in the chapter, most of the larger health care organizations operating today have formal ethics committees to address ethical questions as needed. A typical committee might include the organization's

- patient care services executive
- human resource executive
- finance executive
- medical director
- corporate compliance officer
- managers from specific functional areas as needed

## MANAGEMENT'S RESPONSIBILITIES: A TOP-DOWN OBLIGATION

One need not look far or long to appreciate the presence of a crisis of ethics in American business. Much of the highly publicized unethical behavior is unconscionable and greed-driven, but perhaps some unethical conduct is also owing to the increasingly competitive nature of business. With competition attaining cutthroat dimensions in some industries and with other pressures increasing, some organizations, including many health care providers, are fighting for their very existence. Many employees—including managers at all levels—see themselves as fighting for their jobs or careers or at least struggling to get ahead on an uphill playing field.

A great deal has been published concerning high-profile ethical breaches. Hardly a week passes without news of alleged wrongdoings in high places as CEOs and other leaders apparently seek to enrich themselves by questionable means at the expense of employees and other stakeholders. In classrooms, students of business and the professions hear that ethics should be a vital concern, but outside of school they see that it does not receive a great deal of serious attention in the workplace.

What are employees to think when they see the kinds of behavior typified by the high-profile cases of recent years? Numerous CEOs and others have grabbed up company profits and left their own employees financially devastated. These major scandals have tended to undercut worker trust and whatever loyalty employees might have extended to their employers during these volatile times. Also, scandals at high levels in the government serve to further feed worker distrust.

But the majority of today's ethics problems are not those presented by the high-profile cases. The prominent cases simply feed attitudes that prevail at lower-management and rank-and-file levels. Consider just a few of the numerous ethical decisions many people face from day to day:

- Am I justified in calling in sick when I'm really not ill?
- Do I work the full 8 hours, or do I start late, leave early, spend time socializing, or amuse myself surfing the net or playing computer games?
- What's the harm if I take care of personal business during work time?
- Is it really up to me to point out the error being made by the sales clerk who is giving me too much change?
- Surely it must be all right for me to punch a friend's time card because I've been asked to do so? After all, lots of others do it.

The foregoing are but a few of the ethical breaches occurring regularly in the majority of organizations. These might even be called the smaller breaches; beyond these there are theft, sexual harassment, deliberate discrimination, violations of confidentiality, and cutting corners and jeopardizing safety or quality for the sake of meeting deadlines, schedules, or budgets.

One might reason that taking an unwarranted day off once in a while or fudging a few dollars on an expense report are insignificant acts compared with what some highly placed "leaders" seem to be doing regularly. Up and down the line the reasoning becomes: *They're doing it—why shouldn't I?*

Recall the definition of ethics as *a system or code of morals.* Perhaps this broad definition is itself part of the problem, since moral principles and values differ among people, often significantly. Often the dilemma is a rules-based perspective dictated in laws and policies versus a values-based perspective, that is, one's personal beliefs and individual sense of right or wrong.

It is clear that the strongest examples of unethical behavior are those visible breaches that occur at high organizational levels. The problem is not a lack of rules; most of the larger organizations have a published code of conduct or ethical standards. The problem is in the lack of observance of the code and especially in the absence of modeling behavior.

Every business should have a code of ethics actively modeled by top management. It's absolutely critical that the people at the top be visible models of ethical behavior. Whether they realize it or not—and if they fail to realize it, perhaps they're unsuited for their elevated positions—top management's behavior sets the tone for the rest of the organization.

A business's ethical standards should be written in positive, constructive terms, laying out practical guidelines for ethical practice. This is no place for legalese that can be variously interpreted or ignored as some might choose. All employees should be aware of this code and share an understanding of appropriate conduct. Also, every such system needs features that protect those who report unethical conduct. Ethics has to be taught, actively communicated to employees without assuming that all in the company automatically share an understanding of ethical behavior.

The creation and maintenance of a dedicated and motivated workforce begins with the ethics and character of its leaders. The latter-day catchphrase "walking the talk" has never been as true as it is concerning management's ethical behavior.

### The Department Supervisor's Key Role

It falls to the individual supervisor to ensure that all employees receive, review, and understand the organization's ethical standards of conduct. The ethical standards of conduct should be a regular subject of both new employee orientation and continuing education.

In managing a department or group, the supervisor should strive to model ethical behavior in all aspects of job performance. Thorough orientation and education notwithstanding, there is probably no more effective influence in shaping employee behavior than the supervisor's visible behavior. If the supervisor visibly observes and conscientiously adheres to the ethical standards of conduct, the employees are more likely to do the same. The supervisor's continued demonstration of ethical behavior is one of the most important dimensions of successful management in the modern health care organization.

## BUT IT REMAINS EVERYONE'S JOB

All employees at all levels have the continuing responsibility to display complete integrity in all aspects of their work activity. Integrity influences the reputations of people as individuals, and individual reputations together ultimately determine the reputation of the organization. Indeed, no set of ethical standards can ever replace a balanced combination of sound judgment, common sense, and personal integrity.

---

## REVIEW QUESTIONS

1. Provide an example of how ethical standards can change over a period of time.
2. Why is it necessary for a health care institution to have official written policies for addressing issues of medical ethics?
3. What is ordinarily the function of an institution's ethics committee?
4. What is self-referral and why is it considered unethical as well as illegal?
5. What is the single ethical issue that is—or should be—of broadest concern among health institution employees? That is, which one concern affects more employees than any other?

6. Why is it important for the department supervisor to be a model of ethical behavior?

---

### EXERCISE: WHAT IS APPROPRIATE, WHAT IS NOT

Address the following situations in essay form. In each case describe what you believe is ethically appropriate and what is not, and why. Also, be sure to describe in as much detail as necessary what you believe should be done about each situation.

- A Mr. Smith, visibly upset, visited the hospital administrator's office to register a complaint about comments he heard on a hospital elevator. It seems that two doctors—both young, possibly interns or residents—were discussing a particular case. One described the patient as "imagining things" and "not nearly as sick as she thinks she is." The other laughed softly and agreed, saying, "We might want a psych consult for that one." They left the elevator on the same floor as Mr. Smith, just a few steps ahead of him; they entered the semi-private room housing Mr. Smith's mother and another patient. Without entering the room, Mr. Smith returned to the elevator and went straight to administration.

- Christmas was but two days away. Williams, the director of the human resource department, was in his office when a heavy package arrived. It was an ornate wooden wine crate containing a dozen bottles of relatively expensive wine. A note attached to the crate said, "A little something for you and your capable assistant Ms. Brown." It was signed by a benefits provider who did a small amount of the hospital's insurance business and was regularly proposing to take on more. The same day, one of the hospital's medical chiefs, Dr. Young, dropped in on Williams to wish him Merry Christmas and leave him a beribboned bottle of champagne as he was doing for every department head in the hospital.

---

**NOTE**

1. *Webster's New Twentieth Century Dictionary, Unabridged*, 2d ed. (New York: Simon & Schuster, 1983), 627.

## CHAPTER 17

# Decisions, Decisions

*All decisions should be made as low as possible in the organization.
The Charge of the Light Brigade was ordered by an officer
who wasn't there looking at the territory.*
—*Robert Townsend*

## CHAPTER OBJECTIVES

☛ Establish a direct relationship between the amount of effort going into a decision and the potential consequences of that decision.

☛ Identify the elements of the basic decision-making process and describe the steps followed in rational decision-making.

☛ Define constraints and identify the various forms in which they appear.

☛ Establish perspectives on risk and uncertainty in decision-making.

☛ Discuss the implications of the "no-decision option."

☛ Review decision-making authority and responsibility.

## SITUATION: DECIDING UNDER PRESSURE

Not unusual for a person in a position such as hers, Helen Grove, director of nursing service at 200-bed Community Hospital, found each day to be a bit fuller than her attention could serve and bringing her a few more problems and demands than she could thoroughly address. Helen had long heard of "management by crisis," and on many days she felt that because of forces beyond her control she had fallen victim to exactly that pattern of functioning.

Several times over the recent few months June Weston, the emergency department (ED) supervisor, had mentioned to Helen that the ED had been getting steadily busier and that she needed more help. June's complaints were always general and sometimes delivered "on the run"; her requests, seemingly never stated very strongly, were never more specific than "more help," so Helen, never lacking for problems demanding her attention, had not pursued the matter.

However, early Monday morning this week June came to Helen, actually walking in on a meeting of head nurses in Helen's office, and said with some degree of apparent agitation, "The ED needs one more RN and more clerical help now. I'm tired of waiting and tired of being overworked. If something isn't done about it by Friday of this week you can find yourself a new ED supervisor!"

*Instructions*

As you proceed through the chapter, identify several alternatives that might permit Helen to solve the ED problem and indicate the primary advantages and disadvantages of each. Also, consider what hazards might be presented by the way the "pressure" was introduced, and prepare to describe the manner in which this places the director, Helen, at risk in the situation.

## A FACT OF LIFE

Decision-making is a fact of life for supervisors and nonsupervisors in both working and nonworking situations. We all make decisions every day, sometimes a great number of them. Many of these decisions are small and inconsequential and are made automatically or very nearly so. Some are larger, potentially significant, and require considerably more time and effort.

Generally it is the potential consequences that govern the amount of effort going into the making of any particular decision. This stands to reason; decisions involving appreciable risk usually are not—or should not be—made lightly, nor can they usually be made with speed and ease.

Most people are self-programmed to make some decisions, especially small decisions of little consequence and those decisions made regularly. You probably do not consciously think of yourself as making a decision when you decide what to have for lunch or decide which shoes you will wear to work, but you nevertheless are following the basic decision-making process: you are receiving information, forming and comparing alternatives and selecting one of these, and translating your choice into action.

The more often we make certain kinds of decisions, the better we get at it. For instance, if your job happens to include the ordering of disposable gloves, the first time you were faced with this task you may have gathered information about several brands and carefully evaluated it for cost and other features. This could have taken you a significant amount of time, and you might have switched to a second or perhaps even a third brand later on as you accumulated information based on experience. However, chances are that each time you repeated the ordering process the task became quicker and easier. Eventually you may have reached a point where your decision to order gloves became no more than the simple act of reordering a product that you had already accepted as meeting your needs. Similarly, you become self-programmed to make many decisions that come your way periodically. Regardless of preprogramming, however, and regardless of the existence of comprehensive policies and procedures, as a supervisor you are going to face numerous situations that require you to make original decisions.

Policies and procedures never cover everything. What, then, do you do when you discover that a necessary decision cannot be made "by the book?" What do you do when no one is immediately available to tell you what you should do? When a situation requiring action is left up to you—and there are plenty of these in supervision—you have to take some kind of action. Your supervisory position requires you to exercise judgment as to whether the situation is in fact your problem and to exercise judgment in arriving at a solution.

## THE BASIC DECISION-MAKING PROCESS

The six elements of the basic decision-making process are (1) identifying the problem, (2) gathering information, (3) analyzing information and arranging it into alternatives, (4) choosing an alternative, (5) implementing the chosen alternative, and (6) following up on implementation.

Regardless of the scope or potential impact of any particular decision, most of the foregoing elements are present to some extent in every decision-making situation. In minor situations the problem or need may be self-evident and may require no attention beyond simple recognition. You still gather information, analyze it and form alternatives, and make a choice, although in simple, repetitive situations—again, for instance, consider deciding what shoes to wear to work—your preprogramming may compress these steps considerably. Implementation is always present, and since your decision is nothing without it—you must, for example, put the shoes on. Follow-up is also always present, fleeting though it may be—Do the shoes really match the outfit, and does that little scuffmark show?

As decision-making situations grow in scope and complexity, however, the importance of each element of the process looms greater.

### Identifying the Problem

Before tackling any problem requiring a decision, it is necessary to consider whether you are dealing with the real problem. When confronted with a situation you will have to decide if you do indeed have a problem, something that is based on fact and not the result of opinion, misinterpretation, or bias. Do not simply jump into every apparent problem that comes along; rather, investigate to determine whether it is indeed a problem deserving your attention.

Look also at the nature of the apparent problem. Is it a unique situation, not previously encountered and certainly not covered by existing policies and procedures? Is it a common, recurring problem, one for which specific procedures exist? Is it perhaps self-solving, one of those rare but nevertheless genuine situations that correct themselves when left alone?

Also, be mindful of whether you are dealing with a true problem or simply with a symptom of some hidden problem. Being led astray by symptoms, which are the obvious, surface indications of trouble, is an inherent hazard in supervisory decision-making. Effective treatment of a symptom may lead to immediate improvement. However, the symptom may soon reappear, suggesting that what you thought was the problem might not be the problem at all. If, for example, a backlog occurs in the transcription section of health information management, you may feel the need to do something about it. Perhaps you authorize overtime or give the group some temporary help, and in a few days the backlog is gone and the transcriptionists are current with incoming work. A few days later, however, you notice that a backlog is again growing; there is a 1-day, then a 2-day accumulation of work left undone. You treated a symptom by reducing the backlog; the return of the backlog suggests the problem is elsewhere, perhaps in the staffing itself, the distribution of work, the patterns of physicians' dictation, or somewhere else.

You cannot always tell if a symptom is a symptom until you deal with it once and it returns. However, by scratching beneath the surface indications of trouble, you can often determine where the real difficulty lies before you begin to decide on corrective action.

### Gathering Information

Volumes have been written on this and the next stage of the decision-making process. Elaborate quantitative approaches to decision making concentrate on the collection of information and the arrangement of this information into alternative choices.

Essentially your task is to gather enough information to give you some degree of assurance that you are making a decision consistent with reasonable risks. Your broad objective in gathering information is to gather everything that has a bearing on your decision-to-be, that is, everything you can collect considering the time and effort you can or should devote to the decision. You will be researching and observing with a specific purpose in mind: to get as much information as you feel you need, or can get, to help you make an intelligent decision.

Recognize that often you will never have "enough" information. Further, nobody can tell you in a general sense how much information is enough. We can only suggest that your information-gathering effort should be consistent with the potential impact of the decision you have to make. If you happen to be selecting a new copy machine for the business office, you may spend a considerable amount of time talking with salespeople and studying the prices, operating costs, and features of many different machines. Your activity could consume a number of hours spread out over days or weeks, and this effort may be justified because of the amount of money at risk. However, if you happen to be trying to decide what brand of pencils to buy for the office you should not spend 3 days gathering data about brands and prices.

In gathering information for decisions, work with facts and do not depend on opinions. Much so-called information comes to you directly or indirectly from other people. As you gather your decision-making building blocks, take care to separate the factual from the subjective. Both may well be useful, but the latter will more readily lead you astray.

### Analyzing Information and Arranging It into Alternatives

This, along with gathering information, constitutes a cyclic process. You will find that you are arranging and evaluating bits and pieces of information while you are still collecting more information. You tend to fill in the gaps as you go along, going back for more information whenever questions arise or you discover weaknesses in your data. This cyclic process can go on for quite some time in decisions of considerable impact; you want as much information as you can acquire when the potential consequences are significant.

However, this is the stage in which the process begins to break down in the hands of some so-called decision makers. Projecting the impression of being conscientious, cautious, and thorough, some people continue gathering more and more information and keep refining the alternatives further and further, somehow seeming to take forever getting around to actually making the decision. As already suggested, however, in a decision of importance you will never truly have "enough" information. You may never reach the stage where you are 100 percent comfortable taking a risk based on the information you have in hand. However, you cannot "if" a problem to a solution; somewhere along the way you must take a stand, accept some risk, and decide.

Any number of different kinds of information will greet you when you are researching a problem. When buying a copy machine, you will learn about cost, size, operations, service and maintenance, warranties, color, and a dozen other factors. When buying pencils, you will encounter price, brand, color, hardness, and so on. It is the same in almost every decision-making situation: A number of factors are present, and all may or may not have a bearing on your choice.

The organization's needs, the department's needs, the patients' needs, and your needs and preferences all have a bearing on the decisions you make. However, it is not often possible to achieve complete satisfaction of all needs and preferences. For instance, you might like a copy machine that gives you the lowest operating cost and the longest warranty, but it turns out that machine A has the lowest operating cost and machine C has the best warranty. You then find yourself in the position of having to make smaller decisions along the way relative to your decision factors themselves. You are led to discover that trade-offs are necessary between and among decision factors and that you will settle for less in regard to the factors that mean the least to you for the sake of achieving satisfaction on certain other factors.

Ultimately your decision factors will be arranged into a number of alternatives, the possible choices from among which you will select one. The number of alternatives may be clearly limited and well defined. Sometimes, however, the number of alternatives is up to you. If there are 11 brands of disposable gloves on the market and 23 makes of copy machines available, you should not limit yourself to looking at only one or two possibilities. Neither, however, can you afford to perform an exhaustive analysis of every possible choice. Rather, you will scan the field of available choices using some broad criteria and concentrate on developing perhaps three or four of the more appealing choices as specific alternatives. You may look at several possibilities along the way but discard some because certain constraints rule them unsuitable (more about constraints later).

## Choosing an Alternative

When you are left with several reasonably well-defined alternatives, you should make your decision by picking the one you feel best fills your needs and meets your preferences. It is a matter of comparing the possible choices and taking the one that "comes to the top"—both objectively and subjectively—for you, the decision maker. This becomes your solution (or at least your recommendation), and you should immediately question it from the following directions:

- Does this answer deal with cause (the problem) rather than simply with an effect (a symptom)?
- Does this answer have the effect of creating policy or establishing precedent, and as such should it be formally expressed as a guide for future decisions?

- Will the implementation of this solution have adverse effects on any other aspects of operations?

## Implementing the Chosen Alternative

Implementation is action, putting the decision to work. Without implementation a decision is no decision at all; it is simply an academic exercise in "What if we did this?" A true decision is both choice and action.

From this point forward we could repeat, with added emphasis, most of what was said in Chapter 4 about the basic management functions. Planning, organizing, directing, coordinating, and controlling all come into active play in the implementation of a decision and in the follow-up on that implementation.

## Following Up on Implementation

Follow-up is usually the weakest part of the decision-making process. Employees resist change for many reasons. Old habits persist, new habits are difficult to form, and, most important here, conditions surrounding the decision may change. The moment you obtain specific information and commit it to paper it starts to become obsolete. Needs and preferences change, products change, people change, and the environment changes. Time goes on, and the more of it that passes—and with significant decision-making the lag between choice and complete implementation can be considerable—the more change is likely to accrue. You will need to clarify instructions, assess timing and make adjustments as necessary, and in general supervise the entire implementation effort.

During implementation be open to employee suggestions. Allow yourself to learn from the way implementation appears to be going. Do not be afraid to admit an error; be willing to reverse or withdraw the decision if experience shows it is turning out to have been a bad one. Sometimes through no fault of your own the alternative that appeared best on paper will go sour in practice, and it makes little sense to continue pushing a poor choice. On the other hand, however, if partial implementation only assures you that your decision was the best you could make under the circumstances, then stick to it and see it all the way through.

A comprehensive outline of the generalized problem-solving and decision-making process is presented in Exhibit 17–1.

## CONSTRAINTS

Anything that is constrained is limited in some way. In decision-making, constraints are those limiting conditions that rule out certain alternatives as possible or desirable choices. Once identified, constraints let you know how far you may go in considering certain alternatives; they tell you what is practical and what is not.

The constraints commonly encountered in supervisory decision-making involve time, money, quality, personalities, and politics. Other factors such as limitations of physical space and shortages of various material resources may

### Define the Problem
- Is it genuine?
- How did it come about?
- Is it a problem or a problem symptom?
- Is it a critical issue?
- What are the objectives involved?

### Gather the Facts
- Review available documentation
- Determine what rules and policies apply
- Talk with involved and concerned individuals
- Include opinions and feelings

### Weight and Formulate
- Fit facts together and form alternatives
- Compare alternatives with each other
- Look for other possible actions
- Check against policies and practices
- Consider effects on individuals or groups
- Consider potential effects on productivity

### Take Action
- Is your own authority sufficient to permit implementation?
- Should you take it to your manager as a recommendation?
- Plan the timing of implementation before acting

### Assess Results
- Decide how soon you need to begin follow-up and how often you need to check progress or results
- Watch for changes in quality, output, attitudes, and relationships
- Be alert for the likelihood of regression (as some employees may surrender to old habits and revert to former practices)

**Exhibit 17–1** The Problem-Solving and Decision-Making Process

also appear as constraints; however, since it is possible to build space and buy material, these seeming constraints reduce themselves to limitations of money.

## Time

Everything done in the organization takes time. It takes time to process a laboratory test, to escort a patient to the X-ray department, to order and obtain a new drug, to design and build a new wing on the building, to organize to react to an emergency, to perform a surgical procedure, and to accomplish thousands of other activities. Time may be a critical factor in a decision, or it may matter not at all. If you are still wondering, for instance, about what brand of pencils to buy, it may not matter at all that you need to wait an extra week to get the best deal on the preferred brand. However, if you are deciding on alternative procedures for reacting to a code in the emergency department, you will be limited to considering only those alternatives that can be successfully activated within a tightly restricted amount of time. As it relates to health, safety, and the quality of medical care—as it relates, in fact, to life and death—time is a key constraint in many supervisory decisions made in the health care setting.

In situations when it may not be critical, time can be considered flexible: you may trade off timeliness with other factors. When time does not matter, you may choose to complete a given task more slowly for the sake of greater convenience or lower cost.

It is necessary to assess the decision situation for the importance of time in the outcome. Once realistic timing is determined, the alternatives shaping up as well outside the limit begin to rule themselves out.

## Money

Money—the full cost of implementing a decision—is a common constraint. Often the limits are clear, defined by the amount of money that you know is available. For example, when you go to lunch with just $4 in your pocket you know that all meals costing more than $4 are ruled out by financial constraints. The money constraint can also be put there by someone who is making decisions of another kind or from another perspective. For example, you would like a new computer with increased capacity but your immediate supervisor says, "No, it's not in the budget, we have no money available, and you'll have to make the old one last another year." Although there might be money available in the organization, someone else has made a decision on the relative worth of your proposal versus other uses for the money, so you are fully as constrained as though the money did not exist at all.

In short, any time an otherwise workable alternative costs more than you have or can raise, you are subject to financial constraints and that alternative is effectively ruled out.

## Quality

Quality of care and service is always a primary consideration in the operation of a health care organization, and it can be just as great a constraint as time or money. Generally, when we make decisions affecting the delivery of health care we are faced with the necessity of considering only those alternatives that either maintain or improve quality. Often the "quick and dirty" solution to a problem is clearly the best in terms of time, money, or both; however, if quality is likely to suffer then the solution is inferior and should be considered no further.

## Personalities

Although personalities may not strike you as presenting legitimate constraints on decision alternatives, they nevertheless must be reckoned with. We must try to avoid getting tied too tightly to the belief that "people shouldn't be that way." The fact of the matter is that people *are* "that way," and the constraints presented by personalities can be fully as limiting as absolute financial constraints.

There are managers who will not buy a particular product that analysis shows to be the best available simply because they do not like the salesperson.

Some employees will not work well with other employees because of personality clashes, so an alternative that might otherwise be the best solution may not work at all. Also, some people are more resistant to change than others; some are more solidly attached to old habits or have strong tendencies toward doing things their own way as opposed to anyone else's way.

Although personality constraints are usually not the most powerful forces shaping a decision, they are nevertheless important. People are themselves a key factor to consider in analyzing alternatives. Approval and implementation are accomplished only through people, and people's acceptance of the decision and their ability to work with it are fully as important as the elements of the decision itself.

## Politics

Politics may not strike you as a legitimate constraint in a decision situation. However, the political implications of a decision are fully as real as the personality factors, and they often have far greater impact.

The health care institution is an organization of people with a common purpose. The institution serves a community; this community is itself a body of people having certain wants, needs, and preferences. Within both institution and community are many subgroups organized along various social, economic, professional, vocational, and other lines, and each of these groups has its own desires. Hardly a supervisor has not said at one time or another, "Politics shouldn't matter in running the organization," but in reality political considerations do matter.

Politics (the word carries a negative connotation for many people) is frequently described as "the art of the possible." Specifically in the health care organization it is the art of the possible given the actions and characteristics of all the various groups involved. For instance, a particular decision that serves the financial interests of the institution may alienate the employees. Another decision that may appear good for the health care of a region, for example, a county or a larger area, may be seen as bad for the locality and would thus alienate the local community. Within the organization, a decision that serves the needs of nursing service may at the same time alienate the housekeeping department, or a decision that serves the needs of administration and finance may upset relations with the medical staff.

This is not to say that political considerations should rule or that "pressure groups" should get their way simply because they are larger, stronger, or more vocal than other groups. However, it is necessary to consider political implications because a decision that is made in the face of the strongest opposition, whether that opposition is justified or not, generally requires far more in the way of resources and effort to implement.

## Absolute and Practical Constraints

Constraints may be absolute or practical in nature. An absolute constraint clearly defines a limit beyond which you cannot go. For example, if you are choosing a copy machine and $2,000 is the absolute extent of what you can spend, then $2,000 is the limit for any machine you seriously consider. More often than not, however, constraints present themselves by limiting the practicality of a decision. A certain condition becomes a constraint because it renders an alternative impractical under the circumstances. For example, if you decide it is important to have two particular functions located next door to each other you might be faced with considerable expense for altering physical layout. You may then look at other possibilities: you may have a space available two doors down the hall, another 300 hundred yards away at the end of the wing, another on the second floor of the next wing, and yet another at a satellite facility 5 miles away. You can function under any of these alternatives, but you will obviously do better with some than with others. It may be that the closer together you bring the two functions, the more financial resources you will consume implementing the decision. Given that finances are limited but you are still trying to achieve reasonable operating efficiency, you develop trade-offs and settle perhaps for the second or third most desirable choice. Many constraints, then, are in effect not saying "You absolutely can't do this" but are rather saying "You're going to pass a point where you shouldn't do this because it's no longer practical"—like locating one function next door to another even though it costs a fortune, or locating it 5 miles away only because it is cheap.

We need to assess the constraints inherent in the situation realistically, recognize our limitations, and focus our attention on realistic, practical alternatives. Alternatives that lie beyond the bounds of the constraints we have identified are really not alternatives at all.

## RISK, UNCERTAINTY, AND JUDGMENT

Some decision-making theorists speak of something called "perfect information." This is a state that exists only when you know all there is to know about all aspects of every available alternative. If there truly were such a thing as perfect information there would be no decision at all: the decision would have made itself because the only true alternative would be self-evident.

Because there is no such thing as perfect information, there are always elements of risk and uncertainty in a decision-making situation. Risk is there because something may be lost—be it time, money, effectiveness, or perhaps life itself—if the wrong decision is made. Uncertainty also exists; since you do not know everything about all aspects of the situation and have no guarantees that things will come out right, you do not know in advance whether your choice is the right one.

One of the major objectives of the decision-making process is to minimize risk and uncertainty by learning as much as practical about each decision-making situation. Since risk and uncertainty are always present, there is always the need for judgment in decision-making. Decisions do not make themselves; people make decisions. All of our efforts at gathering and analyzing information, as well as all sophisticated quantitative decision-making techniques, are no more than efforts to reduce the extent of pure judgment required in decision-making. For example, someone lines up three copy machines for you and asks, "Which one do you want?" You might make a purely judgmental decision by pointing and saying, "I'll take the red one." The probability that you have made the "right" decision is literally one third, based on a random choice of three available alternatives, so you experience a two-thirds chance of being "wrong." However, if you analyze all the data you can obtain about the three machines and allow your judgment to be influenced by quantitative information, although you might never be absolutely sure you are making the right decision you could well reduce the chance of being wrong to considerably less than two thirds.

In the last analysis many decisions will be right or wrong because of human judgment regardless of the amount of quantitative information involved. It is not your objective to try to completely eliminate judgment from decision-making. This cannot be done. Rather you must refine that judgment by learning as much as it is practical to learn about the alternatives.

## THE NO-DECISION OPTION

In even the simplest of decision-making situations there are always at least two choices: to decide or not to decide. The no-decision option is the case in which you select the latter choice. In effect what you do is "decide not to decide." This does not have to be a consciously made decision, but it can, and very often does, occur by default through procrastination. Taking no action on a problem amounts to the exercise of the no-decision option.

Appreciate that whether the no-decision option is exercised by choice or through procrastination it is still a decision. Frequently it is the decision with the most potentially far-reaching consequences. All too often we adopt an attitude, either consciously or unconsciously, that suggests: "If I'm really quiet maybe it'll go away." Sometimes it does indeed go away and things get better. However, things usually do not get better. To cite one of the corollaries of the well-known Murphy's Law: "Left unto themselves, things invariably go from bad to worse."

## THE RANGE OF DECISIONS

Decision-making situations may range from the highly, but rarely totally, objective, with plenty of factual information on which to decide, to the purely subjective or totally judgmental decision. The decision-making process described in this chapter essentially applies to all decisions; the differences lie in the kinds of information with which we must deal in developing alternatives.

We can usually be more comfortable with so-called objective decisions. We have facts, figures, and other data to work with. We compare prices, statistics, hours, pieces, or some other specific indicators and make our choices. Orderly approaches to decision-making are possible, and improved facility at making such decisions comes with practice in conscientiously following the steps of the process through decision after decision.

The highly subjective decision is another matter. Little or no data are available. We must make our choices based on rules and regulations, policies, procedures, and precedents, and very often on our basic sense of what is right or wrong, fair or unfair, or logical or illogical. Many personnel-related decisions fall in the area of the subjective, and while the basic decision-making process does not apply nearly as specifically as with most objective decisions, improved decision-making ability again comes largely through experience.

Although decisions may range from the mostly objective to the wholly subjective, the character of any particular decision may be greatly influenced by the conditions under which it must be made. The single circumstance that probably has the greatest effect on the character of any particular decision is the imposition of pressure.

Decision-making pressure is often felt as a limitation of the time available in which to investigate properly and render a decision. It is one thing to face a situation in which you have more than adequate time to develop and assess all workable alternatives; it is another matter entirely to realize that undesirable consequences will result if a decision is not rendered by a deadline—and that this deadline does not leave time enough for reasonable investigation. Unfortunately many supervisory decisions are pressure decisions, and we have to accept the fact that limited time will squeeze us into a less-than-desirable pattern of analysis and action. In this regard, time may constrain not only the alternatives but also the entire decision-making process.

## RESPONSIBILITY AND LEADERSHIP

An anonymous quotation goes, "It's all right to pull decisions out of a hat as long as you're wearing it." While this statement is only partially true (it is *not* usually all right to pull decisions out of a hat) the point about responsibility is well made. If you are assuming the authority to make a decision, you should be charged with equivalent responsibility. In making decisions for your department you are consistent with your charge as a supervisor; you are responsible for the output and actions of your employees. However, it is not your place to make a decision with which employees other than your own or the supervisors of other departments must comply. In accepting a given amount of responsibility you ordinarily acquire decision-making authority consistent with that responsibility. No supervisor's decisions should exceed the limits of designated authority.

Also on the subject of authority, when you are delegating certain decision-making powers to some of your employees, be sure to extend authority and responsibility in equivalent amounts. Authority and responsibility are each weakened, if not negated entirely, by the absence of the other. How much decision-making authority you delegate to your employees will be a direct reflection of your leadership style. Generally the autocratic or authoritarian leader will prefer to retain all such authority while the participative leader will involve the employees in shaping and choosing decision alternatives.

## PROBLEM AWARENESS: OFTEN AN ESSENTIAL PRE-STEP

In addition to presenting a potentially serious management dilemma, the "Situation" presented at the beginning of the chapter holds implications for what was described as the initial step of the decision-making process, identifying the problem. Whether we wish to say it was Helen Grove's fault for failing to pick up on the potentially serious issue behind what June Weston was saying or we choose to blame June for not being specific, Helen suddenly finds herself in a critical position—she is pressured to make a decision when she has insufficient information available to her. It is all well and good to suggest analyzing the apparent problem and deciding it is indeed the problem rather than a symptom of some greater difficulty, but Helen is in no position to do this if she is not even aware there is a problem to begin with. An essential pre–decision-making step, then, is awareness of the likely existence of a problem that causes the decision maker to apply conscious effort to determine what may be wrong.

As to alternatives, Helen has at least the following three possible courses of action immediately identifiable:

1. Helen can simply give June what she is asking for. Although doing so could resolve the problem at once, it also could build in added cost that may not be fully justified, and doing so could suggest to Helen's other direct-reporting supervisors that the way to get anything from her is to become the "squeaky wheel."

2. Helen can call June's bluff, waiting until the week is over to see whether she makes good on her threat to quit. However, this would turn a problem that deserves a collaborative approach into an ego contest. Also, failing to do something during the intervening 4 days to address a potentially serious problem is to encourage a bad situation to become even worse.

3. Helen can acknowledge the problem and the fact that she missed the earlier signals indicating its likely existence and then begin working immediately with June to study the situation. There remains the risk that June may resign anyway, because Helen cannot realistically hope to completely analyze the problem and propose and implement a solution in just 4 days. However, by demonstrating an honest effort now that June has her attention, Helen could draw June into the problem-solving process and this may be enough to take the edge off June's frustration.

The pressure was of course introduced in the form of an employee ultimatum, and what is at risk is Helen's employees' regard for her authority and capability as a manager. If this one employee can blackmail Helen into granting what she wants by threatening her, other staff also may conclude they can use this approach to get what they want. But if Helen digs in her heels and refuses to move, as in the second option above, she is likely to be seen as ignoring a significant problem. Since Helen may be equally criticized for quick action or no action, the only realistic alternative is to act out of an interest in determining the problem's real causes so they may be corrected.

## NO MAGIC FORMULA

It is possible to create valid guidelines for making many decisions. We do it all the time: We generate rules, regulations, policies, and procedures to guide our decisions. However, in spite of what a few determined bureaucratic leaders may believe, it is not possible to anticipate all contingencies and premake all decisions. It is not possible to cover everything with rules that say, in effect, "When this situation arises, apply this remedy." Good supervisory decisions will remain a matter of arriving at a proper emphasis on all decision elements through judgment based on facts and figures, knowledge, experience, advice, intuition, and insight.

## REVIEW QUESTIONS

1. Why does the exercise of the no-decision option sometimes represent the most consequential alternative?
2. With a simple example, explain the difference between a practical constraint and an absolute constraint.
3. What should be the principal determinant of how much time and effort you put into a decision situation?
4. Explain how any of us become "self-programmed" to condense or compress steps of the decision-making process for decisions made regularly.
5. How would you define *risk* and *uncertainty* as separate but related factors in decision-making?

## CASE: THE NEW COPY MACHINE

You have several offices within your responsibility. It is up to you to decide on a new copy machine for general use. The need for the machine has already been established, but you do not yet know which particular machine to select.

You have investigated several machines and discarded a number of them because they do not do your kind of work or because their costs were beyond the bounds of anything you could possibly afford. You are left with three machines from which to choose. All three will give you the kinds of copies you want, and all three will fit within your department's available space and are consistent with available power sources.

Machine A is available for $1,500. It must be purchased outright; it is not available on a lease. It will last at least 5 years in normal operation.

Machine B costs $3,000. It is also available on an 8-year lease at $500 per year. The estimated useful life of machine B is 8 years.

Machine C costs $2,500. This machine is also available on a lease at a cost of $450 per year for a term of 6 years. Machine C has an estimated useful life of 6 years.

### Questions

1. Based on the very limited information you are given above, which of the three machines might you select? Why?
2. Would you alter your decision if you were constrained by the necessity to limit expenditures because of a severe cash-flow problem?
3. What additional information would you like to have before making a decision? (In other words, what important information has been omitted?)

## CHAPTER 18

# Management of Change: Resistance Is Where You Find It

*Have no fear of change as such and, on the other hand,*
*no liking for it merely for its own sake.*
—*Robert Moses*

## CHAPTER OBJECTIVES

☛ Establish a perspective on "change" as an unavoidable feature of the work environment.

☛ Consider the effects of change on the pursuit of health care careers.

☛ Examine some significant potential changes in the supervisor's role driven by the rapidly evolving health care delivery environment.

☛ Identify likely sources of employee resistance to change.

☛ Suggest guidelines for the supervisor to consider in managing change and minimizing employee resistance.

## SITUATION: DELAYED CHANGE OF COMMAND

With full notice to administration and with the knowledge of his staff, the information systems manager left for a better paying position elsewhere. Within the department it was assumed that Mr. Smith, the most senior systems analyst and the departing manager's frequent back-up, would become manager. However, a week passed and no appointment was made.

The initial week became several weeks. The finance director, to whom the information systems manager normally reported, began to make the administrative decisions for information systems. Mr. Smith was left the growing task of overseeing the functions of the group in addition to keeping his regular work under control.

The department became aware that the hospital was advertising for an information systems manager and that the controller was conducting interviews. However, no one was hired. Finally, after six months without a manager, Mr. Smith was elevated to information systems manager and was immediately authorized to hire a person to fill the vacancy caused by his promotion.

*Instructions*

As you proceed through the chapter, think about how you would address the following questions:

1. During the period without a manager, how would you assess Mr. Smith's position from the department's viewpoint? The finance director's viewpoint? Mr. Smith's own viewpoint?

2. How would you assess Mr. Smith's position after he was finally made manager?

## THE NATURE OF CHANGE

### The Only Constant

We have heard it said over and over again that the only constant in this world is change, and often we do feel, with good reason, that there are few permanent features in our everyday world. It is also no secret that much seemingly accelerated change is a product of recent times, so much so that change has become the dominant force in our lives.

Unswerving stability, once the hallmark of our existence, is a thing of the past. No longer can we rely on the same dependable characteristics of living, the same technology and the same social structures and values, from generation to generation. Consider, for example, the technology of daily living. Compare the era of the Roman Empire with the period of Colonial America and consider how little true change occurred in some 2,000 years.

Methods of transportation remained about the same—if one wanted to go somewhere one did so in a conveyance with two or four wheels pulled by an animal. Means of communication differed little, at least in effectiveness if not in availability. (It is true that the impact of the printing press was felt in Colonial America, but its effects were not widespread because the general literacy rate remained low.) Whether one lived in the days of the Caesars or in the days of America's founders, cooking, heating, lighting, and plumbing would have been accomplished in about the same way, and in both societies slavery was an accepted practice. It is perhaps a sad commentary on human development to point out that one area in which noticeable advancements were made was warfare (since gunpowder was introduced along the way and refined in several "practical" uses). It seems we had learned how to end life more efficiently without learning how to improve it appreciably.

### How Times Have Changed

Over the years, technology—our total storehouse of knowledge—remained fairly constant until the late 1820s and the advent of the railroad locomotive. The invention of the locomotive improved transportation and began to draw people closer together in practical terms, thus launching a period of steady technological growth that lasted more than a century. From about 1830 to the mid 1940s—approximately 115 years—total knowledge increased about five times over.

It might seem surprising to learn that knowledge could multiply some five times within 115 years after remaining practically static for thousands and thousands of years. That increase, however, pales by comparison with the rate of knowledge growth experienced since about 1945. With the splitting of the atom concurrent with giant strides in electronics followed by advances in every field of endeavor and the opening up of numerous new fields, technology has literally exploded. Recent technologic growth has been such that it cannot be satisfactorily measured; new knowledge is accruing so rapidly on so many fronts that nothing will stand still long enough to be measured. We need not be overly impressed with the fivefold growth occurring in the 115 years preceding 1945; in the relatively brief time that has elapsed since the mid 1940s, technology, that is, total knowledge, has grown by a factor of thousands!

In few areas of life has the change wrought by technologic advancement been more evident than in medicine. Consider some of the advancements that have occurred within the lifetimes of many who are still in their working years. Penicillin was discovered, giving us the ability to combat many previously uncontrollable infections. The Polio vaccine was developed, closing the door on the horrors of the epidemics of the 1940s. Surgical techniques once thought impossible now regularly save lives. Consider also the implications of technologic change on people employed in the delivery of health care. A standout illustration was provided by Michael Crichton in his book *Five Patients*, in which he described the use of 26 diagnostic tests on a critically ill patient in 1970. Of these 26 tests, 24 did not exist 60 years earlier. Further, 10 of these 24 tests were less than 30 years old, and all 26 tests had been improved on, some of them several times over, within the 30 years prior to 1970.[1] Thirty years can be a significant part of a working career; if you had worked in a clinical laboratory for the three decades from 1940 to 1970 you would have experienced the need to change, learn, and grow to adapt to the constantly changing demands of laboratory technology. Technologies that were not commonly available when this book's first edition was published—for example, magnetic resonance imaging (MRI)—have proliferated and matured and are already being joined or followed by newer technologies that will perform the same functions in improved fashion.

The point to be appreciated is that most of what we must work with, and most of what we have, use, and enjoy, was developed within the lifetimes of the generations now alive. Careers are not stable. We find ourselves faced with constant change as a way of life; we must continually upgrade our knowledge and skills simply to stay even with the advances made in our own fields.

### Is There Any Security?

We tend to equate stability with security. However, we are undeniably among the first generations on earth to experience massive change within our own lifetimes. In the past there was security in being unchanging and inflexible—in adopting a set of values, a pattern of living, and an approach to our work and pursuing these for life. However, this behavior is no longer appropriate. The times in which we live suggest that our security now lies in our ability to be flexible and adaptable.

### INFLEXIBILITY OR RESISTANCE?

Failure to keep up with legitimate change in our fields can severely diminish our effectiveness as producers. If you are in the early stages of your career, chances are that half or more of what you do, or half or more of the tasks your employees perform, will change completely in the next 20 years. Today's methods, techniques, and requirements will give way to new and generally more sophisticated counterparts. It will become more and more likely that the work you are called on to perform in the latter stages of your career will bear little resemblance to the duties you performed when you first entered the health care work force. This suggests that flexibility could be essential to your continued usefulness to the organization.

Most of us are resistant to change to some extent. Sometimes our resistance is rightly founded; restraint is a stabilizer, a needed counterbalance to frivolous disruption and change for the sake of change. However, much resistance has its basis in human nature alone and forces the basic needs of the individual to take precedence over the common good.

Think for a moment of what your own reactions may have been to seemingly wild, "crackpot" ideas, both inside and outside of health care: Actually perform surgery on a living heart? ("Impossible.") Transplant an organ from one human to another? ("Never work.")

Most of us are not instant believers in drastically new techniques or in the workability of marvelous new gadgets. Often it is because we do not have sufficient grasp of the principles on which these advancements are based, and just as often it is because we are reluctant to accept principles or theories that have yet to be proved. Perhaps we fail to appreciate that much of today's technology that we take for granted was, in its day, subject to resistance of almost destructive proportions. When the Wright Brothers were still trying to get their plane off the ground, many supposedly knowledgeable people of the day, engineers and scientists among them, were publicly labeling powered flight as impossible. More than once the telephone was branded an out-and-out fraud, with one critic going so far as to say that "Even if it were possible to transmit the human voice over metallic wires, the thing would be of no practical value." Likewise, the automobile and the railroad locomotive had their detractors. We view such past attacks on today's accepted technology as on the order of someone saying to Columbus: "Don't try it, Chris—you'll sail off the edge." However, when our initial response to a seemingly far-out idea is "It can't be done," we are reacting in the same way.

Consider how many ideas suggested on the job are disposed of on the spot with supervisors' reactions like: "There's no budget for that," "The boss won't like it," "The medical staff would kill me," "They won't let us do it," and "The old way's good enough for me." We have so many ready-made reasons why not that it often requires an extremely compelling why to get through to us.

## CHANGING WITH AN EVOLVING ROLE

As an industry, health care has for some time been accustomed to constant technologic change, and certainly business overall has seen continuing social and legislative change. In addition to these previously visible sources of change, the past few decades have brought a number of additional changes, some approaching traumatic, driven by economic concerns related to the alarming growth of health care costs. The health care industry has been put in a position of attempting to provide all citizens with the best available care from an ever-expanding base of medical technology while holding down the consumption of financial resources in doing so. In other words, the industry is expected to improve access to care, maintain or improve quality, and hold costs down.

Like it or not, old paradigms are falling and health care delivery is changing (see Chapter 1). Thus, the delivery mechanisms, and certainly the organizations that deliver care, are changing as well. This has been increasingly evident in the amount of organizational restructuring that has become commonplace in health care. All forms of restructuring, whether via merger, acquisition, affiliation, downsizing, internal reorganizing, or whatever, as well as the development of completely new delivery models are fraught with change, and for the most part it is change that affects the supervisor.

The ways in which the supervisory role is changing for many may include some or all of the areas listed below.

### Increased Scope of Responsibility

Because of changes in care delivery, changes in organizational structure, and cost-reduction measures, most supervisors can expect to be required to do more than they previously had to do. With the flattening of the organization—the elimination of intervening layers of management (see Chapter 1)—the individual supervisor often finds that he or she must now make decisions that were previously made at a higher level in the structure. Also, the various forms of restructuring usually result in fewer managers rather than more, so invariably the supervisors remaining in place following reorganization find that they have inherited a few functions once associated with positions that no longer exist.

### Increased Span of Control

Usually related to increased scope of responsibility is increased span of control. As the total numbers of supervisors and managers decrease, and as in many cases departments or units are combined, the supervisors who remain discover they now oversee more functions and activities, larger physical areas, and greater numbers of employees. In many cases one's title and compensation will remain the same or very nearly the same, but for all practical purposes the job will have been expanded.

### Shared Management

As more and more formerly independent health care providers come together via merger, acquisition, or affiliation into health systems and other entities, it is becoming more common to encounter supervisors who are shared among separate facilities. The advantages of such restructuring include savings based on economies of scale. Consider, for example, two hospitals in the same community, now merged into one organization, sharing a pharmacy manager or a billing supervisor instead of each having to employ their own. Working in the shared mode places a whole new set of requirements on the supervisor, not the least of which is the necessity to constantly balance the needs of one site with those of the other. Or, on the other end of the shared management phenomenon, the individual supervisor may experience no significant change in job structure but may nevertheless be forced to operate much more independently than before because the manager to whom this supervisor reports is now shared between facilities.

It is stressed elsewhere in this book as well as in this chapter that flexibility is becoming increasingly important in helping a working individual attain some measure of employment security. Flexibility is also likely to be viewed as one of the hallmarks of the successful health care supervisor in the coming decade. The supervisor who is able to flex in the face of a steady stream of change over which the individual has no control is the supervisor who is more likely to be relied upon in the future.

The emerging mode of operation for the health care supervisor involves more overall responsibility, more work to do, more decisions to make, and fewer helping hands and other resources to accomplish this. These circumstances suggest that personal planning, as reflected in the supervisor's approach to the job (see Chapter 7) will become more important. One of the most valuable skills today's supervisor can develop is the ability to effectively reorder priorities "on the run," to achieve a state in which at any given time he or she virtually by nature concentrates on the problems and issues of highest priority.

## WHY RESISTANCE?

People resist change primarily because it disturbs their equilibrium and threatens their sense of security. For the most part we all seek equilibrium with our surroundings, that balance of values, activities, and environment with which we can be most comfortable. To some people that equilibrium is a comfortable, dependable rut; to others, equilibrium is a pattern of change, but it is their change, ordered in their way. With equilibrium we find a measure of security, and we shift and move against daily forces in small ways to reestablish continually and maintain equilibrium just as surely as water continually seeks its own level. However, change coming from outside of the person intrudes, and equilibrium is disturbed and security is threatened, so resistance results.

In work organizations, most instances of resistance can be traced to one or more of the following general causes:

- organizational changes, in which departments are altered or interdepartmental relationships or management reporting relationships are changed
- management changes, in which new management assumes control of an organization or subunit
- new methods and procedures, indicating that people are expected to do new and different work or accomplish old tasks in new ways
- job restructuring, requiring that tasks be added to or be deleted from people's jobs
- new equipment, representing new technology or technological departures from equipment previously used

Brief consideration of these five general causes can give one an appreciation of the effects that the health care industry's emphasis on merger, acquisition, affiliation, and such is having on employees and their tendency to resist change. Look at the general causes of employee resistance, and then look at what happens when, for example, two organizations merge. Significant organizational changes are a virtual given; extensive management changes are likely to occur; and job restructuring and new methods and procedures are expected to follow. And in addition the reality of a merger or other organizational combination can give rise to the fear of job loss on the part of many employees. This all adds up to a maximum threat to employee equilibrium.

If you can accept the claim that change disturbs equilibrium and threatens security, then go a step further and accept one additional factor that seems to be borne out in practice: it is the unknown that people really fear most. It is the unknown that actually disturbs equilibrium and threatens security. When your employees seem to be resisting change it is usually because all of the implications of the change are not known, understood, or appreciated.

However, most available ways of improving supervisory effectiveness also involve changing the way things are accomplished in your department. To have improvement you usually need to have change—change in ways of doing things and especially change in attitude. In the last analysis the success of any particular change depends almost completely on employee attitude.

Our consideration of change, then, brings us once again to consideration of the supervisor's approach in dealing with employees.

## DEADLY DELAYS: REVISITING MR. SMITH

The previous section reviewed a number of the kinds of changes that can upset employees. To each of these we can legitimately add consideration of another element: the length of time that the "unknown" hangs over employees' heads. The opening "Situation" involves a management change, and a management change usually gives rise to fears of changes in other areas including organization, methods and procedures, job restructuring, and the like. Often, changes in management can be the most upsetting kind of change in terms of impact on employees.

Consider the effects of delay in the circumstances in which Mr. Smith finds himself. At the beginning of the period without a manager, most employees in the department would look favorably upon Smith because they would be assuming that Smith is going to get the job. Some might experience growing annoyance with higher management as days become weeks and weeks become months, but as time wears on some will begin to wonder what is "wrong" with Smith in higher management's eyes. As time passes more staff will experience creeping doubt as to whether Smith is right for the job, especially when they learn of the external recruiting efforts.

The finance director's regard for Smith was apparently not sufficiently strong to allow him to comfortably promote Smith in timely fashion. External recruiting reinforces this view; the controller may be thinking that perhaps Smith could do the job but there might be someone better available on the job market. Since the process is allowed to drag out so long with Smith working under continuing uncertainty, the controller could be regarding Smith as a passive individual who will tolerate less-than-normally acceptable circumstances forever without speaking up.

Smith himself is likely to experience growing doubt as the weeks turn into months and as he learns about the outside recruiting efforts. Chances are he will worry increasingly about the regard in which he is held by his superiors.

After Smith is finally made manager, he enters the role "officially" with all of the doubts and uncertainties suggested above and with all the baggage accumulated during the six months. If he is strong enough to rise above the baggage and overcome his deficit starting position, then he could prevail. However, he has to prove himself to an extent that would not have been necessary had the promotion been timely. Because of his deficit starting position, Smith, unless he happens to be exceptionally capable, may well have been set up for failure.

## THE SUPERVISOR'S APPROACH

As a supervisor interested in implementing a particular change, you have three avenues along which to approach your employees. You can (1) tell them what to do, (2) convince them to do it, or (3) involve them in planning for the change.

### Tell Them

Specific orders—commands, if you will—have been described as one of the marks of the autocratic or authoritarian leader. The boss is the boss, a giver of orders who either makes a decision and orders its implementation or relays without expansion or clarification the orders that come down from above.

The authoritarian approach is sometimes necessary; sometimes it is the only option available under the circumstances. However, the "tell them" approach is the approach most likely to generate resistance and should be used in only those rare instances when it is the only means available.

### Convince Them

In most instances, including those in which the change in question is a hard edict from the upper reaches of the organization, you have room for explanation and persuasion. At the very least you should endeavor to make each employee aware of the reasons for the change and the necessity for its implementation. It may be that you have to champion the cause of something clearly distasteful (to you as well as to some employees) because it may be good for the institution overall or good for the patients or even perhaps because it is mandated by new government regulations. Your employees may not like what they are called on to do, but they are more likely to respond as you need them to respond if they know and understand the why of the change.

Your employees deserve information, and information serves you well because it often removes the shadow of the unknown from your employees.

Few if any changes cannot be approached by this "selling" means, and the authoritarian "tell them" approach should be reserved for those occasions when someone clearly cannot be "sold."

## Involve Them

Whenever possible, and especially as it affects the way they perform their assigned tasks, involve your employees in shaping the details of the change. It has been proven that employees are far more likely to understand and comply when they have a role in determining the form and substance of the change. For instance, if you are considering new equipment and have sufficient lead time, get the input of the people who will have to work with the equipment once it is in place. If the institution is to be expanded or remodeled and your department will change its physical space and arrangement, get your employees' opinions on where things should be located and how work should flow. Through involvement, change can become a positive force. Your employees will be more likely to comply because the change is partly "theirs." And there is another potential benefit to involvement as well: Your employees know the work in ways that you may perhaps never know it. You supervise a number of tasks, some of which you may have done once yourself. However, your employees do, in hands-on fashion, those tasks that you only supervise. Thus your employees know the details of the work far better than you and are in a much better position to provide the basis for positive change in task performance.

It is suggested here, as elsewhere, that participative or consultative approaches to management are the best ways of getting things done through your employees. The most effective ways of reducing or removing the fear of the unknown make full use of communication and involvement.

## Guidelines for Effective Management of Change

- Plan thoroughly. Fully evaluate the potential change, examining all implications in regard to its potential impact on your department and the total organization.
- Communicate fully. Completely communicate the change, starting early, and be sure that your employees are not taken by surprise. Make it two-way communication; pave the way for your employees' involvement by soliciting their comments or suggestions.
- Convince employees. As necessary take steps to convince your employees of the value and benefits of the proposed change. When possible, appeal to employee self-interest. Let them know how they stand to benefit from the change and how it may perhaps make their work easier.
- Involve employees when possible. Recognizing that it is not possible to involve employees in all matters—again, for instance, you cannot do much about a mandate from above—involvement is nevertheless possible on many occasions. Be especially aware of the value of your employees as a source of job knowledge, and tap this source not only for the acceptance of change but for the development of genuine improvements as well.

- Monitor implementation. As with the implementation of any decision, monitor the implementation of any change, especially one involving employee task performance, until the new way is established as part of the accepted work pattern. A new work method, dependent for its success on willing adoption by individual employees, can be introduced in a burst of enthusiasm only to die of its own weight as the novelty wears off and old habits return. New habits are not easily formed, and your employees need the help you can furnish through conscientious follow-up.

## TRUE RESISTANCE

Resistance to change will never be completely eliminated. People possess differing degrees of flexibility and exhibit varying degrees of acceptance of ideas that are not purely their own. However, involvement helps, and you will eventually discover, if you have not already done so, that most employees are willing to cooperate and genuinely want to contribute. Beyond involvement, however, communication is the key. Full knowledge and understanding of what is happening and why are the strongest forces the supervisor can bring to bear on the problems of resistance to change. Ultimately you will discover that it is not change that people resist so much as they resist being changed.

---

## REVIEW QUESTIONS

1. Describe your understanding of the differences between *resistance* and *inflexibility.*
2. In the present-day health care environment as you see it, what are the two or three changes that have been most upsetting to employees?
3. Provide an example of a situation in which you must tell employees what to do rather than solicit their input. Explain why you must tell instead of convince or involve.
4. Why is change in the management of a department one of the most upsetting changes that can occur affecting the work group?
5. Explain the statement: *It is not change that people resist so much as they resist being changed.*
6. How can a change that may be considered positive, such as moving into new quarters or acquiring all new equipment, still be upsetting and create resistance from some?

---

## CASE: SURPRISE!

On Monday morning when the business office employees arrived at the hospital they immediately noticed the apparent absence of the office manager. This was not unusual; the manager was frequently absent on Monday. However, he rarely failed to call his department when he would not be there—but on this day he still had not called by noon.

Shortly after lunch the two working supervisors in the business office were summoned to the administrator's office. There they were told that the office manager was no longer employed by the hospital. They, the two supervisors, were told to look after things for the current week and that a new manager, already secured, would be starting the following Monday. All the supervisors were told about the new manager was that it was somebody from outside of the hospital.

## Questions

1. What was right or wrong about the manner in which the change in business office manager was made?
2. What would you suppose to be the attitudes of the business office staff upon hearing of the change?
3. With what attitudes do you suppose the staff will receive the new manager?
4. In what other ways might this change have been approached?

---

**NOTE**

1. Michael Crichton, *Five Patients* (New York: Alfred A. Knopf, 1970).

## CHAPTER 19

# Communication: Not by Spoken Words Alone

*I have made this letter rather long because I have not had time to make it shorter.*
*—Blaise Pascal*

## CHAPTER OBJECTIVES

☛ Review the essential functions of written communication in the supervisor's job.

☛ Provide guidelines for writing clearer, more concise letters and memoranda.

☛ Examine old habits in writing and suggest why some of these habits should be changed.

## SITUATION: THE WILSON LETTER, OR, THE AGENTS OF WORDINESS

Dear Mr. Wilson:

In the past the Board of Examiners has approved credit for courses designed and taught by the Management Services Division of the State Hospital Association. You will find enclosed an outline of a 3-hour seminar, which is designed primarily for boards of directors. We have discovered in the initial presentations that administrators also are extremely interested in attending this course along with their boards of directors. Since many of the administrators involved have nursing home administrator's licenses, and are responsible for long-term care facilities, a request has been made to me to apply for continuing education credit by the Board of Examiners.

Please consider this letter a formal request for approval for continuing education credit by the Board of Examiners of Nursing Home Administrators. If you need further information, I would be most happy to send whatever you require.

I am looking forward to hearing from you, and thank you in advance for your consideration.

Regards,

*Instructions*

At any time you wish while going through this chapter, revise the Wilson letter by cutting out all words that can be considered unnecessary and rearranging thoughts and condensing passages as necessary. When finished, compare the length of your finished letter with the length of the original and explain why your new version represents improvement over the original.

## THE WRITTEN WORD

Letters, memoranda, and other written communications are essential in the operation of any organization. Although it seems at times that we have to put up with far more paperwork than we care to handle—and this is certainly true in health care organizations where the paper tiger has become a beast of considerable proportions—much of this paper is nevertheless necessary. Many organizations function quite well in spite of hefty amounts of paperwork, but just try to run an organization without paper.

Written communications perform several important functions. They are used to advise (or inform), explain, request, convince, and provide permanent records.

However, the written word possesses a serious drawback: A piece of writing is essentially a one-way communication, providing no opportunity for immediate feedback in the development and transmission of the message. As you write you are unable to amend, correct, clarify, or defend what you are writing based on the reaction of your audience.

Because of the one-way nature of this means of communication, the need for clarity in writing becomes critical. However, clarity is the attribute most often lacking in written communications in the organizational setting.

## SOURCES OF HELP

Far too many letters and memos resemble low-grade Thanksgiving turkeys: they are hefty and meaty looking, but when you cut into them you discover they are mostly just stuffing. This chapter will present some guidelines aimed at helping you take some of the stuffing out of your letters and memos. However, although our guidelines will help improve the clarity of your writing, no single chapter in a work such as this will make you a good writer, especially if you experience basic difficulties with grammar, punctuation, and usage. To become a writer of effective business communications you need two things: (1) the desire to improve your writing and (2) the help provided by practically oriented teachers of business writing and good references on writing.

Numerous books on writing techniques are available. Several are described in the bibliography at the end of this book, but if you were to utilize only one of them, give first consideration to *The Elements of Style* by William Strunk Jr. and E.B. White. This book has fewer than 100 pages yet contains more solid, usable advice per page than any other writing book available. It is a great place to start when you decide to get help in improving your writing.

## GUIDELINES FOR BETTER LETTERS AND MEMOS

Conscientious use of the following guidelines will help you improve your writing in a minimum amount of time.

### Write for a Specific Audience

Your letter or memo may be going to one person, or it may be intended for several people. You will need to decide to whom, specifically, you are writing.

The person who will receive your communication, that person for whom your message is primarily intended, is your primary audience. However, you may also have a sizeable secondary audience—others who will receive, read, and perhaps make use of your communication.

Many managers seem to believe they should write in such a way that any-one picking up a particular document will completely understand its contents. However, this is a difficult task at best, and it becomes nearly impossible when there is a sizeable secondary audience including people of widely vary-ing backgrounds and different degrees of familiarity with the subject.

Write specifically for your primary audience. You cannot successfully write for everyone. If you have trouble identifying your primary audience, sift through the likely recipients of the message with this question in mind: Who of all these people needs this information for decision-making purposes? Often your primary audience will consist of a single person, but it could just as well be two, three, or more people. If you are a nursing supervisor writing about the need for specific change in departmental policy, perhaps all of nursing management should be aware of the issue. However, it would be your immedi-ate superior, for example, the director of nursing service, who would be the primary audience because it is in that position where the decision-making authority concerning departmental policy is located. On the other hand, if the director of nursing service is releasing a new policy with which all supervisors are expected to comply, then the memo announcing the policy will have all supervisors as its primary audience.

Use what you know about your primary audience in deciding how to struc-ture your message. Can you do it on a friendly, first-name basis? Must it be a formal letter, or will a brief, casual note suffice? Does this person seem to pre-fer detail, or would a concise overview be enough? Let your knowledge of your primary audience suggest how you should communicate.

## Avoid Unneeded Words

We could fill volumes discussing the subject of unneeded words. However, understanding and exercising one simple concept—that of the "zero word"— will take you a long way toward removing excess words from your writing.

Every word in a given piece of writing can be placed in one of three cate-gories: necessary, optional, or zero.

A necessary word is one that is essential to getting your basic message across. An optional word, as the name suggests, can be used at your option to qualify or modify a necessary word or phrase. A zero word contributes nothing to the message and should be removed.

Consider the following sentence:

*Harvey is certainly an exceptionally intelligent man.*

This sentence contains only three necessary words: *Harvey is intelligent.* Note, however, that even with all zero words and optional words removed, what remains is still a sentence.

The word *exceptionally* is the only optional word in the sentence. It may well make a difference in what you are trying to communicate to say that "Harvey is exceptionally intelligent" rather than simply, "Harvey is intelligent." While this is perfectly acceptable, watch out for the excess use of such modifiers and qualifiers; after a while they not only become tiresome but also begin to lose their impact.

The sentence includes three zero words: *certainly, an,* and *man.* At least they are zero under normal circumstances—assuming that Harvey is a man. Still, if Harvey were anything else, a dog, for instance, we would say so. The word *an* is there for structural reasons, and *certainly* is certainly unnecessary, since in terms of what we are trying to convey, Harvey either is or is not intelligent and *certainly* does not make it any more binding. Zero words abound in most business communication. However, they are relatively easy to get rid of with conscientious editing.

This is not to say, however, that the zero word infests all writing to the same extent. In many uses of written language, writers are attempting to tell stories or create moods or impressions. However, in writing an interoffice memo you are not writing a poem, a novel, or even a textbook. Your primary objective is to get your message across with clarity. A memo can be correct in every sense of grammar and usage although stripped of every zero word.

Select a sample of your writing and go hunting for zero words. If in doubt about a word, sound out the sentence without it. If the sentence remains a sentence and continues to carry the basic message you wish it to carry, then the word is probably a zero word. Chances are you will find a surprising number of zero words, among which you are likely to find many uses of the, that, of, and other simple words.

Often we use unnecessary words in bunches, applying several-word phrases to do the work that could be done by one or two words. This is especially common in business correspondence in which some phrases have reached cliché proportions. Consider these examples:

- the use of "due to the fact that" when the writer could simply say "because"
- saying "be in a position to" when all that is needed is "can"
- saying "in the state of California" when "in California" says the same
- using the stuffy "with reference to" when the job can be done by "about"

Avoid roundabout phrases in your writing. They simply add bulk to your communication without adding clarity. In fact, such words not only fail to add clarity but also can actually harm your message by surrounding and obscuring your real meaning.

## Use Simple Words

Almost every technical and professional field has its own jargon, with jargon being defined in the dictionary as "the technical terminology or characteristic idiom of a special activity or group." However, this is the second definition of jargon carried in several dictionaries—the first is "confused unintelligible language."

It is one thing if you happen to be a laboratory technologist writing to an audience of other laboratory technologists. In this case you can get away with the free use of the language of your field. However, the employees of the health care institution usually include highly educated, specialized professionals, unskilled and semiskilled workers, and numerous levels between. Also, an institution's staff includes people in many different but medically related fields, all of which have their own "languages."

Medical and technical professionals are among the worst offenders when it comes to sprinkling their correspondence with jargon. However, the "in language" of a field should not be allowed to cut across departmental lines to any considerable extent. As already suggested, technologist-to-technologist may be a safe channel for the use of jargon. However, technologist-to-finance director is a channel calling for a completely different approach. Again, consider your primary audience (in this case, the recipient's background and familiarity with your subject) in preparing to write.

If medical and technical professionals are the worst offenders when it comes to jargon, then administrators, administrative staffers, consultants, and other managerial professionals are the worst offenders when it comes to made-up words. Management is cluttered with once-sensible words to which have been appended the suffixes -ize and -wise. So now we stylize, prioritize, and regularize and speak of concepts as timewise or wordwise, for example. Consider, for instance, the increasing number of people in business who show an apparent fondness for the likes of operationalization. Interestingly, the clumsy operationalization has in recent years, through use, become a legitimate word by its inclusion in several dictionaries. However, this legitimacy makes it no less awkward and overblown.

Coined words and barbarisms of legitimate words are much of the clutter that clouds communication. These can also get us into trouble when such a language twist creates an unintended meaning. For example, a young administrative staffer, assigned to study systems and staffing in a pathology department, referred on paper to the staff of the department of pathology as the "pathological staff." The department's director, who was sensitive to the analysis in the first place, flew into a rage after reading the word pathological—literally referring to the department's employees as the sick staff—and it was days before the remainder of the report was read.

### Edit and Rewrite

During editing and rewriting, the zero words, the roundabout phrases, and other verbal stuffing should come out of your correspondence. There are few pieces of writing that cannot be improved by careful editing or perhaps rewriting. Very few people—and this statement includes professional writers—can go from thought to a completely effective finished message in a single try. In fact, professional writers probably do far more editing and rewriting than do most writers of day-to-day business correspondence. Therein lies the problem: much of what is wrong with our writing is wrong simply because we do not put enough time into it. As this chapter's opening quotation suggests, given a particular message to get across it generally takes more time to write a shorter letter than it does to write a longer one.

If you are thinking that better writing is too time consuming, that you would have to double your correspondence time to provide that extra reading through every letter and memo you write, think also of the cost of misunderstanding. Have you ever had to spend valuable time and effort smoothing out some problem that developed because a written message was misunderstood? You can edit many memos in the time it takes to solve a couple of knotty problems arising from missed communication.

## CHANGING OLD HABITS

In our day-to-day writing we are often unconsciously still trying to please dear Mrs. Smith who taught us English "way back when." Even in the 1940s, 1950s, and 1960s, we were taught how to write letters that sounded as though they were lifted from a Victorian secretarial handbook.

Most of what has been said so far in this chapter is "legal" in terms of what Mrs. Smith taught us. However, there are additional practices that would have been guaranteed to get us into trouble with the teacher even though they will definitely help us improve our business writing today.

### Be Friendly and Personal

Feel free to use personal pronouns in your letters and memos. We use *I, you,* and *we* when we talk to each other, so why not use them when we write? However, many of us were taught to avoid personal pronouns, and this warning sticks with us. We were once taught never to say *I.* For clarity and directness, however, *I* is far preferable to archaic affectations such as *the undersigned* or *the author.*

Most of your letters and memos should sound as you sound when you talk. Once you achieve that conversational tone, your correspondence will be direct, friendly, and personal.

### Use Direct, Active Language

Ask direct questions when the situation warrants it. You may have been taught to go out of your way to avoid questions and thus say things like, "Let me know whether or not you will attend." It is much more direct to ask, "Will you attend?"

Keep your statements in the active voice, avoiding the likes of, "The contract was signed by your representative." How much cleaner it is to say, "Your representative signed the contract."

### Use Contractions

Use *don't, wouldn't, can't, shouldn't,* etc., even though the use of contractions may have been taboo in your education. Contractions contribute to the natural, conversational tone you should be working to achieve. Even so, many writers of business correspondence squeeze the contractions out of their writing without realizing what they are doing. The result is a formalistic style, stilted and stuffy, that serves only to create more distance between writer and reader.

### Write Short Sentences

You are not William Faulkner, who could get away with writing an opening sentence of some 180-plus words. Neither are you writing the Great American Novel.

Although it is difficult to lay down any firm guidelines for sentence length, consider that any time you create a sentence much more than 20 words long you are edging into questionable territory. Some teachers of business writing have suggested 20 words as maximum sentence length; others suggest that 14 or 15 words be considered maximum. Regardless, it is safe to say that the longer the sentence, the more opportunities there are for misunderstanding.

### Forget Old Taboos about Prepositions and Conjunctions

It is likely that most of us were repeatedly and sternly warned against committing two terrible "no-nos": ending a sentence with a preposition and starting a sentence with a conjunction.

A story is told about Winston Churchill and the rule concerning prepositions. When reminded that it was improper to end a sentence with a preposition, Churchill replied, "This is something up with which I shall not put." An extreme example, for sure, but it cleanly illustrates how far out of the way you may be led in search of so-called structure. Go ahead and say, "This is something I won't put up with."

A sure-fire way to lose points with many teachers is to begin sentences with conjunctions, especially *and* and *but*. Fortunately this archaic prohibition has been successfully shattered by professional writers. Of course if every other sentence in your letter begins with and, then you will have created a different kind of monster. However, the freedom to open a sentence in this manner can save you from long sentences and needless repetition.

### Say What You Want To Say and Stop

Avoid starting your letter by repeating what was said in the letter you are answering. Also, avoid opening with standard stuffing such as "In response to yours of the . . ."

Simply say what you are trying to say. If the point of your letter is to tell a potential supplier that the bid was not accepted, do not spend two paragraphs describing the evaluation process and building the rationale for the no you deliver in paragraph three. Deliver your answer in the opening paragraph, preferably in the first sentence. Then go on to explain your reasons why, if necessary.

Having delivered your message and explained it as necessary, do not spend another paragraph or two winding down by repeating what you have already said. Simply say it—and stop. Also, watch out for standard closing lines that mean little or nothing. It may be quite all right to say something like, "Call me if you need more information"—if you really mean it. It is thoughtful and it shows that you are interested, but avoid phrases such as, "We trust this arrangement meets with your complete satisfaction." For one thing, you are telling your reader you expect satisfaction to result—you are not just asking. Anyway, if your reader is not completely satisfied you are likely to hear about it.

Consider something else that appears in the last example: the use of the collective *we*. Few words are more likely to make a letter impersonal to a reader than one who is made to feel that the communication is coming from a crowd. The *we* has its place, for instance, when you are writing to someone outside the institution and speaking for the organization. However, rather than being organization-to-person or organization-to-organization, most of your writing will be person-to-person. As long as the thoughts are your own and yours is the only hand pushing the pen, say *I*.

## SAMPLE LETTER

To illustrate the application of some of the guidelines offered in this chapter, a sample letter is presented in before and after versions. The letter in its original form (Exhibit 19–1) was received by the medical records (now health information management) department of a hospital.

Critical comments on Exhibit 19–1 are likely to include the following:

---

**Exhibit 19–1** Sample Letter: Before Editing

---

November 10, 2005

General Hospital
Main Street
Someplace, New York 00000

ATTN: Medical Records

Gentlemen:

         Re: John Doe
            Accident: August 9, 2005
            Someplace, New York

Please be advised that we are attorneys for the above named John Doe. We are enclosing herewith authorization for which please forward to this office copy of medical record of the said John Doe.
Thanking you, I am,

            Very truly yours,
            Brown & Jones
            Attorneys-at-Law

---

- Although the writer used *gentlemen* as a salutation and the overwhelming majority of health information management are not male, we will hedge on the matter of the salutation except to say that with little effort the writer could have come much closer than gentlemen. (Ideally, the writer should have first called the hospital to learn the name of the person to whom to direct the letter.)
- "Please be advised" is one of those bits of stuffing spoken of earlier. It went out of date before most of us even learned it.
- "We are enclosing herewith" suggests more pomposity. Much preferred is *enclosed is*, or simply *here is*.
- "The above named" is right; within-named, also. In fact, the unfortunate Mr. Doe is named three times in one brief letter.
- "Thanking you, I am" is silly. It is made all the sillier by the presence of two names in the signature block following I am (and the letter was received unsigned).

Now take a look at Exhibit 19–2, the same letter after reasonable editing. This letter is simple, straightforward, and to the point. And this is but one of several acceptable ways the letter could be rewritten.

Why all the fuss? You say you got the message anyway, without the criticism and the editing? True, you may have gotten the message. The sample letter is extremely short, so the potential for serious misunderstanding may not be evident. However, the potential for misinterpretation builds rapidly with the number of words in a letter. The body of Exhibit 19–1 contains 48 words. The edited version in Exhibit 19–2 contains 32 words. The difference represents a 33 percent reduction in the number of words used to get the message across, not to mention the mistreatment of the language corrected by the revision.

It has been estimated that most business correspondence contains from 25 percent to 100 percent more words than are needed to communicate effec-

---

**Exhibit 19–2** Sample Letter: After Editing

November 10, 2005

Medical Record Dept.
General Hospital
Main St.
Someplace, New York 00000

Dear _____,

   We are representing John Doe, who was treated at General Hospital on August 9, 2005, following an accident.

   Please send a copy of Mr. Doe's medical record. Proper authorization is enclosed. Thank you.

Sincerely,

T. L. Brown
Brown & Jones
Attorneys-at-Law

tively. Each added word presents another unwanted opportunity for misunderstanding. Also, keep in mind that if every business document you received were properly written, the 2-inch-thick stack of paper awaiting your attention could possibly be one-quarter inch to a full inch thinner.

## ATTACKING THE AGENTS OF WORDINESS

In reference to the Wilson letter presented in the "Situation" at the beginning of the chapter, there is probably no single version that is absolutely "best." However, there are a number of possible variations that are briefer, clearer, and far more effective than the original. One possibility follows.

Dear Mr. Wilson:

I am requesting continuing education approval for the seminar described in the enclosed outline. Originally developed for boards of directors, it also has interested licensed nursing home administrators who would like to receive continuing education credit for attending.

The Board of Examiners has previously granted credit for our courses, and several licensed administrators have asked us to secure similar approval for this program.

Please let me know if you require more information to evaluate this request. Thank you for your consideration.

The foregoing version of the Wilson letter reduces the verbiage by 50 percent and clarifies the message. The fewer words there are in a message, the less reading the recipient has to do. More important, however, is that use of fewer words reduces the chances of misunderstanding.

Note that in the rewritten Wilson letter, style and form have not suffered for the sake of brevity. The rewritten letter is grammatical; whole sentences are used. In urging the attack on the agents of wordiness and a quest for brevity we are not encouraging sentence fragments and a rapid-fire "telegraphese" construction. Rather, we are suggesting that any letter—in fact any document you must produce, whether letter, memo, report, or whatever—is not complete until you have gone through it again to delete the excess words and polish up the meaning. There is considerable truth in the opening quotation from Blaise Pascal; because of the editing and revising it takes a little longer to generate a shorter document, but the results are worth it in terms of improved clarity and the reduced chance of misunderstanding.

## OTHER WRITING

We have been discussing guidelines primarily for writing letters and memos, since these make up a significant percentage of most supervisors' writing chores. However, you may occasionally find it necessary or desirable to tackle larger writing tasks such as informational or analytical reports, educational presentations, speeches, or journal articles.

Many elements of the personal, direct style preferred for correspondence are applicable to other writing. For instance, some speeches or educational presentations can, and should, be handled with the same personal touch. However, some additional rules apply in writing more structured material such as formal reports, and still more rules apply when writing for publication in magazines or journals.

If you have to write a report, get a manual or handbook on the subject and do some studying. Be especially aware of the need to use one of the commonly recommended formats—one that calls for a tight summary of objectives, conclusions, and recommendations early in the report. Also, remember that the first step in preparing to write a report (or a letter, memo, or any other piece of writing) is to get a clear image of your audience.

If you are serious about improving your writing, start with the few suggestions presented in this chapter and go on to the information contained in published sources. Ideally, consider keeping a four-volume self-help library on your desk: Strunk and White's *The Elements of Style*, any other book about writing in general (preferably business writing), a reference book on report writing, and a reasonably current dictionary.

## TECHNOLOGY STRIKES: WHEN THE MESSAGE IS AN E-MAIL

In both business and in our personal lives we are seeing a growing reliance on electronic mail for the transmission of messages. The ease and convenience of e-mail have surely caused a dramatic increase in the numbers of messages moving among people. Surely many of these messages would not be sent at all were it not for the ease of doing so. However, since a significant number of e-mails have taken the place of other forms of message transmission, replacing telephone calls and hard-copy letters and memos, the use of e-mail has brought and continues to bring more communication problems.

Some in business have fallen back on e-mail in place of the telephone for some reasons that are evident and some that are not obvious. You can send an e-mail at your convenience; no need to call on the telephone, perhaps playing telephone tag or juggling voice mail—just tap out your message and click "send." Also, among the not-so-evident reasons, unlike a telephone call, with an e-mail you do not have to discuss the issue, perhaps be asked questions you would just as well not have to deal with. In other words, e-mail lets you dodge various personal contacts. In doing so, e-mail often slows down the communication process because the often-inevitable clarification must occur through subsequent messages.

As a replacement for hard-copy letters or memos, e-mail, as it is frequently used, results in "messages" that look like nothing we would ever allow out of our offices on paper. In the sometimes daily flood of e-mails it is common to find messages that are more ramblings than memos; lacking capitalization and punctuation; and filled with typographical errors, blatant misspellings, poor word choices, and convoluted structure.

As a message, an e-mail has nothing going for it except the words on a screen. Absent are the sender's vocal tone, body language, and facial expression, and absent is the opportunity for immediate feedback and questions aimed at clarification. If those words on the screen are garbled, the message is garbled. Thus it is fully as important to edit, rewrite, spell-check, and otherwise clean up every e-mail message before clicking "send." In an e-mail message the words alone are all you have, so make certain they are able to do the job you need them to do.

## Misuse and Abuse

Probably no modern business technology is more misused and abused than e-mail. E-mail is even more problematic than the next most misused and abused business technology, the photocopier. Many photocopiers, as we all know but frequently choose to ignore, handle a significant volume of non-business copying ranging from cartoons, jokes, and recipes to announcements, schedules, and newsletters for outside organizations. E-mail not only carries a high volume of non-business material, unlike the photocopier it also carries business information that is communicated in a slapdash, generally careless fashion that frequently does more to raise questions than to convey information.

## Getting It Under Control

If you have to spend a third to half of your e-mail time sorting through unimportant communications and personal information before getting into pertinent messages, many of which you must then interpret or question before passing along or acting upon, your e-mail is out of control. To bring it under control, consider the following suggestions for regulating the flow of messages:

- Emphasize deleting rather than reading. In most instances a quick look at the subject line along with your knowledge of the sender will indicate whether a message should be read in full. If a full reading is not needed, then delete it.
- Get to know your frequent senders and what they are likely to be sending. There has never been and never will be a beneficial technology that does not have a downside, and the downside of the personal computer is its appeal to some users as more of a toy than a tool. You should soon learn where many of your important messages come from and who is usually sending junk.
- Similar to the age-old advice about handling each incoming piece of paper only once, try to deal with each e-mail message once and only once. When you open and read a message, reply to it, forward it, delete it, or put it away in an electronic folder. Do not allow messages to accumulate; they fill up your electronic inbox and increase the chances of importance messages getting lost in the clutter.
- When sending a message, use a clear, understandable subject line that tells the addressee in a few words what to expect of the communication.
- Inform your employees of the proper business use of e-mail and train them in handling incoming mail as suggested above. You might also remind them that e-mail is not as private as they might believe; messages

are regularly misdirected accidentally, and it is easy for some computer users to tap into others' e-mail. It helps to imagine that any particular message could conceivably become as public as a bulletin-board notice.

Concerning the seemingly prevalent casual ("sloppy") use of e-mail, at times it seems that e-mail brings out the worst in many writers of business communications. E-mail is such a readily available and easily usable means of interpersonal communication that it is easy to overlook its troublesome shortcomings: no body, facial expression, vocal tone, or opportunity for immediate feedback. An e-mail message is like a letter or memo in that all you have to convey the message are words that must be read and interpreted.

To more effectively use e-mail, start thinking of it as simply one subset of tools in that versatile toolkit known as the personal computer. Like any good tool, to retain its usefulness keep it in good order and use it for its intended purposes only.

## A MATTER OF PRACTICE

Writing is much like any other skill in that the more you work at it the better you get. If you enjoy writing, or feel that you could enjoy it, then you have a head start on the self-improvement process. But if you do not enjoy writing, if every letter, every memo, every report, every performance appraisal narrative looms before you as a painful, distasteful task, you had better examine your attitude toward writing. Is writing tough for you because you truly dislike it? Or is it the other way around—you dislike it primarily because it is difficult for you?

You may not have to write a great deal on your job, but chances are you write enough to make it worthwhile to try a modest self-improvement program. One thing is certain: You will never get better at writing unless you work at it.

---

## REVIEW QUESTIONS

1. Comment on the quotation from Blaise Pascal: *"I have made this letter rather long because I have not had time to make it short."*
2. Would it make more sense to write so that anyone who picks up what you have written will understand it, rather than writing for a specific, possibly narrow, audience? Why or why not?
3. What is wrong with overly wordy writing as long as the important information you want to convey is part of the message?
4. What are the primary advantages of editing and rewriting?
5. Why do a great many people in business "write it out and send it," not concerning themselves with editing and rewriting?

## EXERCISE: THE COPY MACHINE LETTER

Write a letter to Mr. James Ware, district manager of Copyco, Inc., describing the trouble you are having with your copy machine. Include the following information (not all points are of equal significance, and they are not presented in any logical order):

- You are purchasing manager for City General Hospital.
- City General has one Copyco Model-T machine.
- You have had the machine for 10 months.
- You have discovered that the local address for Copyco service is a manufacturer's representative and that the nearest real service agency is 125 miles away.
- The machine has required outside service five times.
- For the last three breakdowns your machine was down for 3 days, 2 days, and 4 days, respectively, awaiting service.
- You bought the machine without a service contract.
- There is administrative pressure on you to replace the Copyco machine with a better-known machine.
- The machine gives off a strong odor when operating.
- The Model-T Copyco was the cheapest machine available.
- The sales representative promised prompt service.

## Additional Considerations

1. Your letter should probably contain complaints (poor performance, poor service, and so on) and threats (to replace, and so on). Before writing, decide which kind of message—complaint or threat—will be the dominant message.
2. You have admitted to yourself that your own organization caused much of the problem when it "bought cheap" (lowest price, no service contract). Carefully consider to what extent—if at all—you might admit this in your letter.

## CHAPTER 20

# How to Arrange and Conduct Effective Meetings

*Meetings: Where you go to learn how to do better the things you already know how to do anyway, but don't have time to do, because of too many meetings.*
—*Anonymous*

## CHAPTER OBJECTIVES

☛ Characterize various types of meetings by the purposes for which they may be held.

☛ Provide guidelines for determining the need for a meeting and for preparing to conduct an effective meeting.

☛ Offer suggestions for leading a meeting in such a way as to obtain maximum benefits from the process while consuming the least possible amount of the valuable time of those attending.

☛ Place meetings in general in perspective as an often misused but potentially effective management tool.

## SITUATION: THE CONFERENCE

There is a conference involving the following five people:

1. Dan Andrews, administrative assistant. He functions in a staff capacity and has no direct employees except for his secretary, Susan. One of his assignments is a long-term project intended to determine some of the reasons for employee turnover. He called the meeting approximately 10 days ago. Two of the other people in attendance he notified by telephone, and the other two people he invited in person.
2. Harry Robertson, personnel director
3. Jane Dawson, director of nursing service
4. Arthur Morey, director of housekeeping
5. Arlette Wilson, director of food service

The meeting was scheduled for 1:00 P.M. in Andrews's office. Andrews returned from lunch at 1:08 to find Robertson and Wilson already there. At 1:12 Dawson entered and Andrews said, "I'd like to get started, but where's Morey?"

"I don't know," somebody answered.

Andrews dialed a number and received no answer. He then dialed the switchboard and asked for a page. A moment later a call came in and Andrews spoke briefly with Morey.

Turning from the telephone Andrews said, "He forgot. He'll be here in a minute."

"Dan, I wish you had a larger office or a better place to meet," said Dawson. "I don't know how we're going to fit another person in here."

"I know it's small," Andrews answered, "but both conference rooms are tied up and I couldn't find another place. Say, holler out to Susan and tell her to find another chair—we're going to need it."

Arlette Wilson said, "Dan, can you open your window a little? It's already stuffy in here."

Dan responded by opening the window a few inches. Then the housekeeping director entered, squeezing into the office with the chair that had just been located. It was 1:18 P.M.

Andrews said, "I guess we can get started now." He shuffled through a stack of papers before him and said, "I've got a copy, if I can, ah—oh, here it is—of a recent turnover survey done by the personnel directors in the eastern region." Looking at the personnel man he asked, "I assume you have this?"

"Yes, I have it. There's a copy in my office, but I didn't know I needed to bring it with me."

Andrews said, "Well, I think what we can get from this thing is ——"

The nursing director interrupted, "Dan, wouldn't it be better if we all could see it? Then you could go down it point-by-point."

Dan said, "I guess you're right. I just have this single copy." He turned toward the door and hollered, "Susan, can you come here a minute?"

Susan entered and Dan instructed her to run four copies of the survey at once.

Turning back to his pile of papers Dan said to the group in general, "The last time we got together there were a number of things we decided to look for. I don't remember just what we assigned to whom, but I've got it here somewhere."

For a half-minute or so Dan leafed through the papers before him. Then he turned to the file drawer of his desk and began to go through folders.

While Dan was looking, Jane Dawson turned to Robertson and said, "Say, what have you been doing about finding that new in-service instructor we need? We notified your employment section three weeks ago, and Eleanor is leaving in another week and we still haven't had any candidates to interview."

Harry Robertson responded. His tone sparked a defensive reaction and a lively discussion began.

Andrews located the paper he was seeking and Susan returned with the requested photocopies. Andrews distributed the copies and fixed his attention on the nursing director and personnel director as he waited for an opening in the discussion, which was now something between a conversation and an argument. At approximately 1:32 P.M. they managed to return to the subject of employee turnover.

"Now, about this eastern region survey," Andrews began.

Arlette Wilson said, "What about the survey? I thought you wanted to start with the things we agreed to do the last time we were together."

"Who cares," said Robertson. "Let's just get started."

The nursing director looked at her watch and said, "We'd better hurry up and get started and finished. I have a staff meeting at 2:00."

The meeting settled down to a discussion of the eastern region survey and the preliminary data each person had gathered since the previous meeting. At exactly two minutes before 2:00, the nursing director excused herself to attend her meeting. At 2:08 P.M. Morey was called over the paging system; he left Andrews's office and did not return.

At 2:12 P.M. Andrews said he felt they had tentatively decided on their next step but required some input from the two parties who had already left. He then started to excuse the other two participants with the suggestion that they get together again after 2 weeks.

At that point Andrews's telephone rang. He answered it himself, his usual practice, and talked for some 4 to 5 minutes before returning his attention to the two persons left in his office. He said, "I guess that's about it for this time around. I'll get back to you and establish a time for the next meeting."

When the last of the participants had left, Andrews's secretary came into his office and asked if they were finished with the extra chair. Andrews indicated they were, and as Susan removed the chair, Andrews thought gloomily of how difficult it was to get anything done in this hospital.

*Instructions*

At whatever point in the chapter you feel comfortable doing so, perform a detailed critique of "The Conference." Make a list of points you consider errors and omissions in the way this meeting was arranged and conducted, and indicate what positive steps could have been taken to avoid each of the errors and omissions.

## "LET'S SCHEDULE A MEETING"

Whenever a meeting of any kind threatens to land on your schedule, your primary objective should be to render most of this chapter's advice unnecessary by finding a way to do without the meeting. Not that you will always, or even frequently, succeed in doing so, but the amount of management time consumed by meetings is more than enough to prompt us to ask of each potential meeting: "Is this really necessary?"

Therefore, when a meeting looms, the proper order of essential steps is (1) to consider possible alternate means of accomplishing what the meeting would supposedly accomplish and (2) having concluded that a meeting is the best way to do what needs to be done, then plan, schedule, and conduct the meeting in such a manner that maximum possible output is obtained with the least possible time and effort.

### Can a Meeting Be Avoided?

For the most part we decry the frequency, number, and length of meetings, yet we continue to hold them and attend them in the same old ways. The majority of managers can be counted on to grumble about meetings, but many of these managers' true attitudes concerning meetings are revealed through their behavior. In true attitude managers in fact range from those who are action-oriented people and obviously impatient with the passiveness of most meeting situations (after all, talking is not doing) to those who seem not to mind sitting and talking for hours at a stretch. The latter probably includes more than a few to whom a schedule full of meetings is a measure of (self) importance.

Before putting a meeting on the schedule, determine whether the answers to a few simple questions might allow you to avoid the meeting.

- Is the intended flow of information strictly one-way, with people to be advised or informed but no immediate feedback to be necessary? If so, consider other means such as letter, memo, voice mail, bulletin board, or such.

- Is there a single, clearly defined topic and a limited number of people involved? Perhaps you can personally contact three or four people to solicit their input and then develop a recommendation that you communicate to them individually. (Voice mail has proven itself useful in reducing the numbers of calls and return calls in this kind of process.)

- Is the topic worth a meeting of its own? Perhaps an issue that legitimately requires a meeting can wait until it can be bundled with other matters at a regularly recurring meeting.

### Is the Cost Worth It?

Meetings are costly relative to other ways of doing business. They are not necessarily costly in terms of out-of-pocket expenditures; their cost is reckoned largely in terms of the expenditure of unrecoverable time. The true cost of most unnecessary or questionable meetings would have to be reckoned in terms of lost productivity. What would these people be doing had they not been involved in a meeting?

Only when it is determined that a meeting is indeed necessary should one be scheduled. And once scheduled, it should be conducted in such a way as to secure maximum value from the time and efforts of the participants.

### MANAGEMENT BY COMMITTEE

Meetings often represent the best available technique for arriving at joint conclusions and determining joint actions. It is often possible to accomplish results in minutes that would require hours, days, or weeks by other means.

Meetings are also essential to consultative and participative leadership styles. Joint decisions and actions take longer to formulate than do unilateral decisions and edicts, since true two-way communication including discussion and feedback requires more time than one-way communication. However, the extra time spent in meetings can represent a small price to pay for the benefits afforded by an honest, open, participative style.

Prevalent in business activities of all kinds, in recent years meetings seem to have become an even greater concern for their frequency and complexity. Certainly the total quality movement and the greatly increased use of employee teams and work groups have added to the impression of endless meetings. And the increased numbers of meetings have led to the increasing impression that it is now groups—committees, if you will—that make decisions, not individuals.

"Management by committee" may be a widespread and not completely unavoidable perception that falls out from the reality of numerous meetings. While a group may provide information and recommendations, however, the ultimate responsibility for any specific decision usually resides with an individual.

## TYPES OF MEETINGS

### Information Meetings

The information meeting is held simply for the transfer of information. You have something to pass along to your employees or others and you choose to do this with a meeting rather than by some other means. The basic purpose of any information meeting is to transfer information to the group, and in this setting the leader may do most or all of the talking. Although there are usually questions and discussion for the sake of clarification, the transfer of information is essentially one-way communication.

### Discussion Meetings

The objective of a discussion meeting is to gain agreement on something through the exchange of information, ideas, and opinions. The essence of the discussion meeting is interchange; the exchange of information must be established between and among all participants.

### Directed Discussion

A directed discussion meeting may be appropriate when a conclusion, solution, or decision is evident. The conclusion has already been determined; yet it is not simply being relayed to the group as straight information. It is the leader's objective to gain the participants' acceptance of the solution. In effect, a directed discussion is a sales pitch.

### Problem-Solving Discussion

This type of meeting is held when a problem exists and a solution or decision must be determined by the group. Although the answer determined by joint action may well turn out to be based on the ideas of a single participant, at the outset it is apparent only that there is a problem with which several parties could reasonably be concerned.

### Exploratory Discussion

The purpose of an exploratory discussion meeting is to gain information on which you or others may eventually base a decision. The objective is not to develop a specific solution or recommendation but rather to generate and develop ideas and information for others (perhaps yourself, but possibly your boss or some other manager) who must make the decision.

### A Special Case: The Staff Meeting

The staff meeting may be an information meeting, a discussion meeting, or both. A staff meeting is usually held for the purpose of communication among the members of a group. Staff members may report on the status of their activities, and thus each may be required to effect the one-way transfer of information to others. This meeting form is also used to solve problems, sell ideas, and explore issues, and, depending on the business at hand, it may take on any or all of the three forms of the discussion meeting.

## MEETING PREPARATION

A few of the following suggestions are most pertinent to discussion meetings convened for dealing with specific situations. Most, however, apply generally to all types of meetings.

### Defining the Problem

To enable a group to begin dealing with a situation it is necessary to establish the nature of that situation. The first step, then, in preparing for a meeting is your identification of what is wrong. Before your invited participants attend the meeting they must understand what they are going to discuss when they get there, so you must be able to supply a concise statement of the problem or other reason for the meeting.

### Confirming the Need for a Meeting

In addition to what was said in earlier paragraphs about determining the need for a meeting, it is also suggested that the decision of whether or not to involve several people in a meeting may not be yours alone. Confirming your thoughts with a few potential participants can be helpful; if, in addition to you, two others believe it can be done without a meeting, you are fairly secure in using other means. However, if you stand alone in your opposition to a meeting, there may be aspects of the situation that you are overlooking.

### Deciding What Should Be Accomplished

Before you convene the meeting you should have a clear idea of what you want to achieve. As your definition of the problem provides your starting point, so your meeting provides your target. As a minimum, and before calling people together, you want to be able to say whether the meeting should give you the solution to a problem, the group's acceptance of an idea, some significant decision-making information, or other such results.

## Selecting the Meeting Type

Based on your determination of what should be accomplished, you should then decide what type of meeting you are going to have. There are some broad differences between information meetings and discussion meetings, but there are also significant differences in emphasis among the subtypes of discussion meetings. Your clear understanding as to whether the discussion should be directed or should be oriented toward problem solving or exploration will assist you in controlling the meeting and keeping the discussion headed toward the result you wish to accomplish.

## Selecting the Participants

Again based on your best determination of what is to be accomplished, next you need to determine who should attend the meeting. This determination should be based on your best assessment of who has the knowledge to deal with the problem and the authority to make decisions and commit resources to solve the problem. Your objective in selecting people to attend the meeting should be to secure the broadest possible coverage of the problem without overloading the meeting.

## Distributing Advance Information

All those invited should receive, along with the meeting notification, all information that would be helpful in preparing for the meeting. If you can give them only a statement of the problem, then let them know this is all you have. If you have background information in the form of letters, memos, or reports, send it to them so they can consider all aspects of the problem in advance of the meeting. Give them also your expectations of the meeting. At the very least, those invited should know both the problem and the objective.

## Notifying and Reminding the Participants

Written notification of the meeting should include time, place, preparations to make or materials to bring, the statement of the problem, and the meeting's objectives. Ideally, you should provide written notification a week or more in advance and plan on telephoning reminders a day or two before the meeting actually takes place. Generally, the more important the topic of the meeting and the busier the people you are inviting, the more advance notice you should provide.

It is also a good idea to clear the date and time in advance with the key people attending. Otherwise you are likely to find yourself having to notify everyone of a change in arrangements although some have already cleared their calendars to attend. Remember that you are not the only busy person in the organization; it may frequently be necessary for you to bend your schedule to accommodate the availability of other people.

## Arranging for Proper Facilities

This step should seem self-evident, but too often a dozen people find they are ready to meet but have no place to sit down. If you need sizeable conference facilities, make sure you secure them for the preferred date and time before your notification goes out. It should also go without saying—but nevertheless must be said, judging from the number of times things go wrong—that you need sufficient space for all persons involved, reasonably comfortable surroundings, and reasonable freedom from interruptions. Also, advance arrangements should be made for needed equipment such as chalkboards, projectors, and other aids.

## Preparing an Agenda

For all but the simplest of meetings you should use an agenda to guide you. If the meeting promises to be long and involved, the agenda should be worked out sufficiently in advance so it can be supplied to all attendees with the meeting notification. Whether or not it is supplied in advance, however, as meeting leader you need the agenda. It may consist of only a few broad points jotted in the corner of your note pad, but the process of writing it forces you to rethink your purpose in calling the meeting and consider how you will get from problem to objective. Although you will not think of every necessary step or essential question ahead of time, with an agenda you can at least remind yourself of certain important points. When the meeting is under way your agenda may well expand as issues are raised and information previously unknown to you is offered. This is all well and good, as long as all agenda additions or digressions contribute directly to moving the group from the problem toward the meeting's objective.

## LEADING A MEETING

### Start on Time

You may want to allow some flexibility in how closely you adhere to a rigid starting time. If the meeting is a one-time affair involving a number of people who are organizationally scattered, perhaps including some who are your superiors in the management structure, you may want to bend a few minutes on starting time. (In a practical sense, you are likely to wait more than a few minutes for a tardy person to show, especially if that person happens to be your boss.) Also, a one-shot meeting is not a regular part of someone's schedule or pattern of behavior. It is perhaps best to give yourself some slack in scheduling; for instance, you schedule a session for 1:30 P.M. although you know full well it will not start until 1:45 P.M. Try not to overdo this practice; it suggests disrespect for those who do show up on time and deference to the latecomers.

In the case of a regularly scheduled meeting (for instance, your monthly staff meeting held at 3:00 P.M. on the third Thursday of each month), begin precisely on time. The more you defer to chronic latecomers, the more likely these people are to remain chronic latecomers. Also, chronic tardiness can often be an indication of other problems, such as hostility, disrespect, lack of interest, or perhaps inflated ego.

Making it a habit of starting on time can go a long way toward curing chronic tardiness. If it is 3:00 P.M. and only half of your staff members are present, start the meeting even though you know the remainder will be trickling in over the next several minutes. Out of respect for those who show up on time, do not repeat what has already been said for the sake of the latecomers. Rather, let the late arrivers know they have to wait until after the meeting to find out what they missed from those who were present. Make it plain, also, that the content of the early part of the meeting is not always filler or "warm up" material that people can afford to miss. Make it a habit to start your regularly scheduled meetings precisely on time, and most chronic latecomers will change their ways as they get the message and become accustomed to your pattern of behavior.

### State the Purpose of the Meeting

First tell the group why they are there and what they need to accomplish. Also, give them your best estimate of the amount of time the meeting should require. Ending time can be fully as troublesome as starting time in some situations. A meeting can be a form of escape for some people who lead busy, hectic working lives, and some people may tend to prolong the session with irrelevancies if progress is not well controlled. (It has been suggested that an effective way to get a one-hour meeting concluded in just one hour is to schedule it to start an hour before lunch or an hour before quitting time.) In short, your first item of business should be to advise those attending why they are there, what they are expected to accomplish, and approximately how long it should take.

### Make Some Assignments

Some of the practical ideas coming out of the total quality management or TQM movement and its emphasis on working with teams include guidelines for running meetings. You may have done everything yourself up to this point, but once the meeting is convened, you are likely to find that you alone cannot do everything that ought to be done. It is time to involve some of the others in moving the meeting along by handing out some assignments. The common assignments for a meeting of reasonable size (say five, six, or more people) are recorder, scribe, and timekeeper.

#### Recorder

The recorder keeps track of what happens in the meeting for the sake of generating meeting minutes or some other written record of what occurs. The recorder may actually do the minutes or the report or simply hand the rough notes over to you to proceed as you will. The point of having the recorder is to relieve you of trying to keep a record of the proceedings while you are also running the meeting; you cannot do both together as well as you could do either alone.

*Scribe*

The scribe serves an important purpose if you have a need to capture points or ideas on a chalkboard or flip-chart. This is "talking material" that may evolve as you meet, so it may not be the same as what you might embody in meeting minutes. In a very small meeting, the recorder and scribe might be one and the same, but the roles are really different and a meeting of as few as three lively contributors could readily overwhelm someone who is trying to fill both roles.

*Timekeeper*

The timekeeper is exactly what the name suggests, a person who keeps track of the time spent on each agenda item and who keeps the group aware of where they stand relative to total allotted time, the clock, and the agenda.

## Encourage Discussion

Do not allow the meeting to move in such narrow lines that valuable input is lost. Ask for clarification of comments that are offered. Consider requesting opinions and asking direct questions, particularly of the few "silent ones" who frequently populate your meetings. Remember, if you have structured your meeting wisely then everyone who is there is there for a good reason. It is part of your job as meeting leader to do everything you can to get those people talking who ordinarily tend to remain quiet.

## Exercise Control: A List of Don'ts

*Of Yourself*

- Don't let your ego get in the way simply because you are the meeting leader and thus automatically in control of the proceedings.
- Don't lecture or otherwise dominate the proceedings. Remember, the setting is a meeting, not a speech or a class.
- Don't direct the others by telling them what to do or what they should say or conclude. This would amount to one-way communication, which is only marginally appropriate even when the purpose of the meeting is purely informational.
- Don't argue with participants. Discuss, yes—argue, never.
- Don't attempt to be funny. What may be funny to one person may not be to another. The best laughs generated at a meeting are those that arise naturally from the discussion.

*Of the Group*

- Don't allow lengthy tangential digressions to pull you away from the subject of the meeting. Granted many legitimate problems are identified through tangential discussions, but, legitimate or not, if they do not relate to the problem at hand they are diluting the effectiveness of the meeting. Should a legitimate problem arise, make note of it but sideline it for action at another time or at another meeting and proceed with the subject at hand.

- Don't allow monopolizers and ego-trippers to take over. Although certain talkative people may have significant contributions to make, their constant presence center stage serves to narrow the discussion and discourage marginally vocal contributors from opening up at all. Overall, your effectiveness as a meeting leader will largely be determined by how effectively you control the discussion of the group.

### Summarize Periodically

Agreement in a discussion meeting is usually not reached in a single, progressive series of exchanges. Rather, agreement accrues as discussion points are sifted, sorted, and merged, and a solution or recommendation begins to take form. Capture this by periodically summarizing what has been said, giving the group, in your own words, a recounting of where you are and where you seem to be headed. If they can agree with your summary of progress—essentially, their thoughts encapsulated and restated in your words—then the meeting is on the right track.

### End with a Specific Plan

When the meeting is over you should be able to deliver a final summary stating what has been decided and who is going to do what and by when. Far too many meetings are frustrating affairs that may feel productive while under way but afterward leave participants hanging with a sense of incompleteness.

No one should leave your meeting without full understanding of the decisions made, the actions to be taken, the people responsible for implementation, and the timetable for implementation. If the subject is sufficiently complex, it may be to your advantage to call for understanding by going around the table, asking everyone for their interpretations of what has been decided and how they see their roles, if any, in the implementation of the decision. In any event, do not let the group leave without a clear understanding of what has been decided and what happens next.

### Follow Up

As far as your authority over the problem extends, it is up to you to follow up to determine that what has been decided gets accomplished. It is also up to you to see that the minutes of the meeting, should they be necessary, are prepared and distributed; provide later assurance to all participants that what they decided has in fact been accomplished; and schedule a follow-up meeting should one be necessary.

## CLEANING UP "THE CONFERENCE"

The errors and omissions in the way the meeting described in the "Situation" at the beginning of the chapter was arranged and conducted are numerous and, in most instances, glaring. For the most part, we know intuitively and through plain common sense that most of these are indeed errors, but nevertheless we often find ourselves allowing many of these to occur because we simply fail to take control of our own meetings.

In most of the following items, identification of the problem directly implies what should have been done:

- Andrews was late for his own meeting. It is bad enough to be late for a meeting at which you are an invited participant, but, in the absence of some dire emergency, being late for your own meeting is inexcusable.

- Dawson arrived late, wasting several minutes of other peoples' time, and then expected events to turn upon her arrival.

- Andrews did not provide written notification of the meeting or reminders as the date neared. When meeting notifications are oral, they often do not make it onto someone's calendar page. Also, for an important meeting that is scheduled more than a few days in advance—say more than a week ahead of time—reminders are in order.

- A reasonable meeting space was not arranged in advance, and insufficient seating caused an added delay. Overall Andrews used an inadequate space with inadequate ventilation.

- The meeting began 18 minutes late. Need we reiterate the necessity of beginning scheduled meetings at the scheduled time?

- Andrews should have had his meeting material available and ready, rather than having to shuffle papers and search for the proper documents.

- Andrews should have planned for meeting handouts, having them copied and ready in advance, rather than wasting time trying to secure copies.

- There were apparently no minutes taken at the previous meeting, and apparently no one had kept track of who had agreed to do what. The file Andrews sought, the finding of which created another delay, should have been out and available before the meeting began.

- The participants permitted a digression of topic that threatened to become highly disruptive.

- The group lost considerable time in disagreement over what they were expected to be doing.

- Although Andrews was in no position to stop those who left when the meeting had barely gotten started, he let them go with no indication of what they should be doing concerning this group's mission.

- Andrews took a telephone call while people remained in his office, putting them in an awkward position and wasting their time as well.

- No advance consideration was given to scheduling the next meeting. The best time to set a follow-up meeting is when you have all or most of the intended participants—and, we would hope, their calendars—in the same room at the same time.

- Apparently no decisions were made at this meeting, and no specific tasks were assigned, rendering the meeting useless for all practical purposes.
- In his gloomy thoughts about "how difficult it was to get anything done in this hospital," Andrews seemed to have missed all consideration of what it was that made the meeting useless: people and, in this instance, primarily Dan Andrews.

## USE OR ABUSE?

As with any other management tool or technique, meetings can be overused, underused, or used ineffectively. They can be expected to do far too much— meetings are certainly no substitute for effective individual decision-making in the presence of proper authority and responsibility—or they can be denied the opportunity to serve their purpose appropriately.

Whether the meetings you call are used or abused is largely up to you, the supervisor. Meetings are often an unwieldy way of doing business, and as such it is easy for them to become wasteful and ineffective. However, the properly conducted meeting remains one of the most effective available ways of accomplishing certain tasks. Whether meetings are effective or ineffective revolves on the issue of control: If we fail to control our meetings, our meetings control us.

---

## REVIEW QUESTIONS

1. Describe how you would suggest "drawing out" a particularly silent participant at a meeting you are chairing.
2. What is always the first question that should be asked, or the first decision that should be made, when you are considering convening a meeting for some purpose?
3. What do you see as the primary advantages of conducting business in the context of a meeting? The disadvantages?
4. Recognizing that many meetings take far too long and accomplish too little because they wander over a variety of subjects, suggest how to keep a meeting on track while still ensuring that any essential issues that arise are not lost forever.
5. What are the final points to be covered or actions to be taken at the end of a meeting?
6. Comment on this quotation from C. Northcote Parkinson: *"The amount of work accomplished by a committee is inversely proportional to the number of members on the committee."*

## CASE: YOUR WORD AGAINST HIS

You are at a meeting chaired by your department head. Also present are another department head and four other supervisors. The subject of the meeting is the manner in which the hospital's supervisors are to conduct themselves during the present union-organizing campaign.

Your department head makes a statement concerning one way in which supervisors should behave. You are surprised to hear this because earlier that same day you read a legal opinion that described this particular action as probably illegal.

You interrupt with, "Pardon me, but I don't believe it can really be done that way. I'm certain it would leave us open to an unfair labor practice charge."

Obviously annoyed by the interruption, your department head responds sharply, "This isn't open to discussion. You're wrong."

You open your mouth to speak again, but you are cut short by an angry glance.

You are certain that the boss is wrong; he had inadvertently turned around a pair of words and described a "cannot-do" as a "can-do." Unfortunately you are in a conference room full of people and the document that could prove your point is in your office.

### Questions

1. Recognizing that you are but an attendee at the meeting and that your immediate superior is running the meeting, what should you—or what can you—do to ensure that the other participants do not act on critically incorrect information immediately after the meeting?

2. What fundamental requirements of effective meeting leadership appear to have been ignored in this meeting?

## CHAPTER 21

# Budgeting: Annual Task and Year-Long Implications

*A budget is a means of telling your money where to go—*
*instead of wondering where it went.*
—*Anonymous*

## CHAPTER OBJECTIVES

☛ Introduce the basic concepts of budgeting and establish the importance of budget preparation to the individual supervisor.

☛ Describe the advantages of participative approaches to budgeting.

☛ Define operating budgets, capital budgets, and cash budgets.

☛ Provide a step-by-step illustration of the preparation of a budget for an individual department.

☛ Describe the process of developing an institution's annual budget from the budgets of individual departments.

☛ Illustrate the fundamentals of the process of monitoring expenditures against budget allocations.

## SITUATION: "WHAT'S A BUDGET BESIDES LOTS OF WORK I DON'T HAVE TIME FOR?"

Following is the essence of a lunchtime conversation between Mary Regal, recently hired as Wilson Hospital's director of food service, and Eva Perry, business office manager, Mary's friend, and a long-time Wilson employee.

Mary: "I've barely been able to get my feet on the ground learning the department and meeting with all my people individually, and now I've got this big thick pack of stuff I'm expected to do for the budget."

Eva: "I know it seems like a lot, but we've all got to do it. However, it does seem like this once-a-year task comes around a lot more often than that."

Mary: "But I don't know why they have to put us through all that. My budget's going to be what finance wants it to be, so why don't they just tell me and get it over with?"

Eva: "You don't want to have any input into your own budget?"

Mary: "Look, I was at County General for three years and at John James Hospital for a long time before that. At General, my budget was handed down from somewhere upstairs and I was expected to meet it. Nobody ever asked what I thought I needed. At John James things were even worse because I had to play the budget game every year."

Eva: "The budget game?"

Mary: "The budget game. Pad and cut. You learned quickly that you'd better have some fat in your first draft because there would always be one or two rounds of mandated cuts. After the first submission every department head was always told to cut some percentage—maybe 2 percent, maybe 5 percent, once even 8 percent. And it was always across-the-board, every department. Cut this percent out and resubmit. Before I wised up I got stuck, turning in an honest budget and then having to reduce it. I learned quickly enough to leave myself some slack."

Eva: "Maybe slack isn't the right term. I know it pays to start with an optimistic budget—one that would allow you to do everything you feel is needed. Then you've got room to trim a couple times if necessary, down to an austerity budget that just serves absolute essentials."

Mary: "Then you could say that every year at John James we had an austerity budget, because that's where we wound up. And every year we'd hear administration and finance moan about how tight the money was going to be, and in the last quarter we were always pressured to cut or stall expenditures. Then came year-end and somehow we managed to finish with a modest surplus. Some used to claim the finance director had hidden reserves so he could move numbers around and make the year come out okay."

Eva: "You're bound to feel pressure to keep expenses down wherever you work in health care today or at least in any hospital. There's just not enough money coming in to do everything we'd like to do. I've never yet seen a budget process where the first round showed that expected income wasn't smaller than anticipated spending. Adjustment is always necessary."

Mary: "That may be, but if they know how much we'll have to work with why don't they just tell us at the start, instead of putting us through all this work?"

Eva: "Don't you think it's helpful to have a voice in determining what your budget looks like?"

Mary: "A voice? At County General we were handed our budgets, already done. At John James it was even worse because we had to go through all those gyrations to get to where they'd already decided we should be. Then there were the monthly reports—about as easy to interpret as Latin code. They'd just accumulate in a stack until someone dared to throw them out."

Eva: "You didn't use your monthly budget reports for anything?"

Mary: "No. Trying to figure them out just wasted more time, and anyway we could always expect to be nagged about spending too much no matter how the month's results were coming out."

Eva: "Well, whether you're looking forward to it or not, it's that time of year again. I hope you find that budgeting here works better than it did at your other jobs."

Mary: "I hope so. All a budget has been to me is a bunch of useless work that I don't have time for."

*Instructions*

As you proceed through this chapter, consider how you would comment on the dialogue above. Prepare to comment on the manager's participation in budgeting, the overall management of the budgeting process, and the value of the process to the manager and the department given that financial resources will always be capped at a certain level.

## INTRODUCING THE BUDGET

There are likely to be considerable differences in the ways supervisors approach this chapter. In some institutions, individual supervisors have been actively involved in the budgeting process for years. In other institutions, however, the budget remains a mysterious collection of numbers assembled by higher management and finance with no supervisory involvement whatsoever.

If you have often been directly involved in the preparation of departmental budgets, you will find little in this chapter that you have not encountered in practice. However, if your budget preparation experience is minimal or non-existent then you could benefit from this elementary view of budgeting.

This chapter provides an overview of the budget and the budgeting process and offers some specifics in a manner intended for consideration by supervisors who do not have backgrounds in accounting and finance (certainly the vast majority of supervisors).

A budget is a financial plan that serves as an estimate of future operations and, to some extent, as a means of control over those operations. It is a quantitative expression of the institution's expressed operating intentions, and it translates these intentions into numbers.

A budget can be several things to the institution and to the individual supervisor. Used as a control mechanism, it can be a cost-containment tool that helps keep costs in line with available resources. It can also be a basis for performance evaluation, since performance against a budget provides an indication of how well you utilize the resources under your control. Further, a budget can be a means for directing efforts toward productivity improvement —since performance against budget, in revealing how well resources are utilized, can give you the basis from which to work for better utilization.

### Participative Budgeting

In some hospitals and other health care organizations the budget is still prepared "upstairs" and handed down for supervisors and department heads to live with. This practice leaves a great deal to be desired, since it requires the supervisor to implement a plan without having participated in the plan's development. The supervisor may remain ignorant of many of the whys and wherefores of the budget and thus be in a position of weakness when it comes to translating the department's financial plan into action.

Fortunately, however, more and more health care institutions are bringing their supervisors into the budgeting process. The team approach to budgeting, requiring active participation of managers at all levels, calls for close coordination of a multitude of diverse inputs and activities. It takes considerably more time and effort to assemble a budget in this manner than it does simply to allow administration and finance to get their heads together and issue a budget, but the results of the team approach are well worth the extra work. The participative approach to budgeting has several distinct advantages:

- The end item of the process, the budget, is usually a far more realistic and workable plan than any that could be developed by some other means.

- The involvement of individual supervisors in the process breeds their commitment; they are more likely to believe in the budget and strive to make it work because they took part in its development.
- The interdepartmental and intradepartmental activities and interpersonal contacts pursued during the process tend to strengthen supervisors in their jobs.
- A spirit and attitude of teamwork is created in getting managers at all levels to work together toward a common goal. Teamwork is, to a great extent, one of the keys to the successful operation of an organization.
- The encouragement of more realistic planning serves to sharpen the focus of management's efforts and produce more appropriate results a greater part of the time.

Involving you, the individual supervisor, in the creation of the budget helps to define clearly the authority you possess and the responsibility you are charged with in the operation of your department. Quite simply, you created your budget, so you are responsible for operating according to that budget.

Although the responsibility for draft budget preparation may lie with the supervisor, there is no reason for involvement not to extend below that level. As you will discover in this chapter, there are certain budget-related activities (such as the accumulation of operating statistics) in which some of your employees could participate. Employees who understand the nature of the budget and the reasons behind its preparation are more likely to share actively in the objectives of the department.

### Accounting Concepts

Before we discuss how a budget is structured, explanations of a pair of simple but important concepts are in order: the fiscal year and fixed versus flexible budgets.

The fiscal year is simply your institution's 12-month accounting year. This may be any consecutive 12-month period established for accounting purposes; for instance, May 1 of this year to April 30 of next year. This means that for accounting purposes your institution's "year" begins on May 1. However, your fiscal year is just as likely to be coincident with the calendar year beginning January 1. The governments of several states have encouraged health care institutions to use the calendar year as their fiscal year if they were not already doing so.

Within the accounting year are a number of accounting periods. It is common practice to keep track of payroll and certain other expenses on a basis of one, two, or four weeks and to accumulate this information on the basis of the 4-week "accounting period." Thus, there are 13 such accounting periods in the year. However, other important facts and figures are accumulated by month, either because it is necessary to do so, or because this is clearly the best data collection period available. Accountants and others speak of the "monthly closing," the act of determining the financial results of operations for a given month.

One of the biggest headaches encountered in budgeting involves differences in the length of the periods for which some data are accumulated. Payroll data are almost always kept in two- or four-week periods; many other expenses and various operating statistics are accumulated by month. In developing a budget, and especially in examining the results of operations after the fact, it is frequently necessary to manipulate some of the figures by "adding in" or "backing out" certain numbers at either end of a given period so you have complete information for the period you are interested in.

The idea of fixed versus flexible budgeting refers to the structural character of the budget relative to activity throughout the year. A fixed budget, by far the simpler of the two, assumes a stable level of operations throughout the year and spreads all budgeted costs evenly across the 12 months. A flexible budget, however, recognizes that certain costs can vary as the level of operations varies and attempts to account for this variation in the budget. A flexible budget may treat certain costs as fixed because they are in fact fixed or because this is simply the best way to handle them, but it will also attempt to identify and allow for costs that vary as departmental activity varies.

## THE TOTAL BUDGET

There are several parts to the institution's overall budget, some calling for the supervisor's involvement and some that the supervisor will rarely be concerned with. The parts and subparts of the total budget described in the following paragraphs are each properly identified as budgets in their own right, so if it seems as though we are saying "a budget is a part of a budget" we are doing so in the sense in which these financial plans have always been described.

### The Operating Budget

The operating budget usually consists of three parts.

*Statistical Budget*

The statistical budget is made up of projections of activity for the coming budget year. Usually based on a combination of past activity, current trends, and some limited knowledge of future conditions and circumstances, this is the organization's best estimate of work activity for the coming 12-month period. These estimates are projections of statistics such as admissions or discharges expected, patient-days expected, likely number of laboratory tests or X-ray procedures, number of meals to be served, pounds of linen to be processed, and so on. These may be prepared as gross, fixed estimates of a year's activity, or they may be projected by month based on certain knowledge suggesting variations in activity.

When getting ready to prepare the budget for the institution, the accounting department will generally compile and summarize the most recent historical data and projections available and supply this information to the other departments. However, it is often necessary for the departments to refine these figures into detailed estimates of activities for the coming budget year.

You accomplish this refinement the same way the accounting department makes its projections—based on past activity in your department and your particular knowledge of future operations.

## Expense Budget

The expense budget attempts to anticipate costs of operations for each department individually and for the organization as a whole. In a true participative budgeting process, the departmental expense budget is the primary area of supervisory involvement in the budgeting process.

The expense budget is made up of projections of personnel costs and all other costs. The cost of anything acquired or consumed in the operation of the department and directly attributable to the department will ordinarily appear in that department's budget. Some elements of expense that cannot readily be directly associated with the department (for example, heating, lighting, and building depreciation costs) will be budgeted for the facility as a whole. Most elements of personnel cost will be budgeted in the department, although in many organizations it is accepted practice to budget employee benefits as a percentage of payroll for the organization as a whole.

There are some important determinants of personnel cost that lie partially beyond the scope of this elementary treatment of budgeting. The most important of these, the question of how many staff members are required to operate the department, is briefly addressed in a later section, "Staffing and Scheduling Considerations."

A simple step-by-step illustration of the preparation of a departmental expense budget is presented following this discussion of budget components.

## Revenue Budget

Usually prepared by the finance department, the revenue budget is a projection of the income likely to be received by the institution during the budget year. Keeping in mind that revenue ultimately must cover all costs of operation, the revenue budget must attempt to consider the impact of numerous factors beyond the simple earning of income from services. A revenue budget may, for instance, attempt to reflect the impact of a new service coming into being during the budget year; the effects of a service being deleted or curtailed during the year; additions to or departures from the medical staff that have a direct bearing on number of admissions; and the effects of changes in reimbursement regulations introduced by the major third-party payers.

The bulk of health care institution revenue comes from third-party payers (major insurers such as Blue Cross and government programs such as Medicare and Medicaid) or from the patients themselves. There are also other sources that may include general donations, United Fund allocations, taxes (in the case of government institutions), research grants, investments, school operating revenues, television and telephone charges, purchase discounts, cafeteria, and other miscellaneous income.

Certain legitimate or potential deductions from revenue need to be considered as well and include free care (such as hospitals are required to render in certain amounts if they accepted money under the federal Hill-Burton program), outright charity care, discounts to employees, and bad debts.

## The Capital Budget

A capital budget is prepared to account for potential expenditures for major fixed and movable equipment. Fixed equipment (a building, a boiler, or a new roof) and major movable equipment (copy machines, hospital beds, X-ray machines, and computers) represent those costs that must be capitalized. These costs apply to operations for considerably longer than just the coming budget period, so they must be spread out over a number of periods.

Sometimes the boundary between capital purchases and items that can be allocated to operations in the budget period is hazy. However, consistent with legal guidelines for determining what must be capitalized, the institution usually has its own guides for determining what should be called a capital purchase. The institution's guide may be expressed as some specific amount of money, some useful-life criterion, or a combination of these. For instance, your institution may have decided that any purchased item having a useful life longer than 1 year and costing more than $200 must be capitalized. Thus a $250 typewriter would be capitalized but a $150 calculator would not, although both will clearly last longer than 1 year.

As a supervisor, you should make it a point to learn your institution's guidelines for identifying capital assets. You may either ask for a certain item in your capital budget request or attempt to secure it through your departmental expense budget according to where it fits by your organization's definition.

In capital budgeting, requests for purchases often outrun the money available. Requests may come from all directions: from the medical staff, who would like certain equipment to work with; from the public, who would like to see certain services and facilities available; from supervisors and department heads, who would like to have newer and better equipment; and from the government, which may tell your institution there is something you need to buy to enable you to conform with some code, regulation, or requirement.

Development of the capital budget may also involve the development of short-range and long-range capital plans as the institution attempts to determine best what new and replacement equipment will be required for future operations. This involves looking at all equipment and listing each piece along with its age, original cost, and estimated replacement date. When looking at capital equipment within your own department, you should at least list all items according to projected replacement date and then go on to add your ideas of what new equipment you may require in the foreseeable future.

Capital budget requests usually receive close scrutiny, and the request for a substantial capital expenditure must usually be accompanied by the following:

- a realistic assessment of the urgency or priority of the purchase
- a detailed projection of all costs involved in the acquisition
- a full description of the project and the rationale (justification)
- a statement as to whether the requested item represents an addition, replacement, or improvement
- the impact, in the case of a revenue-producing department, of the proposed acquisition on revenues

Most capital budget requests are ordinarily subject to several levels of review and approval. As a supervisor you may have been assigned a certain dollar limit for capital purchases for your department, but this amount will usually be low when reckoned against the cost of desired capital purchases. However, it is just as likely, perhaps even more so, that you personally will have no capital budget approval in your department. Your immediate supervisor, or perhaps the chief executive officer (CEO) or finance director, may retain the authority to approve minimum capital purchases up to a given amount. Many capital expenditures, however, must be authorized by the board of directors. A certain hospital in the eastern United States, a not untypical institution of approximately 200 beds, permits its CEO or finance director to approve capital purchases not exceeding $2,500. Purchases from $2,500 to $10,000 may be approved by the finance committee of the board of directors, and purchases exceeding $10,000 must be approved by the full board.

### The Cash Budget

The cash budget is prepared by the finance department and is usually done last in the budgeting process. It consists of estimates of the institution's cash needs as compared with projections of cash receipts over the term covered by the budget. The pattern of cash-in versus cash-out examined in the cash budget is extremely important to the institution because of the need to remain financially solvent in the short run. That is to say, it does little good to appear rich on paper—to have impressive amounts of money owed to us—if we do not have sufficient cash in the bank to pay today's bills or meet a payroll.

The cash budget holds clear implications for everyone concerned with the management of receivables and payables. Should cash be in extremely short supply for a given period we may turn more attention to the aggressive collection of accounts receivable, or we might delay a few payables until we are in a better position to make payment. A lack of cash can also lead to short-term borrowing. This sometimes results in not inconsiderable difficulties in obtaining credit and leads to still more operating expense because of today's significant interest rates.

### ILLUSTRATION: THE DIAGNOSTIC IMAGING (X-RAY) DEPARTMENT EXPENSE BUDGET

By way of illustration we will briefly examine the expense budget for the diagnostic imaging department of a 200-bed hospital. (Although still popularly referred to as "X-Ray," the newer title for the function has taken over as this activity has spread to include newer forms of imaging and scanning.) This budget covers the following:

- personnel expenses (salaries and fringe benefits)
- X-ray film
- other supplies
- fixed expenses

- equipment repairs
- staff education

## Statistics and Projections

From the projections assembled for the institution (the statistical budget) we start with the following information for the hospital:

- projected outpatient visits—41,000
- projected patient days—51,500

We know from past experience and analysis that:

- inpatient tests per patient day = 0.2226
- outpatient tests per visit = 0.3437
- standard worked hours per test = 1.2913
- nonworked hours per test = 0.1761

Therefore, we determine that the department may perform:

11,464 inpatient tests
<u>14,092</u> outpatient tests
25,556 total tests

Multiplying the hours per test by the total number of tests to be performed, we determine that performance of the department's projected workload will require

33,000 worked hours
<u>14,500</u> nonworked hours
37,500 hours of personnel time for the budget year

With projected pay increases figured in, personnel time for the department in this illustration is estimated to cost $15.00 per hour for the budget year. (The determination of personnel expense can be far more detailed than this approach suggests. For instance, it is possible to consider each employee and each position, one by one, and apply actual pay rates and add the effects of increases at the precise points where they will occur.)

The next step involves determining personnel expense for the budget year:

- $15.00 ¥ 37,500 hours = $562,500 personnel cost

Moving to elements of cost other than personnel, analysis of film cost and consumption has revealed that an average of 2.40 film units are consumed for each test performed. With a projected price increase being considered, film is expected to cost $2.82 per unit. Therefore

- 2.40 units per test ¥ 25,556 tests = 61,334 units
- 61,334 units ¥ $2.82 = $172,962
- $172,962 / 25,556 = $6.77 per test

As for other supplies (perhaps film developer, paper, pencils, labels, film jackets), variable supply cost analysis shows these costs to amount to $1.00 per test. We expect a 5 percent increase in supply costs, so:

- $1.00 ¥ 1.05 = $1.05 per test for other supplies

Fixed expenses attributable to the department (perhaps a maintenance contract, leases on some of the equipment, and other items that will not vary with activity) have been established through analysis as $18,500 per year.

Furthermore, it has been determined that equipment repairs have historically been costing the department an average of $0.60 per test. We estimate a 5 percent increase in the cost of repairs but no change of repair frequency, so:

- $0.60 \times 1.05 = $0.63 per test repair cost

Staff education (travel, fees, and other expenses associated with sending employees to educational programs outside of the institution) has been projected at a total of $2,000 for the budget year.

### Personnel

One way to handle the personnel portion of the budget is demonstrated in Table 21–1. This method assumes uniform distribution of worked hours at so many per day and assumes distribution of nonworked time on a basis sug-

---

**Table 21–1**  Budgeted Personnel Cost Distribution

| 33,000 worked hours @ $15.00/hr. | = | $495,000* |
|---|---|---|
| 4,500 nonworked hours @ $15.00/hr. | = | 67,500* |
| | | $562,500* |

| Month | Days | Proportion of Nonworked Time** | Projected Cost Nonworked | Projected Cost Worked | Total |
|---|---|---|---|---|---|
| January | 31 | 0.0765 | $5,163 | $42,611 | $47,774 |
| February | 28 | 0.0479 | 3,233 | 39,918 | 43,151 |
| March | 31 | 0.0518 | 3,496 | 44,278 | 47,774 |
| April | 30 | 0.0641 | 4,327 | 41,906 | 46,233 |
| May | 31 | 0.0707 | 4,772 | 43,002 | 47,774 |
| June | 30 | 0.0935 | 6,311 | 39,922 | 46,233 |
| July | 31 | 0.1129 | 7,621 | 40,153 | 47,774 |
| August | 31 | 0.1295 | 8,741 | 39,033 | 47,774 |
| September | 30 | 0.1116 | 7,533 | 38,700 | 46,233 |
| October | 31 | 0.0602 | 4,064 | 43,710 | 47,774 |
| November | 30 | 0.0842 | 5,684 | 40,549 | 46,233 |
| December | 31 | 0.0971 | 6,554 | 41,220 | 47,774 |
| | 365 | 1.0000 | $67,499* | $495,002 | $562,501* |

*Totals differ because of rounding
**Determined from historical data modified by expected vacation time

gested by past practice and knowledge of some future events (such as vacation scheduling). You could conceivably do a more accurate job of spreading the personnel budget if you had some knowledge of a pattern of fluctuation in department activity such as that appearing in institutions subject to seasonable fluctuations.

### Film, Other Supplies, and Equipment Repairs

The month-by-month projections of these three items of expense that are reasonably believed to vary with workload are listed in Table 21–2. Thus, a month with 30 days will absorb a slightly smaller portion of such expense than will a month with 31 days.

### Fixed Expense

The $18,500 of fixed expense for the year is spread evenly by simply assigning one twelfth of that total to each month of the budget year.

### Staff Education

The $2,000 for staff education is spread evenly across the budget year. This amount is not likely to be consumed in the same pattern in which it is budgeted, but as long as the education money is spent throughout the year with that budget limit in mind the results will be satisfactory. This could be budgeted more accurately if we had information about expected patterns of attendance at programs, for instance, like the department that always sends two people to the same annual conference in the same month each year, but again the results should prove satisfactory as long as the year's expenditures remain within the total. Note also that this amount of money is completely

**Table 21–2** Film, Other Supplies, and Equipment Repairs

| Month | Total Tests | Film Cost @$5.64/Test | Other Supplies @$1.00/Test | Repairs $0.704/Test |
|---|---|---|---|---|
| January | 2,185 | $14,792 | $2,294 | $1,377 |
| February | 2,048 | 13,865 | 2,150 | 1,290 |
| March | 2,310 | 15,639 | 2,426 | 1,455 |
| April | 2,228 | 15,084 | 2,339 | 1,404 |
| May | 2,206 | 14,935 | 2,316 | 1,390 |
| June | 2,300 | 15,571 | 2,415 | 1,449 |
| July | 2,034 | 13,770 | 2,136 | 1,281 |
| August | 2,057 | 13,926 | 2,160 | 1,296 |
| September | 2,017 | 13,655 | 2,118 | 1,271 |
| October | 2,104 | 14,244 | 2,209 | 1,326 |
| November | 2,009 | 13,601 | 2,109 | 1,266 |
| December | 2,058 | 13,933 | 2,161 | 1,297 |
| | $25,556 | $173,015 | $26,833 | $16,102 |

manageable by the supervisor since it is usually at the supervisor's discretion that employees are permitted to attend outside programs.

## The Diagnostic Imaging Department Expense Budget

Exhibit 21–1 is the expense budget for the X-ray department for the year. We need not be reminded at this point that a departmental budget is far from precise. Examine this illustration closely and you will note some holes. For instance, predicting equipment repairs as a function of number of tests is a questionable practice at best because there is little solid evidence to go on. We might just as readily have spread repair costs evenly across the 12 months. Note, however, that manageable items of cost, such as staff education, are better highlighted by the budget and placed before you where you can control them in relation to the way you see other expenses going.

Consider also those expenses that are partly manageable, such as personnel. There are a number of management actions you can take when actual costs and activity begin to move one way or the other. For instance, you may wish to permit or even encourage the heaviest use of vacation time during periods when workload falls off. Also, by highlighting all elements of cost in the department, the budget affords you an ongoing awareness of supply expenses and other variable costs. If you see the cost of supplies suddenly exceeding the projected amount, then you are alerted to the need for investigation and possible action. Without a budget, certain costs could run unex-

**Exhibit 21–1** Diagnostic Imaging Expense Budget

| Month | Salaries | Other Film | Fixed Supplies | Repairs | Expense | Educ. | Total |
|-------|----------|-----------|----------------|---------|---------|-------|-------|
| January | $47,774 | $14,792 | $2,294 | $1,377 | $1,542 | $167 | $67,946 |
| February | 43,151 | 13,865 | 2,150 | 1,290 | 1,542 | 167 | 62,165 |
| March | 47,774 | 15,639 | 2,426 | 1,455 | 1,542 | 167 | 69,003 |
| April | 46,233 | 15,084 | 2,339 | 1,404 | 1,542 | 167 | 66,769 |
| May | 47,774 | 14,935 | 2,316 | 1,390 | 1,542 | 167 | 68,124 |
| June | 46,233 | 15,571 | 2,415 | 1,449 | 1,542 | 167 | 67,377 |
| July | 47,774 | 13,770 | 2,136 | 1,281 | 1,542 | 167 | 66,630 |
| August | 47,774 | 13,926 | 2,160 | 1,296 | 1,542 | 167 | 66,825 |
| September | 46,233 | 13,655 | 2,118 | 1,271 | 1,542 | 167 | 64,986 |
| October | 47,774 | 14,244 | 2,209 | 1,326 | 1,542 | 167 | 67,262 |
| November | 46,233 | 13,601 | 2,109 | 1,266 | 1,542 | 167 | 64,918 |
| December | 47,774 | 13,933 | 2,161 | 1,297 | 1,542 | 167 | 66,874 |
| Totals | $562,501 | $173,015 | $26,833 | $16,102 | $18,504 | $2,004 | $798,959 |

plainably high for perhaps months without your becoming aware of the situation.

A budget, remember, is a plan. As such it attempts to look into a time that is not yet here, and it is necessarily based on estimates and projections. In no way is it ever to be regarded as a preordained, concrete picture of future events. Rarely will you budget precisely as you feel you should have budgeted, and rarely will the results be exactly as predicted. In this respect the budget is much like any other management tool: it cannot do the management job for you, but chances are you will do a better management job with it than you would do without it.

## STAFFING AND SCHEDULING CONSIDERATIONS

### Definitions

In practice, the terms staffing and scheduling are sometimes used together to refer to a general process; often they are used separately to mean essentially the same thing. Although they are as closely related as the two sides of a coin, there are practical differences as follows:

- Staffing is determining how many people of what specific skills are needed and making them available.
- Scheduling is determining who, by name and skill, will do what work and when (specific time period).

As they relate to the basic management functions, staffing is largely a part of organizing and establishing the framework within which the work will get done, while scheduling is essentially a refined component of planning. Just as a budget is a quantitative plan for a future time period, a schedule is a quantitative plan for a coming period of time.

### Elementary Staffing Concept: The Full-Time Equivalent

The term full-time equivalent (FTE) simply means the amount of labor input equivalent to one full-time employee. Assume, for example, that the basic work week in your organization is 40 hours; in your department 40 hours of personnel time constitutes one FTE. These 40 hours may belong to a single scheduled employee who works 40 hours per week, two part-time employees who each work 20 hours per week, or some other combination of hours and people that adds up to 40 hours per week. All these variations represent one FTE.

Staffing calculations ordinarily begin with a determination of how many FTEs are required to cover a particular activity. Later, scheduling will determine how many people working how many hours are needed to provide this coverage. Consider a hypothetical department in which complete coverage requires the input of 600 labor hours per week. This need could be filled with 15 people, each working 40 hours per week; 30 people, each working 20 hours per week; or any combination of full-time and part-time employees adding up to 600 hours. Whatever combination is used, the staffing requirement in this example remains 15 FTE (600 hours needed divided by 40 hours per week).

Forty hours cannot always be used to determine FTEs. What must be used is the organization's (or the department's) official workweek. While this frequently is 40 hours, in some organizations it can be 37.5 hours per week or even 35 hours per week. It is how many paid hours a full-time employee works in a week that defines the divisor used to determine FTEs.

The concept of the FTE is convenient in calculating overall staffing requirements, especially in a setting such as a hospital where an 8-hour day shift of Monday through Friday applies only to a portion of the work force.

What, then, of positions that are covered more than 40 hours per week? Consider a medical-surgical unit nursing position that is covered 24 hours a day, 7 days a week. To cover each shift for 7 days requires Monday through Friday coverage for 8 hours a day, or one FTE, and 8 hours for each of Saturday and Sunday or 16/40 = 0.4 FTE. Therefore, covering a single position one shift for 7 days requires 1.4 FTE, and covering it for three shifts for 7 days requires 4.2 FTE. Using the same sort of calculation, the following can be derived:

- A position covered two shifts per day, 7 days a week requires 2.8 FTE.
- A position covered for two shifts Monday through Friday and one shift on Saturday and Sunday requires 2.4 FTE.
- A position covered 12 hours per day, 5 days per week requires 1.5 FTE.

## Staffing Standards

The determination of the number of FTEs required to staff a given function at a certain level of activity lies largely beyond the scope of this budgeting discussion. This determination requires a staffing standard. This is a number that reasonably relates required staff to the department's basic unit of output. It is sometimes expressed in terms of a fixed component and a variable component, and sometimes in terms of a simple variable element alone. The fixed component covers labor requirements that do not change with normal activity fluctuations, such as department supervision, secretarial support, and other fixed costs. The variable component fluctuates with activity volume. When a variable figure is used alone as a standard, the so-called fixed elements of input are spread over all of the activity, rendering the single-part standards somewhat less accurate. For example, the two-part productivity standard for a hypothetical health information management (formerly medical records) department might appear as 22.8 hours per calendar day + 1.746 hours per discharge, while a simple one-part guideline might be 2.20 hours per discharge.

Where do such standards come from? Productivity standards are arrived at through stopwatch time studies and predetermined motion times, which are time consuming and thus relatively costly; work sampling, which is time consuming and moderately costly; and the use of published guidelines, benchmarks, or targets, which are generally provided by various external organizations. These kinds of indicators can be adequate but sometimes they are unreliable because they are broad and do not account for legitimate differences in procedures from one organization to another. However, they are the most commonly used of the three because they are economical.

Ordinarily the department manager must work with a guideline or benchmark standard or none at all, beginning the budget process by assuming that the present staffing level is the starting point and attempting to adjust upward or downward depending on anticipated changes in activity. This process, of course, is contrary to the notion of zero-based budgeting in which it is assumed that nothing is in place and a case must be built for what will be needed to accommodate the expected volume. But zero-based budgeting requires some form of staffing standard, some known, reliable relationship between input and output for the function in question.

In the absence of a program of engineered work standards, the department manager would do best to adopt a staffing guideline or benchmark from a similar organization and modify it as necessary to accommodate the department's unique needs.

## THE BUDGETING PROCESS

### Responsibilities

The responsibility for preparing the budget rests in part with several individuals and groups. The *board of directors* is ultimately responsible for everything in the budget and thus retains the authority for final approval of the budget. Although the board will not likely become involved in the details of budget preparation, this body will probably rule on proposed capital expenditures item by item and review and approve the principal parts of the budget. The board's role in the approval of the budget is consistent with the directors' legal responsibilities as trustees of the resources of the organization.

The *administrator or CEO* must ensure that the budget being submitted to the board is consistent with the goals of the organization and is realistic and workable in the light of current knowledge of expected revenues and expenses.

The *finance director* has an active role in preparing the cash and revenue budgets and assembling all pieces of the operating budget into a total budget for the institution. Like the CEO, the finance director must ensure that budgeting guidelines are followed and that the resulting plan appears to be workable and realistic in terms of what is known about the coming budget year.

*All supervisors and department heads*, at least under a participative budgeting approach, are responsible for assembling the expense and capital budgets for their own departments. In accounting or budgeting terms, the smallest organizational unit for which a budget is prepared is usually identified as a "cost center." A cost center—an organizational unit for which costs are identified and collected—is usually provided with expense and capital budgets prepared by the supervisor. In the case of middle- or upper-level managers who may have charge of several cost centers, the task also includes assembling individual cost-center budgets into a budget for their total area of responsibility.

A *budget committee* may be established each year to facilitate the preparation of the budget. This committee will usually consist of the CEO, the finance director, the director of nursing service and other major department heads, and perhaps a member of the finance committee of the board of directors. It is the role of the budget committee to establish and distribute the guidelines for budget preparation, to decide how particular problems should be solved and certain issues dealt with as they occur, and to keep all stages of budget preparation activity moving toward completion.

## The Budget Coordination Meeting

The budget coordination meeting is generally seen as a "kickoff" for the year's activity in putting together the budget. If the target for presentation to the board should be some time in October, the budget coordination meeting may take place in June or July. Convened and conducted by members of the budget committee, the coordination meeting should include all managers who have an active role in budget preparation. At this meeting the most recent volume factors are introduced, policies affecting budgeting are reviewed and any changes are noted, planned organizational changes likely to affect budgeting factors are reviewed and clarified, and trends of likely future activity are discussed. In short, any known or suspected factor that may have a bearing on budget preparation is reviewed.

Many institutions use a budget manual, a book of informational and instructional documents assembled under the guidance of the budget committee for the current year's budget preparation activity. Given to each person who must prepare and present a budget for one or more cost centers, this manual contains all information, instructions, and forms necessary for budget preparation.

The budget manual describes the full scope and purpose of the budgeting program; outlines all procedures for preparation, review, and revision of budgets; and defines the duties and authority and responsibility of all persons involved in the process.

## The Budget Calendar

The preparation of the budget for a sizeable health care institution is an exercise in timing. Budgets for dozens of individual cost centers must be put together, and these must be assembled into budgets for larger organizational units and eventually into a budget for the total institution. If two or three pieces of the build-up are missing, the total budget is delayed. Also, the cash budget cannot be properly prepared until the operating and capital budgets are complete.

The budget calendar displays deadline dates for all steps in the budget preparation process. The calendar will let a supervisor know when the department's draft budget must be submitted, when it is likely to be returned following initial review, when the revision must be submitted, and how much time must be allowed for the approval process.

Much of the trauma that can be encountered in the annual budgeting exercise is due to matters of timing. We often tend to get things done at the deadline or perhaps a little late, and our planning rarely anticipates all contingencies. As a result, it is often necessary to go through the whole process again, perhaps several times, on the way to a realistic, workable budget for the entire institution. Dozens of supervisors can enter the budgeting process with the best of intentions; yet the results may be unsatisfactory the first time around because the key persons assembling the final budget simply do not know exactly where the totals are going to fall until all the pieces are put together for the first time. We then get into back-and-forth activity as efforts are made to shift resources in more appropriate directions and allow us to come up with a budget that is realistic under the circumstances.

## Review and Coordination

When all of the individual departments' draft budgets are submitted, the finance division will prepare the total budget for approval of the estimates. As already suggested, the budget may go through several drafts before the budget committee believes it has a document appropriate for submission to the board of directors.

## Adoption

A summary of the total budget will be presented to the board of directors for discussion and approval. This summary generally includes the following:

- a narrative description of the budget and some of its key elements and the reasons behind its preparation in this manner
- a condensed income statement for the budget period
- a summary of capital expenditure requests
- a cash analysis covering the budget period
- the key factors used in forecasting
- estimates of the impact of this budget on the institution's services and finances

The board of directors will either approve or reject the budget in whole or in part as the trustees see fit. Necessary elements of the process are repeated until the board approves a budget for the coming year.

## "FINISHED" IS JUST BEGUN

A budget should be a live, working plan. For it to serve in this capacity requires timely and accurate reporting of operating results.

Reporting the results of operations is generally a responsibility of the accounting department. Timeliness is essential; it stands to reason that the more recent the feedback received on results, the more valuable the budget is for highlighting the need for management action. The information received each month—a comparison of operating results for the period with the budget projections for the period—allows you to make adjustments for those aspects of operations that are wholly or partly under direct supervisory control.

Reporting is often done in a way that highlights exceptions. That is, the reporting system, built on recognition of the likely presence of natural variations between operating results and budget projections, will specifically flag items that appear to be out of line beyond normally expected variations.

## A Sample Budget Report

Exhibit 21–2 is a sample budget report, identified as an operating expense schedule and taken from the personnel department of a hospital in the 400- to 500-bed range. In two sections it deals separately with personnel expenses (technician and specialist labor and clerical and administrative labor) and nonlabor expenses (all costs of running the personnel department other than salaries and wages). Absent from consideration are employee benefit costs, which are budgeted separately for the entire hospital in a benefits cost center.

From left to right the columns on the schedule represent identifying numbers of the individual accounts; the department using the accounts; actual expenditures charged to each account for the month under consideration; the amounts budgeted for the month; the variances for the month—the differences between actual and budget—in terms of both absolute dollars and percentage of budget; and for the year to date the actual expenditures, the budgeted amounts, and the variances for each account.

In the actual columns the occasional minus sign after a dollar amount indicates a credit to an account. In Exhibit 21–2 the negative amount for account 901, Dues and Subscriptions, reflects a refund received upon cancellation of a prepaid subscription service.

The minus signs in the variance columns have a clearly different meaning. A minus sign after a variance dollar amount indicates a favorable variance, a condition of being under budget by that amount. Thus a minus sign after a variance percentage also indicates a favorable variance—the account stands at that percent under budget.

A caution is in order regarding the use of minus signs in budget reports. Their use is not always consistent from organization to organization. But minus signs carry a generally negative connotation for many people that is often the reverse of their meaning in a budget report. In Exhibit 21–2, and indeed in many organizations' budget reports, the minus sign attached to a variance is good in that it means "under"—a condition of being under the budgeted amount.

In analyzing a budget report it is best to begin with the obvious. In the case of Exhibit 21–2, the obvious consists of accounts for which there are charges but no budget.

Often charges appear against a "zero" budget—that is, an account for which the department has budgeted no expenditures—because people in the department make errors filling out requisitions and other forms and because people filling out forms may not provide sufficient detail, leaving others to place the charges in specific accounts. In the exhibit, the charge to account 711, Miscellaneous Food Items, was found to be an outright error; another department should have been charged.

The supervisor should ensure that all the department's employees who trigger expenditures and charges supply full charging information, which usually includes both department number and specific account number. Considering the exhibit again, the $152.39 incorrectly charged to account 769 came from paperwork that indicated only department 937 in the "Charge To" space; someone in the accounting department made a guess as to the account. (The

**Exhibit 21–2** Sample Budget Report

| Department-937 | | THIS MONTH | | | | YEAR TO DATE | | | |
|---|---|---|---|---|---|---|---|---|---|
| | | Actual | Budget | Variance | Pct | Actual | Budget | Variance | Pct |
| 502 Personnel Dept | Technician & Spe | 10,812.03 | 10,758.09 | 53.94 | 1 | 31,543.27 | 31,663.16 | 119.89– | 0 |
| 506 Personnel Dept | Clerical & Admin | 8,814.42 | 8,715.30 | 99.12 | 1 | 25,915.60 | 25,650.86 | 264.70 | 1 |
| | | 19,626.45 | 19,473.39 | 153.06 | 1 | 57,458.87 | 57,314.02 | 144.85 | 0 |
| | | | | | | | | | |
| 545 Personnel Dept | Prof Serv Purch | 0.00 | 83.30 | 83.30– | 100– | 0.00 | 249.90 | 249.90 | 100– |
| 571 Personnel Dept | Emp Ed & Train | 390.00 | 499.80 | 109.80– | 22– | 1,233.61 | 1,499.40 | 265.79– | 18– |
| 711 Personnel Dept | Misc Food Items | 98.47 | 0.00 | 98.47 | 0 | 98.47 | 0.00 | 98.47 | 0 |
| | | | | | | | | | |
| 759 Personnel Dept | Books & Film | 58.50 | 63.53 | 5.03– | 8– | 78.45 | 186.43 | 107.98– | 58– |
| 763 Personnel Dept | Office Supplies | 167.88 | 152.46 | 15.42 | 10 | 258.52 | 447.48 | 161.96– | 36– |
| 769 Personnel Dept | Misc General Sup | 152.39 | 0.00 | 152.39 | 0 | 221.00 | 0.00 | 221.00 | 0 |
| | | | | | | | | | |
| 787 Personnel Dept | Inv Chg-Inst, Med | 0.00 | 0.00 | 0.00 | 0 | 4.26 | 0.00 | 4.26 | 0 |
| 789 Personnel Dept | Inv Chg-Dietary | 2.03 | 25.41 | 23.38– | 92– | 15.61 | 74.58 | 58.97– | 79– |
| 794 Personnel Dept | Inv Chg-Forms, P | 129.91 | 127.05 | 2.86 | 2 | 196.52 | 372.90 | 176.38– | 47– |
| | | | | | | | | | |
| 796 Personnel Dept | Inv Chg-Office S | 65.68 | 50.82 | 14.86 | 29 | 173.68 | 149.16 | 24.52 | 16 |
| 797 Personnel Dept | Inv Chg-Paper Go | 2.43 | 2.12 | 0.31 | 15 | 6.57 | 6.20 | 0.37 | 6 |
| 798 Personnel Dept | Inv Chg-Miscella | 47.99 | 4.24 | 43.75 | 32 | 97.38 | 12.41 | 84.97 | 685 |
| | | | | | | | | | |
| 805 Personnel Dept | Prevent Mtc Cont | 0.00 | 125.70 | 125.70– | 100– | 233.75 | 363.75 | 130.00– | 36– |
| 809 Personnel Dept | Misc Repair | 0.00 | 20.95 | 20.95– | 100– | 0.00 | 60.60 | 60.60– | 100– |
| 867 Personnel Dept | Photocopy Charge | 64.30 | 100.56 | 36.26– | 36– | 251.35 | 291.00 | 39.65– | 14– |
| | | | | | | | | | |
| 901 Personnel Dept | Dues & Subscript | 170.00– | 263.97 | 433.97– | 164– | 597.25 | 763.85 | 166.60– | 22– |
| 907 Personnel Dept | Postage | 5.87 | 8.47 | 2.60– | 31– | 15.62 | 24.86 | 9.24– | 37– |
| 913 Personnel Dept | Public Relations | 2.00 | 49.98 | 47.98– | 96– | 5.75 | 149.94 | 144.19– | 96– |
| | | | | | | | | | |
| 931 Personnel Dept | Misc Other Expen | 17.62– | 0.00 | 17.62– | 0 | 6.00– | 0.00 | 6.00– | 0 |
| | | | | | | | | | |
| | | 999.83 | 1,578.36 | 578.53– | 37– | 3,508.79 | 4,652.46 | 1,143.67– | 25– |
| | | | | | | | | | |
| | | 20,626.28 | 21,051.75 | 425.47– | 2 | 60,967.66 | 61,966.48 | 998.82– | 2– |

accounting manager might concede that the clerk could have called the personnel department to learn the correct account number. The manager could also claim, however, with some justification, that the size of his staff would have to increase significantly to be able to call for every missing account number.) The difficulty could have been avoided in the first place if the initiating personnel department employee had simply entered 937-763 under "Charge To."

Occasionally, charges to an account for which there is no budget may be legitimate. If the account in question appears to be the most logical place for a particular charge but there happens to be no budget, this should serve as a flag to consider that account as a legitimate line item for the coming budget year (if it appears as though such charges may occur again).

The supervisor is often provided with guidelines for analyzing the budget report and answering for variances. Such guidelines are usually expressed in terms of a variance threshold beyond which answers are expected. For example, the guidelines for the manager of the personnel department of Exhibit 21–2 are as follows:

- For personnel costs, explanation or justification must be provided for variances beyond plus or minus 2 percent or plus or minus $1,000 for total departmental labor costs for the month.
- For nonpersonnel expense, explanation or justification must be provided for variances beyond plus or minus 10 percent or plus or minus $50 for any specific account for the month.

Answering to variances under budget is almost as important as answering to variances over budget. Being under budget for a period does not necessarily mean that money is being saved or that a favorable condition is emerging. It can often indicate that expenditures are occurring in a pattern inconsistent with the budget allocation, and it can sometimes indicate that certain necessary or desirable expenditures have been overlooked.

Under a thorough financial control system supervisors are usually expected to answer to their immediate supervisor for budget variances. Exhibit 21–3 is a portion of a sample budget variance report for the personnel department in Exhibit 21–2; it shows the manager's response to the first several items of concern on Exhibit 21–2—the first items that fall beyond the plus or minus 10 percent or plus or minus $50 threshold for the month.

In addition to being provided with a monthly report of expenditures versus budget, the supervisor usually receives detailed backup about the individual

**Exhibit 21–3** Budget Variance Report

| Dept:<br>Account | #937—<br>Personnel<br>Variance | Manager: *J.W. Johnson*<br><br>Reason | Responsible V.P.: *R.B. Jay*<br>Action/Anticipated<br>Outcome |
|---|---|---|---|
| 545 | 100% under | Account for temporary help. No expenses yet this year. | No use anticipated until vacation coverage (July). |
| 571 | 22% under | Behind schedule on sending staff to conferences. | To reach zero variance by June 30 with charge for personnel seminar. |
| 763 | 10% over (should be 110% over) | First-quarter supply order billed in March. April expense to be minimal. With error in 769 fixed, should show 110% over for month and –2% YTD. | 2% under for year to date. Should finish year about 15% under. |
| 789 | 92% under | Charges occur unevenly during year. Heaviest use yet to come (fall). | No action necessary. |
| 796 | 29% over | Unusually high use rate for pads, pens, etc. | Altering procedure to have department secretary issue (as well as order) supplies. Should see change in a month if any of usage is "leakage." |

charges made to each account. This backup makes it possible to assess the validity of most charges.

When working with budget reports you should make it a habit to question all details that you do not fully understand. Learning month by month where all of the department's budget dollars are going will eventually enable you to alter patterns of expenditures at least partially in a way that may improve unfavorable trends that appear to be developing.

## LOTS OF WORK? CERTAINLY

In the "Situation" that started the chapter, count it as unfortunate timing that Mary Regal has started in a management position in an organization new to her at just the time when managers are expected to assemble their budgets for the following year. It is surely unfortunate as well that most of Mary's past experience with budgeting has been negative. However, Mary is far from the first manager who has been circumstantially conditioned to view the budgeting process as an intrusive load of largely useless work that they have no time for. On the positive side, however, although Mary may be hard pressed to see a positive side just yet, enough comes through Eva's commentary to suggest that Mary might now be in an organization where budgeting is truly participative.

Mary may believe that her budget will be what finance wants it to be, and there may be some truth in this as far as resources available overall are concerned. But no person in finance will be nearly as capable as Mary in distributing that amount over her budget categories. She may ultimately be limited in total dollars, but she has some flexibility in where to spend them.

Budgets "handed down from upstairs" per Mary's experience at General portray budgeting as a secret process and one with which the department managers cannot be trusted. Also, budgets so handed down are not likely to have the managers' support as would budgets done participatively.

A bit less frustrating than budgets done "on high," but still a nuisance to the manager, is the process involving repeated padding and cutting. Doing a budget in this mode invariably results in the necessity for an additional iteration or two, and the mandated across-the-board cuts can catch the unwary who do not know the unwritten "rules of the game." It is best, of course, to go in initially with an honest budget, with no deliberate padding but incorporating a few features that might later be adjudged frills. A subsequent iteration might result in the loss of some frills and some necessities being trimmed a bit; yet another iteration might result in an austerity budget.

Eva was quite right in some of her comments. In a hospital setting there's usually pressure to keep costs down, and in the first round of the budget process expected income is usually less than anticipated spending. These are both good reasons for the individual manager to take the process seriously and submit a realistic budget request.

Mary Regal should assume that she now has a voice in the budgeting process and participate accordingly. As far as all of the budget reports are concerned, if the reports at Wilson Hospital are also "about as easy to interpret as

Latin code" Mary needs to seek out assistance and learn how to read and interpret these reports. The budget is not an annual phenomenon to be left behind until another year has passed. Rather, it is a live, quantitative plan that requires ongoing attention throughout the year.

## CONTROL: AWARENESS PLUS ACTION

Preparing a budget and working with it throughout the year heightens your awareness of how the department's resources—for which you are responsible—are used to fulfill the department's responsibilities. Reports of actual results versus budget projections provide all-important information on which to base corrective action when needed. For instance, when productivity problems occur and the relationship between worked hours and the volume of work begins to change unfavorably, you can take positive steps that might include effective use of overtime, application of call time, scheduling of vacations and other time off, and routine scheduling of personnel for day-to-day coverage.

Viewing the budget and feedback on actual operations from the perspective of a complete organizational unit, whether a small department or an entire institution, consider what is obtained from the process: at any time you know where you are relative to where you thought you might be, and you also know where you must look for improvement.

---

## REVIEW QUESTIONS

1. What is the primary purpose of having supervisors participate in building their own budgets?
2. Explain what is meant by *flexible budget.*
3. Explain the implications of the following statement: *"What the statements say is only secondary; what's most important is our cash condition. Cash is king."*
4. Since a budget is a plan and as such always deals with the future, why bother with all the work of budgeting if we know that the future is bound to be somewhat different from what our plan assumes?
5. What do you believe should be done with your organization's budget if your operating statistics change dramatically in mid-year? Why?

---

## EXERCISE: "JUGGLING" YOUR BUDGET

You are the administrative supervisor of the diagnostic imaging department. You recently submitted your draft expense budget for the coming year (Exhibit 21–1, "Diagnostic Imaging Expense Budget"). Following initial review of the draft, you received the following information from the finance office:

- Since projections were issued (2 months earlier), the estimated cost of X-ray technician labor for the coming year has been increased to $15.50 per hour.
- At midyear (July 1 of the budget year), the price of X-ray film will be increasing again, going from $2.82 per unit to $3.00 per unit.
- The $18,500 per year in fixed expenses attributable to your department was found to be in error. This figure should actually be $15,000 per year.
- Your earlier request for additional funds for staff education has been approved, increasing your budget for this item to $3,000 for the coming year.

**Instructions**

Revise the "Diagnostic Imaging Expense Budget" in Exhibit 21–1 to reflect the new information throughout.

## CHAPTER 22

# Quality and Productivity: Sides of the Same Coin

*Quality never costs as much money as it saves.*
*—Anonymous*

*We are not at our best perched at the summit;*
*we are climbers, at our best when the way is steep.*
*—John W. Gardner*

## CHAPTER OBJECTIVES

☛ Identify the differences between the total quality movement and traditional concerns for quality in the health care organization.

☛ Identify the conditions necessary for the success of a total quality management program.

☛ Review the progression of the concern for productivity in health care organizations and reinforce the need for attention to continuing productivity improvement.

☛ Interrelate the concerns for quality and productivity as dimensions of the same overall concern for organizational efficiency and identify these considerations as an ongoing part of the supervisory role.

## SITUATION: CAUGHT IN THE ELEVATOR

You are a department manager in a large hospital. Administration has recently announced the introduction of a total quality management (TQM) process that will eventually involve all employees in all departments. You have been appointed as one of 18 members of the TQM steering committee, a group comprised of employees from all levels—rank-and-file to executive management—who will guide the TQM implementation.

You have been advised at an early meeting that the word about the TQM process is out throughout the hospital. Since you have been identified as a steering committee member, you can expect to be asked, perhaps frequently, "What's this TQM stuff all about?" Furthermore, you can expect to be asked literally on the move. It is therefore necessary to have in mind a clear, concise response that can be delivered in very little time.

Accordingly, you are expected to prepare what is often referred to as an "elevator speech," a brief response you can deliver in full even in the limited time available between elevator stops.

*Instructions*

As you proceed through the chapter, decide how you would concisely describe a TQM undertaking to a colleague who asks as you step into the elevator, "Is there anything to this TQM stuff besides another waste of time and energy?" In other words, create your "elevator speech."

## THE TOTAL QUALITY MOVEMENT: JUST "EXCELLENCE" AGAIN?

*Quality* became a fashionable business during the 1990s, in the way that *excellence* was fashionable during the 1980s. Although the total quality movement and the excellence movement of the recent past had somewhat different origins, so far the effects of the quality movement have been much the same as the visible results of the excellence movement: A basically sound and well-intentioned philosophy has been and continues to be adopted, adapted, promoted, and implemented with extremely mixed results.

The excellence movement was sparked by one very good, highly readable, phenomenally successful nonfiction book, *In Search of Excellence*.[1] This book was so successful that being concerned with excellence in the conduct of business activities of all kinds suddenly became fashionable. It also quickly became apparent that almost anything labeled with that newly popularized word would be immediately noticed by a great many people, some of whom would buy. Overall the fundamental message of *In Search of Excellence* was copied, reworked, repackaged, and supposedly expanded upon by countless authors, consultants, trainers, and others. Business organizations of all sizes began to claim excellence as a goal that they had attained or were on their way to attaining.

Many of the organizations that attempted to adopt excellence as a guiding philosophy of operations ran into the same problem that has stopped many otherwise effective organizations in their tracks: how to instill a *philosophy* in people so that it will eventually drive them to behave in a desired manner.

Between the philosophy, which may initially be accepted by a few members of management at or near the top of the organization, and the actual practice, which involves many employees living out the philosophy, there lies a matter of process. There has to be some process available to transfer the philosophy from the few to the many.

A great many people never see past the process and never truly adopt the philosophy. They simply go through the motions, appearing to do what they perceive top management wants them to do. Invariably, when a philosophy is proceduralized—that is, when a process is superimposed upon something as ethereal as a concept, theory, or belief—something is lost. And those who simply adopt the process as part of the job without buying into the philosophy will not truly reflect the philosophy in their behavior.

When a philosophy of management is overproceduralized, overpromoted, overpublicized, and overpraised, it becomes a fad. It becomes fashionable for its own sake. In this manner *excellence* went down the same path traveled years earlier by *management by objectives* (MBO). We have reason to wonder, therefore, whether the quality movement, which continues to flourish, although perhaps not as strongly as a decade ago, may be just another management fad destined to go the way of MBO and excellence.

## Quality Control, Assurance, and Management

For decades many industries, largely those involved in manufacturing, have applied what is referred to as *quality control*. Quality control ordinarily concentrates on finding defects, rejecting defective products, and providing information with which to alter processes so they produce fewer defects.

For some time health care organizations have had what they call *quality assurance*. This consists largely of record scrutiny under which errors consisting of departures from some dictated standard are counted, providing information with which steps can be taken to try to reduce the frequency of recurrence of the same kinds of errors.

In addition to correcting the processes that produce the errors, both quality control and quality assurance are often responsible for instituting more frequent quality checkpoints so that errors might be caught earlier. However, the most important similarity between quality control and quality assurance is that both focus primarily on finding errors after the fact. Both have always been retrospective processes.

It has been only in the recent one-and-a-half to two decades, using philosophical grounding and methods exported from the United States to Japan decades earlier and later brought back as "new, revolutionary management techniques," that the emphasis on quality has been shifting from "catch errors before they go out the door" to "avoid making the errors in the first place." Thus we have the basis of the quality movement, as embodied in labels such as *total quality management* (TQM) and *continuous quality improvement* (CQI).

## Old Friends in New Clothes?

Many of the tools and techniques utilized under the TQM umbrella should look familiar to some people who have been in the work force for a few years. Many of the "current" tools and techniques have been around for quite a while, some for decades. They have been resurrected and revitalized, and in some instances renamed.

For example, a number of TQM-implementation case histories mention the acronym TOPS, standing for *team-oriented problem solving*. As the name suggests, workers who have active concerns with various aspects of particular problems approach problem solving as a team, with a common goal and purpose. These problem-solving teams espoused under TQM look, sound, and function the same as the *quality circles* promoted during the brief popularity of "Japanese management."

Also essentially renaming quality circles are other TOPS look-alikes such as *self-directed work teams* and *team-oriented process improvement*. These particular labels are but two of several similar designations that have emerged as representing a significant part of the path to continuous quality improvement.

Quality circles were themselves nothing new when they were so named. In years past, many work organizations utilized what were called *work simplification project teams*, which were in function and intent essentially identical to quality circles and the problem-solving teams of TQM. Written about in the 1950s and earlier, work simplification teams found their way into hospital methods improvement work as early as 1956.[2,3]

Even many of the specific tools used by today's TQM problem solvers go back 50, 60, 70 or more years. Industrial engineering techniques already existing for decades scored a number of modest, if not long-lasting, successes when implemented in hospitals from the second half of the 1960s to the mid 1970s. However, industrial engineering in the health care field—renamed management engineering, probably owing to a general aversion in health care to anything perceived as "industrial"—has fallen far short of its potential value.

It is ironic that that which failed to have a lasting impact in health care is now cited as part of the solution to today's problems in health care organizations. Consider the following:

The pioneers of quality improvement have left a rich heritage of theory and technique by which to analyze and improve complex production processes, yet until recently these techniques have had little use in our health care systems. The barriers have been cultural in part; physicians, for example, seem to have difficulty seeing themselves as participants in processes, rather than as lone agents of success or failure. The techniques of process flow analysis, control charts, cause-and-effect diagrams, and quality-function deployment, to name a few, are neither arcane nor obvious; they require study, but they can be learned. Many will be as useful in health care as they have been in other industries.[4]

Some of the techniques referenced in the foregoing passage date back to the late 1800s, and serious managers who believe in the potential of total quality management are finding that these techniques are fully as valuable today as they have ever been.

## The Common Driving Force

Regardless of how many previously popular techniques are returned to the spotlight or how many genuinely new wrinkles are added, one ingredient remains fully as essential to TQM as it has been to any other approach by any other name. That crucial ingredient is top management commitment. This should come as no surprise; top management commitment to new ideas and approaches has been a prerequisite to complete success for as long as organized enterprise has existed. Without sufficient top management commitment most organized endeavors are destined to, at best, generate results that fall short of intentions or, at worst, fail altogether and cause harmful results or leave residual damage.

One cannot imagine any rational top manager openly avowing opposition to the principles of quality improvement. Ask any top manager whose organization has espoused TQM if he or she is truly committed to it—or, for that matter, ask any top manager at all if quality, period, is a personal commitment; surely each will state unwavering commitment. We know that many such endeavors fail because of insufficient top management commitment, but since almost all managers will voice commitment there is but one conclusion to be drawn: Top management commitment is a matter of degree. And it is the degree of commitment that is critical.

None of today's total quality programs will work as intended unless top management is actually involved and actively promoting the concept. Superficial, lip-service-only commitment at the top results in similar weak commitment at lower organizational levels. Beware of the skyrocket commitment of the top manager who gets all fired up over TQM, distributes information to everyone, creates a TQM steering committee, advisory committee, or similar body, and chairs the first meeting or two or three—but then starts missing meetings because of "pressing business" and before too long transfers the guiding role to subordinates.

A total quality program also will not work if managers, especially first-line supervisors, will not let go and truly delegate to employees. This means not simply giving employees the responsibility for doing different tasks or determining more efficient methods; it means also giving them the authority to make the decisions necessary to implement their own solutions. Furthermore, letting go also means accepting what the employees decide and living with it.

Letting go to the extent just described is difficult for the majority of managers. A great many managers, far more than would be able to see it in themselves, possess a recognizable streak of authoritarianism. Upon reflection, the reasons for a fairly strong presence of residual authoritarianism are understandable. Modern management—true open, participative management—is a phenomenon of the recent two or three decades. While steady, its spread has been gradual; there remain many areas of organized activity in which employees have yet to experience any management style other than straightforward "bossism."

Managers learn about management mostly from other managers, and especially from those organizational superiors who, for good or ill, were by virtue of position role models for those newer to management. At one time virtually all management everywhere was authoritarian; even now, management that is at least partly authoritarian predominates. Most management role models thus convey at least a modicum of authoritarianism. Subtle proof of the existence of the authoritarian streak can be experienced by the manager who might ponder his or her reaction to being pushed abruptly into a fully participative management situation—the manager may feel that participative management exhibits weakness, and that delegating decision-making authority to subordinates is somehow abrogating one's responsibility.

It remains clear, however, that changes in management style and approach may have to occur in order for a quality management program to be successful. In most instances the manager will need to shift from being the boss—from planning, telling, instructing, and controlling—to being the leader of a team—being counselor, teacher, coach, and facilitator.

Management's commitment, then, can be seen as a total commitment not only to participative management and employee empowerment but also to intra- and interdepartmental teamwork and improved communication throughout the organization.

### Will Total Quality Management Prevail?

Total quality management has a reasonable chance of working where previous and perhaps partial efforts undertaken under other names have failed. There is a great deal going on with TQM; activity undertaken in the name of quality improvement has at times been so widespread that the impression that "everyone is doing it" has placed considerable pressure on those who have yet to undertake quality management. With so much happening in the name of TQM we will find that, in some organizations, top management commitment is real and lasting. Also, some organizations' genuine successes will inspire others to try following a similar path.

Have there been many genuine successes? Therein lies the rub. An informal survey conducted at the height of TQM activity in the 1990s reported that only about 35 percent of organizations implementing TQM processes could report significant improvement in their overall effectiveness. Another informal assessment suggested that only about 20 percent of such organizations had shown tangible results from their TQM activities.

Some significant obstacles to TQM's success are presented by the volatility of the present day health care environment. Few people in health care have to be told that the environment in which they function is in a constant state of change, much of it drastic in that whole organization structures are severely affected by mergers, acquisitions, downsizings, and even closures. A well-mounted TQM process generally takes two to three years to mature and begin to deliver its true potential. However, many organizations have found that those two to three years can bring changes that negate the effects of TQM before they are realized. And some changes can quickly destroy the employee enthusiasm and motivation that took so long to develop. Consider a "reengineering" effort, with its attendant changes including layoffs, which followed a full-blown TQM undertaking by about two years. The TQM process said to employees: *You are all important and your input and participation are valued.* Then the subsequent reengineering effort said, in part: *Some of you are no longer needed.* When this severe contradiction occurs, many if not all of the positive effects of the TQM effort are negated. In the present environment, how many health care managers can say with certainty that the coming two or three years will not bring layoffs or other belt-tightening?

Within health care it will be difficult to completely avoid quality management because of growing pressure from accreditation and regulatory bodies. The Joint Commission on Accreditation of Healthcare Organizations (Joint Commission) has made it clear that monitoring and evaluation standards are shifting the emphasis of quality assessment and improvement activities away from a department and discipline and direct-care approach to an approach that will harness the professional instinct for continual improvement. In other words, there will be continued external pressure on health care organizations to demonstrate that they are always trying to improve quality and that whether called TQM or CQI or known by some other name, quality improvement is not a "project" or one-time fix, but rather a permanent philosophy of operation.

The Joint Commission's *Accreditation Manual for Hospitals* includes the following standard: "The hospitals' leaders set expectations, develop plans, and manage processes to measure, assess, and improve the quality of the hospital's governance, management, clinical, and support activities."[5] At the very least, quality management will prevail in health organizations to an extent sufficient to fulfill all accreditation requirements.

### More Than Just a Job

For total quality management to work, the majority of employees in the organization need to experience sufficient commitment to their employing institution to see it as more than just a place to work. This can be a tall order indeed in these times of staff shortages, increasing patient loads, shrinking reimbursement, and growing regulatory pressure, especially since a growing number of health care workers seem to believe that quality is presently being sacrificed to reduce costs.

It seems clear, however, that as health care organizations wrestle with increased price competition and declining revenues, the tools and techniques of TQM offer workable means of reconciling concerns about quality and cost. Once again it comes down to a matter of commitment: if employees at all levels are sincerely committed to the organization, its mission, and its patients, there is a reasonable chance that TQM will work.

For reasons suggested throughout these pages some attempts to implement TQM will fail and, for some people, quality will gather dust in the old-management-approach graveyard along with all the other techniques that were tried, half-heartedly applied, and discarded. Some attempts, however, will succeed. And those organizations that are successful implementing TQM will find themselves among the stronger, more adaptable institutions in the health field for years to come.

### PRODUCTIVITY "RECYCLED"

A one-page advertisement for a publication dealing with the topic of productivity claimed, "The most pressing problem you face today is how to meet your community's growing health care needs with shrinking resources." The advertisement and accompanying sample publication had much more to say about the necessity of improving productivity and of doing more with less in the delivery of health services.

Another source advised, "Continual improvements within the hospital are necessary, not only because of the worthiness of hospital goals, but because of the economic impact of hospitals upon all people, collectively and individually. The magnitude of this impact may be seen by examining the economics of hospital facilities, operation, and utilization in the United States."[3(p.2)]

The foregoing passages sound much like the legitimate concerns of today as those who operate health care organizations struggle to make each dollar work harder while others both internal and external to health care try to slow the growth of health care costs. The fact of the matter is, however, that these concerns were voiced more than a quarter-century apart; the advertisement appeared in 1991 while the second passage was written in about 1965. Health care productivity, it would seem, has been a concern for some time.

But has the concern for health care productivity been consistent? And have efforts been consistently applied to improve productivity?

### Fad and Practice

Similar to the likes of motivation, commitment, and quality, productivity is a concept labeled with a single word that is frequently misused. Productivity is one of the different-shaped gimmicks in the management tool box that every once in a while is pulled out, polished up, and examined in a supposedly new light.

In health care, productivity became a magic word during the latter half of the 1960s. During the 1960s health care costs began to climb dramatically, fueled by the mid-decade establishment of Medicare and Medicaid along with advancing technology and ever-intensifying modes of treatment. Productivity improvement quickly became much of health care's supposed cure for many of its own ills. The challenge of productivity improvement soon became a challenge of measurement; if the results of a particular human activity were to be improved, there would have to be a means available for measuring those results both before and after the improvement intervention. In short, the apparent need was for measures of output.

There was a great deal of activity concerning measures of output, or so-called "standards," during the latter half of the 1960s and into the 1970s. Much of the activity was grant funded, supported at least in part by government, foundations, and various not-for-profit organizations such as state and regional hospital associations. All measures of output were based in some way on the work measurement techniques of industrial engineering. Various approaches included the following:

- the "Michigan Methodologies," a series of manuals developed at the University of Michigan consisting of detailed predetermined time standards applying to various hospital operations, including separate manuals for a number of clinical and support activities
- the "CASH-LPC" (Commission on Administrative Services to Hospitals-Labor Performance Control), a California development, like the Michigan methodologies a compilation of predetermined time standards and time-standard "building blocks" from which one could synthesize standards for similar activities
- the work of various hospital management engineering programs, including programs of the Hospital Association of New York State (HANYS), Massachusetts Hospital Association (MHA), Chicago Hospital Council, New Jersey Hospital Association, Ohio Hospital Association, and a number of other programs

Hospital management engineering came into prominence. No more than industrial engineering under another name, due primarily to the resistance within health care to anything "industrial," management engineering emerged in two forms: in-house engineering and shared management engineering services.

Some hospitals employed their own management engineers and even established management engineering departments. Many other hospitals participated in the establishment of shared management engineering programs through membership in various associations. These programs were often established as fee-for-service adjuncts of hospital associations; that is, an association service that was paid for not by the general membership through dues but by the actual users of the service.

Cost escalation and productivity were of sufficient importance in the 1960s that steps were taken to encourage the formation of shared management engineering programs that would operate on a not-for-profit basis. Foundation grants were provided to start a number of programs under the auspices of various hospital associations. Other grants went to fund the development of productivity measurements in the manner previously described.

Once started, management engineering programs proliferated dramatically. For a few years productivity was "in." It was a broad-spectrum cure for the apparent ills of the health care industry. However, by 1975, through mergers and dissolutions the number of active hospital management engineering programs throughout the country had fallen significantly, and many surviving programs found their staffing and activity levels greatly reduced. Productivity improvement was no longer promoted as a universal solution. By 1975, in fact, some programs were turning away from promoting improvement through management engineering and turning toward improving hospitals' operating results through reimbursement rate appeals and otherwise "gaming" the growing number of reimbursement regulations so as to ensure maximum reimbursement under the prevailing system.

### The Government Speaks Up

It was not health care alone that saw productivity improvement as an urgent need from the mid-1960s to the mid-1970s. In the late 1960s much was made of apparently declining national productivity, to the extent that in 1970 a National Commission on Productivity and Work Quality was established. The commission comprised seven major committees, one of which was the Hospital and Health Care Committee made up of nearly 75 people from about 20 health-related organizations. Issued in 1975, the Hospital and Health Care Committee's report made a number of recommendations.[6] The following comments highlight the report's ten primary recommendations and briefly describe what might have occurred concerning each in the decades since the report was issued.

1. *Development of a reimbursement system with built-in incentives to include comprehensive coverage for ambulatory care services.* Considerable change has occurred in this area since 1975. Whether this change is seen as progress might well depend on whether one is on the paying or receiving end of the reimbursement dollar. The pressures of reimbursement have been diverting more and more activity to the outpatient side,

and although positive incentives were offered to encourage more reliance on outpatient care, much change has been forced by the negative incentives associated with the continued use of inpatient services.

2. *Expanded implementation and continued evaluation of health maintenance organizations (HMOs) and other comprehensive fee-paid health plans.* Such approaches were seen in 1975 as offering options to the public and physicians alike while taking advantage of economies of scale. Progress has been significant in this area, and although the movement to these managed care programs has slowed in recent years, in many parts of the country these plans account for the overwhelming majority of covered individuals.

3. *Increased use of management engineering services and techniques, preferably through statewide shared services programs.* As was the case in 1975, only about one fourth of hospitals utilize management engineering services. The committee recommended sharing of such services because many hospitals were seen as not large enough to operate their own services economically. However, the number of shared management engineering programs has steadily decreased to a point at which they are nearly nonexistent. In many instances, in-house management engineering services have been an early target for elimination when fiscal belt-tightening has been necessary.

4. *Promotion of the formation of multi-institutional mergers such as those in the investor-owned and religious sectors of the health care industry.* In the early 1990s, it appeared that the greatest number of merged institutions remained those in the proprietary and religious chains. However, this is certainly no longer the case. A significant and increasing number of nonprofit community hospitals are merging into larger systems, while many others are working together in various other forms of affiliation. Overall, the commission's recommendation for multi-institutional mergers continues to be realized, although the primary driver behind health care's efforts along these lines appears to be the restrictions placed on provider reimbursement by the third-party payers.

5. *Expansion of shared services programs by hospitals.* The sharing of certain services, foremost among them being purchasing and laundry, has long been a practice and continues to expand. Additional services such as medical waste disposal and biomedical engineering are expanding in the shared-service arena. It appears, however, that "sharing" as such, as far as it involves clinical services, is coming about more through organizational mergers and the development of multi-institutional systems than through services shared by separate corporate entities.

6. *Development and expansion of hospital employee incentive programs.* Bonus and incentive programs for upper management personnel have been gradually spreading throughout the industry. Incentive programs involving all employee levels have been still slower in catching on. There remain some legal barriers in that certain nonprofit institutions can place their tax-exempt status at risk by paying bonuses. Also, in the

highly regulated states, the issue of incentive or bonus payment frequently vanishes in the presence of a negative operating line.

7. *Continuing education programs for middle management personnel in health care facilities.* This is as much of a need today as it was in 1975. If anything, today's need for continuing management education is far more acute than previously. In addition to productivity issues and other issues that remain, with recent years' proliferation of laws affecting employment we are now faced with dramatically increased needs for management education about issues of discrimination and employee rights.

8. *Expansion of the role of the hospital chief executive in the policy making of the institution.* Little appears to have changed since 1975; only a few top administrators are voting board members.

9. *Expansion of the role of the business sector of the nation's economy in the delivery of health care.* The committee rightly pointed out that business is a large purchaser of health care and suggested that business needs to learn more about health care and use its expertise to help improve health care productivity. Business has clearly become more interested and involved but in perhaps a somewhat different way from that envisioned by the commission. Business is reacting with an increasing sense of urgency to the dramatically increasing cost of health insurance coverage. By increasing employees' share of health insurance premiums, increasing deductibles and co-payments, and cutting back on benefits, business is concentrating on cost control rather than productivity improvement. Because of the large amounts of money paid for employee benefits, business has been able to pressure third-party payers into limiting reimbursement increases and has furthermore been able to encourage the movement into managed care.

10. *Increased involvement and/or responsibility of physicians in both the general and the financial management of health care institutions.* At the time of the commission's report, there were relatively few short-term nongovernmental hospitals having physicians on their governing boards. It has long been felt that since physicians prescribe care and services and heavily influence hospital expenditures, they should be both involved and accountable. Indeed, active physician participation is presently increasing. Anecdotal information suggests that physicians are becoming more active on governing boards, but a greater amount of physician involvement appears to be occurring within the framework of physician practice associations that are forming in support of new health maintenance organizations and other managed care alternatives.

The foregoing suggests a fairly mixed collection of responses to the committee's recommendations of 1975, but overall in 30 years not much has happened in terms of impact on health care productivity. That there was little follow-up at all to the committee's report might suggest that the problems of shallow commitment were fairly widespread.

## Why Be Concerned about Productivity?

It is reasonable to ask why we should be concerned about productivity, especially in the face of reimbursement systems that only indirectly encourage concern for productivity. Productivity deserves attention because:

- It is simply good management to want to apply available resources to best effect.
- It is possible, in an organization as varied and complex as a modern hospital, to redistribute resources from areas of savings to other essentials.
- The inflationary spiral affects all business entities, and when resource inputs grow at a rate faster than system outputs the costs to the consumer increase. Exhibit 22–1 illustrates the effects of the inflationary spiral.
- We should wish to maintain a voluntary system, and to do so the costs of health care cannot continue to rise out of proportion to all other sectors of the economy.
- There is increasing external pressure to hold costs down while continuing to produce quality health care.

Furthermore, concern about productivity needs to be ongoing. One of the common errors prevalent in productivity's heyday was to regard productivity improvement as a one-time effort that could sweep through an organization and make it more efficient for all time. This is not so. Some of the larger, more obvious corrections are one-time changes, but the need for attention to productivity is continuing. When left unto itself, an activity will be subject to creep-

**Exhibit 22–1** The Inflationary Spiral

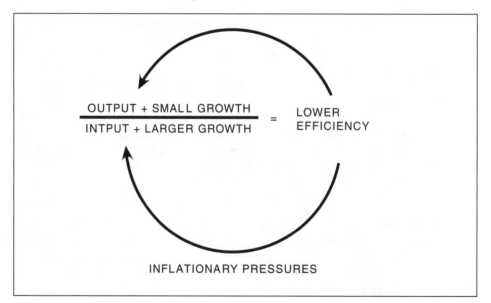

$$\frac{\text{OUTPUT} + \text{SMALL GROWTH}}{\text{INTPUT} + \text{LARGER GROWTH}} = \text{LOWER EFFICIENCY}$$

INFLATIONARY PRESSURES

ing inefficiencies that eventually accrue to a significant problem. Left unto themselves, most human activities will suffer diminished productivity, so regular attention is needed to keep them tuned and running efficiently.

## A Return to Favor?

The National Commission on Productivity and Work Quality came into being in 1970 because American productivity had declined in the late 1960s and had yet to show signs of recovering. But recover it did; productivity statistics indicated gradual recovery through the 1970s, so many people probably assumed the problem had gone away. However, the problem has "gone away" a number of times and returned just as often. Productivity should always be a concern, but sometimes more of a concern than at other times.

A July 1991 news story from the Associated Press carried the headline, "U.S. Standard of Living Falls for First Time Since '82."[7] The story reported that Americans' standard of living declined slightly in 1990 "as the country fell further behind in its ability to compete internationally," according to the Council on Competitiveness. Specifically, "The council said in its fourth annual competitiveness index that America lost ground in such key areas as living standards, productivity, and investment."

On the bright side, in the third quarter of 2003 the productivity of America's workers soared by the largest amount in 20 years, at an annualized rate of 9.4 percent.[8] However, one year later, the third quarter of 2004, the annualized rate of productivity growth was a mere 1.9 percent.[9] When productivity growth exceeds the rate of inflation, as in the third quarter of 2003, the economy gains; when productivity is less than the rate of inflation, as in the third quarter of 2004, the economy loses. The point is that overall productivity is affected by many diverse factors, and variations in productivity are to be expected. Thus productivity is always a concern in the macro sense—that is, nationally—but it should likewise always be a concern in the micro sense, that is, in each individual organization.

Although much of the concern over runaway cost inflation in health care is reflected in the direct efforts of some businesses and third-party payers to simply pay less, there will inevitably be renewed close examination of operations for potential improvements in productivity. If an institution is to have to do more with the same resources or do the same with less, it follows that responsible management will seek all reasonable ways of improving productivity.

## SIDES OF THE SAME COIN

The TQM movement has necessarily brought with it a renewed concern for productivity at a time when many environmental factors are also pointing toward the need for improved productivity. The quality issue is inextricable from the productivity issue; one has direct implications for the other, and there is a direct relationship between quality and productivity.

In the coming years, however, concern for productivity will not be limited to just the methods-improvement, cost-cutting, staff-reduction activities frequently associated with management engineering. Although work measurement may play a large part in productivity improvement, the view of productivity, and the scope of future effort, will likely be broader than past efforts.

In any activity, productivity is represented by a relationship between input and output; that is:

$$\text{Output/Input} = \text{Productivity}$$

It is a simple relationship: the output of any activity divided by the input, that is, the resources that went into completing the activity, equals the productivity, or, as often expressed, the "efficiency" of the activity.

Any process or activity has associated with it a level of quality, broadly describing quality as the relative acceptability of the output. Any change in productivity involves changes between and among all of these factors. Thus productivity may be said to be improved if:

- Output is increased while input is held constant or decreased and quality is held constant (doing more with the same or less).
- Input is decreased while output is held constant or increased while quality is held constant (doing the same or more with less).
- Quality is improved while input and output are held constant or reduced (doing better with the same or less).

It follows, then, that productivity is reduced if the opposite of any of the foregoing changes occurs; for example, if output decreases while input is held constant.

Productivity may have received more or less attention at various times, but the concept of productivity and the need for constant attention to it have always been with us. The overall objective of productivity improvement efforts will remain the enhancement of the accomplishment of work by doing things in less time or with less effort or at lower cost while maintaining or improving quality.

The principal factors influencing productivity, and thus quality, are as follows:

- capital investment
- technological change
- economies of scale
- work methods, procedures, and systems
- knowledge and skill of the work force
- the willingness of the work force to excel at what they do, and in all instances to do the right things in the best possible way

Given the direction from which most of the forces urging organizational improvement are coming, we will likely hear more about quality than we will hear about productivity. However, these concepts remain two sides of the same coin, and the supervisor's tools that have traditionally been associated with productivity improvement (see Chapter 24) are also the tools of total quality management.

## QUALITY VERSUS COST AND OUTPUT

Within health care it is not uncommon to hear reactions to expressions of the need to do more with less such as:

"We can't reduce costs without adversely affecting quality," or,

"We can't cut costs without losing output."

These reactions are founded on an implicit assumption that present methods are already as productive and cost-effective as they can be. This, however, is nearly always an erroneous assumption; there is room for improvement in most human activities, and it is often even possible to increase both quality and output at the same time by improving productive efficiency. Consider the simple illustration of Exhibit 22–2.

Say an activity is functioning such that quality and output are at point A in Exhibit 22–2. Does point A represent the most efficient performance of the activity? It might, but chances are there remains room for improvement. In this simplified example, we are assuming room for improvement to point B at which both quality and output have improved. Note, however, that beyond point B quality decreases as output increases; there will always be this often-difficult-to-identify point beyond which continued effort to increase output will negatively affect quality (perhaps point B might be identified as the "haste-makes-waste" threshold).

**Exhibit 22–2**  Quality Versus Output

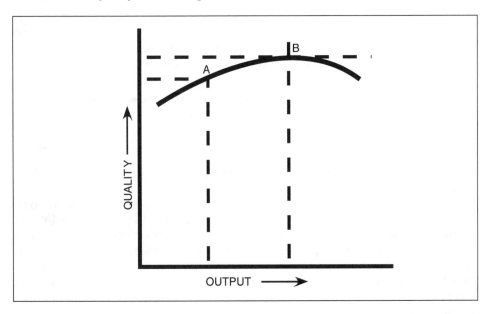

## AN "ELEVATOR SPEECH"

The objective of the "elevator speech" is to be able to describe the organization's TQM (or other) program in a clear, concise form in a brief amount of time, sometimes literally in the time it takes to ride two or three floors on an elevator. The following is one possible response to, "What's this quality stuff all about?"

"It's about doing things right the first time, never settling for second best when we know we can do better. It's recognizing that everything we do can be improved upon, and that we owe it to our customers, internal as well as external, to give them the very best we're able to give. It's about bringing all of us together into a cohesive team and making this place a true customer-focused organization that's known as this community's most effective health care provider."

---

## REVIEW QUESTIONS

1. Comment on the statement: *Quality must be built into the product; it cannot be inspected into it.*

2. As far as involvement is concerned, what does total quality management (TQM) include that earlier approaches like management by objectives (MBO) did not encompass?

3. Although "productivity improvement" is commonly viewed as cost-cutting by many employees, there are actually multiple ways of changing the relationship between and among input, output, and quality. Cite at least two of the relatively simple ways of doing so.

4. Profitability can be increased by increasing revenue or reducing expenses. Describe the effects on the bottom line of an increase in revenue and of a reduction in expenses (remembering that it takes money to make money, and that not all changes fall directly or fully to the bottom line).

5. Name one primary advantage and one significant shortcoming of motivational programs such as TQM.

---

## EXERCISE: IN SEARCH OF— ?

Select one actual application of a "new management approach" for analysis and study. This could be an application of management by objectives (MBO), some formal program or process emanating from the "excellence" movement, a quality circles program, an organized methods improvement program, or any other change-oriented mechanism intended to improve organizational success. The ideal choice would be an application in which you were personally involved, but lacking such involvement you may use any application of which you have some knowledge.

For the application you chose to study, answer the four following questions:

1. Expressed in no more than one or two sentences, what was the guiding philosophy of the program?

2. In your view, was the program's guiding philosophy successfully translated into practice? How was this done or not done?

3. Do you believe that overall the program succeeded or failed? In either case, identify what you believe to be the three most important reasons behind the outcome.

4. What do you consider to be the single most important lesson learned from the organization's experience with the program?

---

**NOTES**

1. T.J. Peters and R.H. Waterman, Jr., *In Search of Excellence* (New York: Harper & Row, 1982).

2. Kjell B. Zandin and H.B. Maynard, eds., *Maynard's Industrial Engineering Handbook*, 5th ed. (New York: McGraw-Hill Companies, Inc., 2001).

3. H.E. Smalley and J.R. Freeman, *Hospital Industrial Engineering* (New York: Reinhold Publishing Corporation, 1966).

4. D.M. Berwick, "Sounding Board: Continuous Improvement as an Ideal in Health Care," *New England Journal of Medicine* 320 (1989): 53–56.

5. Joint Commission on Accreditation of Healthcare Organizations, *Hospital Accreditation Standards* (Oakbrook Terrace, IL: Joint Commission, 1991).

6. National Commission on Productivity and Work Quality, *Report of the Hospital and Health Care Committee* (Washington, DC: GPO, 1975).

7. The Associated Press, "U.S. Standard of Living Falls for First Time Since '82," *Democrat and Chronicle* (Rochester, NY), July 10, 1991.

8. The Associated Press, "Productivity Makes Big Gain," *Democrat and Chronicle* (Rochester, NY), December 4, 2003.

9. The Associated Press, "U.S. Worker Productivity Slows," *Democrat and Chronicle* (Rochester, NY), December 2, 2004.

# Teams, Team Building, and Teamwork

*Man's greatest discovery is not fire, nor the wheel, nor the combustion engine nor atomic energy, nor anything in the material world. Man's greatest discovery is teamwork by agreement.*
*—B. Brewster Jennings*

## CHAPTER OBJECTIVES

☛ Differentiate between types of teams: ad hoc or special-purpose teams versus departmental teams.

☛ Review the composition and structure of ad hoc or special-purpose teams.

☛ Review potential legal problems associated with employee teams and suggest how legal entanglements can be minimized or avoided.

☛ Review the problems encountered by teams functioning in a company environment in which recognition and reward systems are based on individual performance.

☛ Introduce the concept of team building within the context of the departmental group.

☛ Introduce the stages of team building, from original formation to continuing maintenance.

☛ Identify individual employee motivation as the primary driver of team performance.

☛ Identify the leadership qualities necessary for successful team building, and provide guidance for the team-building department manager.

## SITUATION: CAN YOU BUILD AN EFFECTIVE TEAM FROM THE "ENEMY CAMPS?"

Helen Williams, hired from outside the hospital as business office manager, believed strongly in the power of a unified departmental team. In her previous position she had inherited a disorganized collection of individuals who openly competed among themselves for high evaluation scores and the manager's favor, and she made them into a cooperative team that became a model for the institution.

Helen accepted her new position even though she strongly suspected it was something of a "hot seat." She was the fifth person in that position in 3 years.

Although Helen did not know the reasons behind the short stays of her predecessors, after a month she decided that the atmosphere in the department was decidedly unhealthy. Her staff appeared divided into two distinct rival camps that she began to think of as "Camp A" and "Camp B." (Actually, she had heard members of each group refer to the other group as "the enemy camp," but she did not use "enemy" in her descriptions of these groups.)

From her first day on the job it was apparent to Helen that many of the problems in the department stemmed from poor intradepartmental communication and lack of cooperation among staff members. She was surprised to learn that her immediate predecessor never held department meetings but instead met occasionally with groups of two or three to deal with specific problems.

Helen instituted the practice of holding a weekly 30-minute meeting for all employees in the department. She made it plain that everyone was expected to attend.

After four months of staff meetings it seemed to Helen that the atmosphere of rivalry between the camps had scarcely diminished at all, and it was still evident that the group was divided on many matters. It also seemed to Helen that Camp A was slightly more supportive of her than was Camp B, and this seemed to make Camp B all the more difficult for her to deal with.

Helen's initial assessment of the department was that productivity was low relative to the number of people available to do the work. In the patient billing section, for example, the average time lapse between discharge and third-party billing was the longest Helen had ever seen. Helen had come to the job vowing to increase the department's productivity, but at the 6-month mark in her employment she had to admit that little had changed. Camp A and Camp B still went their own ways and at times seemed to be doing their best to undermine each other.

*Instructions*

As you proceed through this chapter, consider what actions Helen might take to improve the level of cooperation and productivity in her department and to point her employees in the direction of becoming a functioning departmental team.

## TYPES OF TEAMS

There are two general types of teams to be encountered in the work force, and it is not always immediately clear what type is being referred to when one speaks of team building. It is therefore appropriate to begin by differentiating between team types to establish the direction for this chapter.

One type of team is characterized by the group that is assembled for a specific purpose, perhaps including people from a number of different departments or disciplines. This kind of team may be ad hoc, assembled for a specific one-time task, or it may be ongoing in that it consists of permanent or rotating membership and handles a certain kind of business or problem on a regular basis. These are the teams of team-oriented problem solving in total quality management; these are the teams that at one time may have been referred to as quality circles; and these are the teams of the form taken by your organization's safety committee or product evaluation committee and other such groups. This type of team, often referred to as a project team or an employee team, is the focus of the first major section of this chapter.

The other type of team, the focus of later sections of the chapter, is the departmental team. The departmental team is simply the group of employees and the single supervisor or manager to whom they report. We say "simply" because the team composition is indeed simple; most people readily understand the relationship between the supervisor and the direct-reporting group, and most understand that everyone in the group has a job to do and together this accomplishes the work of the group. Such a group can, of course, continue to operate as a number of individuals doing their jobs for a common purpose, but when these individuals are united into a true team the potential of the group is expanded dramatically.

## THE PROJECT OR EMPLOYEE TEAM

### Team Organization

The organization of a project or employee team can be relatively simple; a decision is made to pull together a number of people with the appropriate knowledge, experience, perspective, or whatever to address a particular problem, provide input on particular issues, undertake productivity improvement projects, or address certain ongoing concerns such as safety, quality, education, and so forth.

Team organization is addressed in Chapter 24, "Methods Improvement: Making Work—and Life—Easier," in the section titled "An Organized Approach to Methods Improvement". The compositions of both the ad hoc and ongoing team are described. Most of these kinds of teams consist of both managers and rank-and-file employees, and because there are nonmanagerial employees on teams, often constituting the majority of team membership, there are potential legal problems depending on the kinds of problems or issues addressed.

Effective people management is of course important to the success of any form of team; however, fully as important for many of these kinds of teams is sensitivity to the potential legal pitfalls of team operation. Whether through total quality management or simply out of a sincere desire to solicit employee participation, a number of organizations have discovered, much to their dismay, that a team can easily stray into questionable territory.

### Getting Maximum Value from Employee Teams
### While Keeping Them Legal

*"Let's Form a Team"*

In these days of increasing employee participation and involvement, department managers are increasingly likely to hear suggestions similar to the three that follow:

1. "Let's pull an employee team together and find out what the work force thinks about this issue. After all, there's nobody who knows the ins and outs of most of our jobs better than the people who do them every day."

2. "We have no real idea what the work force thinks about our benefits package. If we pull together a group of representative employees we might learn something that will help us do a better job of allocating our limited benefits resources."

3. "Let's give this problem to a hand-picked group of employees to see what they can come up with. There's no danger, because all they can do is recommend. As management we're free to accept or reject what they suggest."

Each of the foregoing suggestions does contain some fairly conventional management wisdom fostered by experience and supported by common sense. It can be summarized as follows:

- In most instances nobody knows a given job better than the person who does it every day.
- It only makes sense to try to account for employees' needs and desires in designing a benefits program.
- Management is indeed free to accept or reject employees' suggestions (as long as they remain aware that the responsibility always resides with management).

Participative management and employee involvement have been talked about for decades and have been practiced in an increasing number of work organizations since the human relations approach to management began to make inroads into the authoritarian management of the past. The recent popularity of total quality management (TQM) programs spurred even greater emphasis on participative management, and it is tending to bring more employees further into self-determination on the job. More and more is being done with the involvement of employees by way of employee teams.

There are, however, areas of employee involvement in which teams are seen as intruding on the territory of labor unions. There is a constant risk that a given employee team could be adjudged an illegal labor organization under the National Labor Relations Act (NLRA). The three suggestions advanced previously, all well-intended ideas for employee involvement, could all readily lead to groups that could be considered as infringing on the rights of collective bargaining organizations.

*Old Problem, Different Emphasis*

The problem has actually existed since the NLRA became law in 1935, but it was brought into sharp focus by the Electromation decision of December 1992. During 1989, Electromation, an Elkhart, Indiana, manufacturer of electrical equipment, established several employee committees. One was created to investigate bonuses, another to look at premium pay, one to study absenteeism, a group to examine employer-employee communications, and one to deal with a no-smoking policy. Management defined the subjects, set the number of members for each committee, appointed managers to all of the committees, and paid workers to participate. When Electromation's five employee committees were challenged, the National Labor Relations Board (NLRB) agreed with the challenge. The NLRB said the five employee representation committees were essentially employer-dominated labor organizations that discussed wages and other terms of employment. The NLRB said that the company was not simply dealing with quality, productivity, or efficiency, but was creating the impression among employees that their differences with management were being resolved bilaterally.[1]

The NLRB's reason for the ruling suggested that in establishing the NLRA years ago, Congress prohibited employer interference with labor organizations to ensure that such groups were free to act independently of employers in representing the interests of employees.[2]

Following the Electromation case and citing that ruling, the NLRB ordered the DuPont Company to disband seven labor-management committees, six created for safety issues and one for recreation. The NLRB said these committees were dominated by management and were dealing with issues that should have been bargained with their union, the Chemical Workers Association, Inc. These committees, the NLRB said, were intended to bypass the union. They were found unlawful because the employer retained veto power over their actions, established and controlled agendas, and decided membership and dictated the structure and purpose of each committee. The NLRB also said that these committees discussed what could be called "conditions of work." The committees' activities supposedly produced changes and benefits that the union had sought but failed to obtain through collective bargaining.

In a case similar to the DuPont situation, the Polaroid Corporation was forced to disband its long-standing employees' committee after the Labor Department determined that it was actually a "labor organization" and its "election procedure was undemocratic."[3]

### For What Does the NLRB Look?

Generalizing from the experiences of Electromation, DuPont, and Polaroid, and expanding on pre-Electromation information, an employee team or committee might be considered an employer-dominated illegal labor organization for any of a number of reasons. First and probably foremost among these reasons is whether the group is dealing with wages, hours, benefits, grievances, or other terms and conditions of employment. These are, of course, among the issues most frequently subject to collective bargaining and are seen (at least by the NLRB) as the exclusive province of unions.

An employee team or committee also might be seen as an illegal labor organization if committee suggestions or recommendations result in management decisions but the group itself does not have the power to make the decisions, and if employees are elected to the group as representatives of larger bodies of employees. The team is also at legal risk if employees see the group as a means of resolving their concerns with management and if meetings appear to involve "negotiation" between employees and members of management.

Many in business consider the NLRB's decision in the Electromation case an unfortunate occurrence. To cite one insightful response: "The NLRB's rigid reading of the law carries forward the Depression-era assumptions that relationships between employees and employers must be adversarial."[4(p.101)] The strongly pro-labor position of the NLRB works against the establishment of a healthy employee relations climate in an organization. It seems that whenever an organization tries to persuade workers that a union is not necessary, someone (in this instance the NLRB) is always ready to suggest that the organization is in some way behaving immorally or unethically for trying to treat workers fairly and equitably without being forced to do so.

Experiences since the Electromation case was decided seem to suggest that a violation will most likely be found if an employee team is actually set up during a union campaign (this can attract an unfair labor practice charge), participation in a committee is made mandatory, and the employer picks the members or controls the method of their selection.

## *Not the Last Word*

It seems to be a matter of individual opinion as to whether "quality" committees or committees established to serve as communications channels to improve quality are labor organizations under the law: "The point at which a committee's work on quality, productivity, and efficiency crosses the line and concerns or impacts 'conditions of work' is defined by the Board, making this defense (that these are 'quality committees') risky."[4(p.103)]

Probably the worst-case consequences of sanctioning a committee that is actually an illegal labor organization occur when the committee itself votes to affiliate with an outside union. If, by dealing with a committee and accepting some of its ideas and recommendations, the employer has already recognized the committee as representing employees, that representation cannot be withdrawn just because the committee decided to affiliate with a union. The employer may be legally forced to recognize the union and deal with it without an election by employees.[4]

It is doubtful, however, that a non-union employer would likely be subject to NLRB charges concerning employer-dominated labor organizations unless active union organizing was occurring.

## *Avoiding "Committee Paralysis"*

Because of what happened with Electromation there may be a tendency for some organizations to shy away altogether from teams or committees that include rank-and-file employees. Some justify a diminished emphasis on teams by pointing out that, following the Electromation decision, attacking employee committees has become an active tactic of unions that are either in place or seeking acceptance.

However, Electromation did not open up any truly new issues; it simply surfaced some that had existed for years. Long before the Electromation decision it was recognized that: "The more effective the committee is, the more likely the NLRB is to find that the committee is an illegally dominated and supported 'company union' in violation of Section 8(a)(2) of the Taft-Hartley Act"[5] (Taft-Hartley being the Labor-Management Relations Act of 1947, amending the NLRA).

The Electromation decision and related difficulties should not be allowed to deter completely the use of employee teams. The active use of employee participation and input via teams or committees lies at or near the heart of every total quality initiative. If management believes what is said to employees about the value of their input, about "empowerment" and about "owning your job," then management had best make maximum use of participative processes including teams.

The Electromation decision should not receive all the blame for rendering teams less effective than they might otherwise have been. Completely aside from labor law implications, employee teams or committees are not without a variety of other problems.

## Shortcomings of Teams or Committees

A sufficient number of problems surface from time to time to suggest that individuals and the organization itself can stifle a committee or dramatically limit its effectiveness.

Some team members, especially managers serving on teams with nonmanagers or others of perceived lesser rank, are unwilling to set aside position and power for the sake of the team. Also, unequal levels of knowledge and ability among team members can lead some to dominate and others to become overwhelmed or "lost in the crowd."

Some extremely important and potentially highly disruptive effects on teams lie in company reward and compensation systems that continue to focus on individual effort, not on team performance. This has been a frequently encountered barrier to successful total quality implementations as organizations have tried to alter how they do business without first—or at least concurrently—changing the systems by which they do business. "Current reward systems support individual performance to such an extent that they discourage teamwork."[6(p.153)]

Performance appraisals that do not account for team performance also present barriers. In fact, an organization's performance evaluation process is one of the major business support systems that has to change dramatically for successful total quality implementation. It is not nearly enough to simply change the language of the appraisal; it is necessary to change employees' concept of evaluation from a focus on the individual ("I had my evaluation today") to emphasis on the team.

In addition to the foregoing, lack of top management commitment to the process is a sure means of destroying effectiveness. It should go without saying that the top management that fails to "walk the talk" will be recognized as insincere. Members will quickly come to see their teams as do-nothing or rubber-stamp bodies if the participative process has no visible effect on top management.

Some problems with teams lie in the labels in use for these bodies, labels such as self-directed, autonomous, self-managed, and the like. These names are misleading in that they convey the belief that these groups are independent and free to act as they choose. No effective teams in business really provide all of their own direction. Each team should be directed by its specific charge or mission and by the goals of the organization. As such, all teams are actually interdependent with other organizational elements.

Effective teams require clear direction, comprehensive guidelines, and open, nonthreatening leadership. Efforts to encourage employee participation with self-directed work groups will not succeed without serious attention given to the development of strong, appropriate leadership for participative management.

## What to Avoid When Using Employee Teams

Considering the issues surfaced via Electromation, plus common sense organizational concerns for participative activities, we can enumerate five potential obstacles to avoid when forming and working with employee teams:

1. Never allow an employee team to deal with terms and conditions of employment, such as wages, hours, benefits, grievances, and such. Even consideration of "working conditions" in general should be avoided. As a member of management who might be part of a team, do not deal with other team members—specifically nonmanagers—concerning terms and conditions of employment. If a team's activities take it from a legitimate topic into the realm of terms and conditions of employment, its direction should be altered.

2. Do not solicit complaints, grievances, or suggestions about terms and conditions of employment from teams. If such issues arise on their own, refer them to the proper point in the organization (for instance, refer health insurance issues to the benefits manager).

3. Do not let team meetings degenerate into gripe sessions in which members simply complain about aspects of their employment.

4. Do not mandate employee participation, ask employees to represent other employees, or sanction employee elections to choose representatives.

5. Do not allow an employee team or committee to exist and function without a clear, understandable mission or charge and without fully and plainly delineated limits on its authority and responsibility. In other words, the group must know exactly what it can and cannot do.

## For Effective Employee Teams

Short of actually establishing teams or committees to wrestle with certain issues, there are a number of steps that can be taken to encourage employee participation. It is possible, and frequently advisable, to consider bringing together loosely defined groups of managers and employees to simply brainstorm ideas, gather information, and help define problems, as long as no proposals are offered or recommendations made. It also is proper to assemble an employee group to share information and observations with management, again as long as no proposals or recommendations are made.

Beyond one-time or limited, informal gatherings and in the realm of actual teams or committees it is important to keep the following seven points in mind:

1. When establishing a team or committee, identify it up front as not intended as an employee channel to management. Have a clear mission or charge in place before soliciting team membership, and have the team's functions and limits identified before any team activity begins.

2. Keep the team focused on work improvement topics only. This requires clear guidelines and plenty of continuing vigilance. It is difficult to talk

about quality, efficiency, productivity, and such without conditions of employment becoming involved, so be constantly aware of the potential need to redefine the team's boundaries periodically.

3. Staff teams with volunteers, or use rotating membership selected by some means that is not management dominated.

4. If a team is empowered to make a final management decision (that is, the team decides in place of management, not just recommends to management), it can be seen as acting as management. This is acceptable. In fact, it has been suggested that the ultimate protection against being ruled an illegal labor organization exists when the team can make final decisions in its own right. "The only true safe harbor is vesting the [committee] with the responsibility of making final management decisions."[4(p.104)]

5. If an issue is sufficiently narrowly defined that all persons affected by it can be included in a single group, a "committee of the whole" including everyone is usually legally safe. In such an instance nobody can be seen as "representing" anyone else.

6. For standing committees or long-lived teams, maintain a majority membership of managers. A committee or team composed of a majority of managers stands less chance of being adjudged illegal. However, a significant drawback of such teams should be obvious; a team composed mostly of managers is far less likely to be seen as a legitimate vehicle for employee participation.

7. Rather than always creating teams or committees that tend to develop a continuing existence, consider establishing specific problem-solving or work improvement ad hoc groups, each with a specific, well-defined charge and a specific problem to solve; disband each group after its goal has been attained. Such ad hoc groups can much more safely consist of a majority of nonmanagers than can "permanent" teams or committees. However, for teams composed largely of rank-and-file employees it is legally safest to have management representatives serve as observers or facilitators, without the power to vote on proposals or dominate or control the group.

For collaborative group problem solving and participative decision making in general, it is always appropriate to bring into the group those people who have the skills needed for dealing with the group's charge. It is necessary, however, to recognize that they have skills pertinent to the problem at hand and will likely have greater influence on group decisions.

Recognize also that teams or committees become unwieldy as they grow in size. Small groups are generally better; active participation in tasks seems to decrease with increases in group size. In fact team participants tend to rate small groups as more satisfactory, positive, and effective than larger groups.[7]

## Team Up for Success

As to the critical factors concerning the establishment of employee teams, it may help to remember that the highest legal risk involved in establishing groups is probably encountered while active union organizing is occurring. A modest amount of risk exists if teams are established in the presence of existing union contracts. The least risk occurs when there is neither organizing nor an active union presence.

Common-sense advice would suggest that employee teams or committees should not be established while organizing is occurring. It could be extremely helpful to have had some productive employee participation in place beforehand, but after the organizers arrive is no time to jump into employee teams. Even if such teams are legally established and operated they will foster incorrect perceptions concerning their creation. Rather, with or without a union in place, and as long as active union organizing is not occurring, employee teams can be employed legally and productively.

Employee participation may well be the key to continuing increases in quality, efficiency, and productivity. Employee participation is essential. As noted earlier, nobody knows the inner workings of a job better than the person who does it day in and day out. Also, there are few if any problem solutions that are not enhanced by multiple viewpoints and inputs. A team brings to the problem the power of the group. To cite a highly pertinent quotation from an anonymous source: "I use not only all the brains I have, but all I can borrow."

## THE DEPARTMENTAL TEAM

As far as the health care department manager is concerned, ongoing project teams experience their periods of inactivity and ad hoc teams come and go; however, the departmental team is—or should be—a constant presence.

As is often the case, a department may be treated as a collection of individual performers whom the manager must organize and guide in a common direction for a common purpose. If the individuals and the manager are conscientious, well motivated, and honestly share a common purpose, this collection of individuals can be reasonably effective. However, a collection of individuals working as individuals cannot achieve the level of performance possible from a well-functioning departmental team even if they are each doing their jobs well. Unless they are able to tap the potential of true teamwork, their output will rarely amount to more than the sum of their individual efforts.

When we speak of team building, we are speaking primarily about building and maintaining an effective, productive departmental team, a working group dedicated as a body to continuing superior performance through teamwork.

## TEAM BUILDING AND ITS PURPOSES

We can describe team building as an organized, systematic process of unifying a group of employees with common objectives into an effective and efficiently functioning work unit. The ongoing challenge of team building is to encourage a diverse collection of people to think and behave as a single entity rather than as a collection of individuals.

What is sought in a properly functioning team is a synergistic effect, a total effect and resulting output that is greater than the sum of individual contributions. The synergistic effect is literally the team effect in which the whole is decidedly greater than the sum of the individual parts.

Like it or not, the trend of today, indeed the wave of the future, in health care is the necessity to accomplish more with less. Therefore, it is not surprising to find that much of today's effort toward improving productivity is directed at improving the performance of work groups. True team building can

- foster increased productivity while maintaining or improving quality
- improve work climate, enhance work relationships, and increase employee satisfaction

Team building is, by its very nature, a continuing process. It is essential to understand that it is a long-term strategy, an activity that is never complete. A supervisor who manages the activities of a few people has a choice. He or she can provide the employees with what they need to do their jobs, insert new employees into the gaps inevitably created by turnover, and accept the work that each employee turns out as long as it meets or exceeds minimum standards. Or the supervisor can take the longer view, focusing on people and their needs and capabilities and striving to build and maintain a functioning unit rather than trying to influence individual productivity.

## RECOGNIZING EMPLOYEE POTENTIAL

The supervisor who would endeavor to build and maintain an effective team must first and foremost ascribe to an optimistic view of employees overall. This has to be a genuine belief in people and their capabilities, a Theory Y approach to the management of people as opposed to a Theory X philosophy (see Chapter 10). The Theory X manager will ordinarily not trust employees to do a proper job unless they are watched, pushed, and regulated. The Theory X manager is a "boss"; people are viewed primarily as producers of output. Accompanying lack of trust we will ordinarily find lack of respect as well, and the manager who neither trusts nor respects the employees will in turn be neither trusted nor respected by the members of the work group.

Yet mutual trust and respect are fundamental to the creation of a fully effective team. The manager who would build and maintain an effectively functioning team must harbor the belief that the majority of employees want to apply more of their abilities to their work, and when they are not allowed to do so their work is less satisfying than it could be.

Thus team building requires the following:

- shared power and authority
- increased employee participation

These requirements lead us back to what has been said about effective people-centered management in earlier portions of this volume (especially Chapter 5 and Chapters 9 through 14). It is fundamental to successful team building that the leader holds a generally positive view of employees and their potential.

### Toward Strengthened Motivation

The majority of workers will put forth a sustained effort to do a good job when and only when—they want to do a good job. Some workers will do a good job in the short term out of fear or apprehension, but quality that is forced or coerced is not sustainable and is usually delivered with resentment. How, then, does the manager inspire a group of employees to the extent that they are willing to do their best consistently?

Recall from the material concerning motivation that it is not possible for the manager to motivate employees directly. All true motivation is self-motivation, so the best the manager can do is foster conditions under which the employees will become self-motivated. Among the actions the manager can take to improve the motivational climate in the department are the following:

- Get serious about proper delegation (empowerment), using the process not to shift work around or shed unpleasant tasks but rather to provide some opportunity for employee learning and growth.

- Consider decentralization of certain tasks when appropriate, giving people at what might be scattered workstations complete control over work that might otherwise flow through two or more employees.

- Look into the possibility of job enhancement, appreciating that a mix of more tasks and more varied responsibility can provide greater interest and thus improved job satisfaction.

- Try cross-training when possible, with a goal of eventually having all employees of a given job grade able to do all jobs pertinent to that grade. This can greatly increase the flexibility of the work group while increasing interest and challenge for individuals.

- Remain conscious of every opportunity for increased participation by employees and take their contributions seriously. This will strengthen mutual trust and respect in addition to opening up some productive avenues the manager might never think of alone.

- Allow employees who have proven themselves responsible to take on special assignments, especially those over which they can exercise complete or nearly complete control.

- Constantly utilize enhanced feedback on performance. Recall that one of the job-related factors that mean the most to employees is the full appreciation of work done. When praise is deserved it should be immediate, sincere, and specific. When criticism is unavoidable it should be immediate, diplomatic, and constructive.

Will absolutely every employee respond positively when so treated? No, of course not. There will always be some who cannot be reached in this manner and some whose preference, whether they could admit it or not, is to "check their brains at the door" and put in their 8 hours in the same old way. However, enough people can be reached to make a difference; enough can be reached so the conscientious manager can build a team and create an environment that puts the resistors on the spot and causes most of them to move in one of two directions: (1) buying in and moving with the team or (2) removing themselves from the group.

## THE STAGES OF TEAM BUILDING

Although a continuous process, team building occurs over the following separately identifiable stages:

- formation
- disequilibrium
- role definition
- maturity
- maintenance

### Formation

It is not often that a departmental team has to be formed from the ground up with all new participants. However, there are significant events occurring that disrupt the balance and composition of a team to an extent that the resulting configuration is essentially a new team. One such event is turnover in team leadership, especially when the new supervisor or manager is a complete unknown. Another is a new departmental configuration such as that resulting, for example, from an inter-organizational merger that throws two or more groups together under common leadership that is new to many of them. These and similar changes in composition throw the team into the formation stage as the participants work to reestablish common ground and build what amounts to a new team.

In the formation stage, individual commitment is tentative; a number of people are likely to adopt a "wait-and-see" attitude, especially where new leadership might be involved. A new leader, even one who is philosophically similar to the previous leader, will have his or her own approach to different facets of the job. New relationships must be established, and until this has been accomplished much team communication will be cautious and guarded. Trust and confidence will not be extended in full until the new leader or, in the instance of a merger, the new group has acquired a level of comfort with this new combination of personalities.

### Disequilibrium

In this second stage of team building most of the people in the group are having their effects as individuals according to their own needs, desires, and capabilities. They may be doing their jobs well, but they are doing them as individuals. Many do not yet see themselves as part of a team. With each other they tend to be competitive more than cooperative; some members fear loss of credit to others, and some may strive to be the ones who are "on the good side" of the manager. Some will view the portion of the work they do as their exclusive territory, and they will become protective of that domain.

Some groups never go appreciably beyond this stage, forever remaining in a state of disequilibrium. The work can and does get done in this stage, at least at a minimally acceptable level, but it is the aggregated work of individuals, not the output of a functioning team. When a group is in a state of disequilibrium there can be no synergistic effect; in this state, at best the whole is no more than the sum of the parts.

Whether a group is to move beyond disequilibrium is dependent on the skill, determination, and desire of its leadership. The purely production-centered manager may have difficulty moving a group beyond this stage; complete and successful team building requires a people-centered focus.

## Role Definition

As mutual trust and respect build among the members of the group, and as individual roles are clarified and the interrelationships of these roles are established, cooperation begins to build and a team identity begins to emerge. Distrust is rare, and mutual respect is high. Communication becomes more open as participants begin to behave less like competitors and find a level of comfort in relationships with other members of the group. Individuals understand their place in the larger picture, and they have essentially taken on the objectives of the group as their own.

Relatively stable departmental groups, especially those consisting of people who have worked in harmony for a considerable time, will be at least at this stage for the majority of the members. What is needed most for a group to move beyond this stage is the appropriate leadership of a manager who sees himself or herself as part of the team as well as the catalyst that moves the team, and who can honestly equate personal success with team success.

## Maturity

Maturity of course describes the mature, functioning team. The mature team will exhibit high levels of cooperation, mutual trust and support, and productivity. The mature team will experience normal or below-normal turnover, and most of the turnover that does occur will be driven not by dissatisfaction but by other, more positive forces such as career advancement or forces beyond departmental control such as disability or death. For the most part, the members of the mature team will experience pride in team accomplishments and exhibit high levels of job satisfaction.

## Maintenance

In team building, maturity is not a fixed destination. Rather, it is a state of existence that must be maintained or it will deteriorate. Nothing remains stable; system inputs change in character, the environment changes, subtle and not-so-subtle changes in organizational mission and direction occur, and the team that does not continuously adapt will fall behind.

Because nothing remains stable, team maintenance requires a regular infusion of new ideas, novel approaches, and challenges to maintain team effectiveness. The mature team, if it is to remain fully effective, must change as the circumstances that surround it and the demands made on it change.

Another important dimension in which a team must be conscientiously maintained is the manner in which new team members are assimilated. All too often new employees are thrown into a job with inadequate orientation and incomplete preparation. When this occurs, one of two results are likely to follow: (1) the new employee feels adrift and uncomfortable to the extent of resigning shortly after placement or (2) the new employee catches on in bits and pieces, fits and starts, by guesswork, by asking coworkers, and so on, and develops as an individual performer, not as a team player. Team maintenance places a high priority on bringing in new members appropriately. Education in the organization's mission and objectives and the departmental team's role in pursuing them; thorough orientation to the functioning of the departmental team; direct mentoring, perhaps teaming a new employee with an experienced person for as long as it takes to achieve comfortable assimilation; regular coaching; and encouragement are what it takes to bring a new person completely up to the status of a fully functioning team member.

## THE POWER OF THE TEAM: THE INDIVIDUAL

A great deal has been said up to this point about the departmental team as a functioning unit. This should not be allowed to communicate an incorrect impression of the individual's place as part of a team; people are not absorbed into some form of "group mind" and robbed of their individuality. Quite the contrary, individual identity and individual motivation must be perpetuated as the heart of an effective work team. Motivation always remains individual; recall the contention that all motivation is self-motivation. Also, we can go so far as to claim that individual motivation is the point at which all human productivity begins.

As to what motivates or, more correctly, what causes most people to self-motivate, the sources of motivation come in the form of opportunity, specifically the opportunity to achieve; learn; do interesting, challenging work; do meaningful work; assume responsibility; and become actively involved in deciding how the work is done (for more detail see Chapter 11).

What teamwork actually accomplishes is focusing the efforts of individuals on common goals and objectives and the process of reaching them. Teamwork itself is not a goal; rather, teamwork is simply a means of harnessing the individual efforts and contributions of the people who make up the team.

To maintain team effectiveness it is essential that individuals work together in pursuit of team objectives, with the aim of accomplishing together something larger than any of them could accomplish alone. A team objective should consist of the same elements as an organizational objective or an individual objective. But individual, team, or otherwise, the statement of an objective is not complete unless it includes an expression of what is to be done, how much is to be done, and when it must be done. For example, a possible objective of an accounts receivable section of finance might read: Reduce the number of days outstanding in accounts receivable (what) from the present 68 days to 60 days (how much) by September 1 of this year (when).

## TEAM BUILDING AND LEADERSHIP STYLE

The department manager's leadership style is the greatest single determinant of successful team building. The development and maintenance of a mature, functioning team requires an open, participative, people-centered approach to management. The difference between success and failure at team building is as fundamental as the difference between participative management (genuine leading) and authoritarian management ("bossing"). The manager who would build an effective team cannot set himself or herself above the group, but must rather be an integral part of the group. Consider the following differences between the old-fashioned authoritarian (called "boss" for this comparison) and modern participative manager ("leader" in this comparison):

- The boss wields authority, whereas the leader cultivates good will. The leader possesses authority but does not openly flaunt it.
- The boss tells people how things should be done, whereas the leader, in so far as possible, shows how things are done.
- The boss pushes people, whereas the leader coaches, counsels, and encourages.
- The boss has an "I" orientation—my department, my staff, my accomplishments, etc.—but the leader has a "we" orientation—our department, our group, etc. The appropriate focus for a team's leader is always "we," "us," or "ours," and never "I," "me," or "mine."
- The boss, in effect, simply says "Go," and watches as the group moves toward a goal; the leader in effect, says "Let's go," and moves toward the goal as part of the group.

## GUIDANCE FOR THE TEAM BUILDER

Under this heading we could perhaps insert an entire educational program in supervisory practice or people-centered management, or at least a dozen or so chapters from this book. The paragraphs that follow may duplicate a few points made throughout those other chapters, but in the briefest possible form they are meant to provide a picture of the approach to be taken by the department manager who truly wishes to develop one of those exceptionally effective teams of which we see far too few.

What we are suggesting for the team-building supervisor is a people-centered leadership approach based on mutual trust and respect of all concerned. Certainly the employees will always see the manager as the manager; we are not trying to immerse the manager in a totally egalitarian situation. The employees know that the manager has the authority of the position, regardless of how directly or indirectly that authority is exercised. Also, the employees know that the manager is in charge; however, it is how this charge responsibility is fulfilled that makes the difference. It has been said on multiple occasions that a truly effective leader sets himself or herself above the staff in only one dimension—the acceptance of responsibility. The manager is not paid more than the staff because he or she is smarter, better educated, or in some way superior to the others; the manager is paid more for bearing the burden of responsibility.

To enhance the likelihood of building and maintaining an exceptionally effective team, the department manager must do the following:

- Be continually aware of what employees want from their employment (refer to Demands on the Organization in Chapter 11), and take these expressions of need seriously. Of particular importance in building an effective team is the acceptance of each person as a full-fledged member of the group and recognition of each as a contributing partner and not simply a servant of the system.

- Be seen as identifying more readily with the department than with that higher-level collective known as "management." The manager whose focus is clearly upward is likely to be viewed by the staff as an outsider, one of "them" (management), while the manager viewed by the staff as an insider, a member of their group, is far more likely to inspire the cooperation needed to build an effective team.

- Be readily visible and available to the department's employees. Visibility and availability reinforce the manager's commitment to the group and provide assurance that support and assistance are always close at hand. The manager who is frequently gone or consumed by meetings, special assignments, external conferences, and such will not be viewed by staff as a true team member. An absentee manager cannot be the catalytic agent the manager must be in building an effective team.

- Be serious about practicing proper delegation (empowerment), and give all capable individuals the opportunity to gain experience that might open new opportunities to them.

- Offer to all staff the opportunity to learn and grow, and work to develop those employees who seriously take advantage of this opportunity.

- Consistently practice the use of deadlines and follow-up in assigning work. Any task worth doing at all deserves a specific deadline (not ever "when you get a chance"); never let a deadline pass unanswered without following up.

- Practice true participative management. Be ever aware that the department's employees can be a nearly bottomless well of improvement opportunity; after all, no one knows the detailed ins and outs of a task like the person who performs it every day.

- Encourage team participation in decision making. The successful team-building manager will recognize that giving employees a voice in decision making does not indicate weakness or abrogation of responsibility; rather, doing so indicates just the opposite—strength and sufficient confidence in the employees to bear the ultimate responsibility for the decisions made jointly.

## ATTITUDE AND COMMITMENT: EVERYONE'S

All that has been said about the behavior of the seriously intended team-building manager is directed toward securing employee commitment to the process of creating and maintaining a fully functioning departmental team. There is a direct and undeniable relationship between employee commitment and an employee's sense of being part of a team. Employee commitment cannot be mandated or manipulated into existence; it must be inspired by the manager's own commitment and continually reinforced by the manager's attitude and behavior.

Attitude, especially the manager's attitude, can be an extremely powerful force. Attitude, whether positive or negative, is invariably contagious. And the leader's attitude can affect the entire group for good or for ill. It can sometimes be the most difficult task a manager can undertake to convey a positive attitude in the face of difficulty and often downright hardship, but without a positive attitude concerning what can be accomplished there will be little chance of building a fully functioning, productive team.

In the foreseeable future health care management will likely continue to experience constant pressure to accomplish more with less. One of the few ways of doing so is through the improved productivity possible from an efficient and effective departmental team.

## HELEN HAS HER WORK CUT OUT FOR HER

Referring to the "Situation" introduced at the beginning of the chapter, Helen Williams surely has her hands full—a formidable task lies before her. There is no magic formula that will instantly dissolve the barriers and merge the "enemy camps" into a unified staff. However, since she had a sense of the "hot seat" nature of the position, Helen probably went into the department knowing she could be facing a significant challenge.

Helen will have to take a number of actions over a period of time to erase the boundaries of the enemy camps, and she will have to exercise considerable patience because the kinds of behavioral change required of her employees will not come quickly or easily. The camps are essentially social groupings that have developed within the work group. They may have been formed in part under the influence of where people are physically located, what group or section they happen to be part of, how long they have been employed, who they are closest to in task relationships, and such. It lies with Helen to break up these camps. Yet this is not easily accomplished because they are primarily social groupings cemented by friendships and perhaps by distrust of the "others."

Helen's use of regular staff meetings is certainly appropriate. Staff meetings should occur as scheduled and be conducted in such a manner that all employees can expect to attend every meeting and to participate actively from time to time. Also, beyond staff meetings, it would be advisable for Helen to meet one-on-one with every staff member over a period of time.

Referring to the possibility that "Camp A was slightly more supportive than

Camp B," Helen should be extremely wary of any perception of favoritism. She cannot afford to have either group "on her side" if doing so increases the resistance of the other group. Helen's behavior should reflect equal regard and fair and equal treatment concerning all of the department's employees.

Once Helen has a solid feeling about the problems and knows who the informal leaders are, she can begin to take steps aimed at dissolving the separate camps. A thoughtful combination of cross-training, job enhancement, decentralization, and proper delegation—all accomplished in a way that supports task performance as well as rearranging people—will change the social groupings within the department. Some will resist these changes because they break up the prevailing social group; some will welcome these changes because there is task work variety and expanded responsibility and thus more challenge and potentially more job interest.

Helen needs to be mindful, however, that new camps can form within the rearranged department. Therefore, she needs to prevent this occurrence by addressing the needs and capabilities of the department's informal leaders (and there will be informal leaders; social groupings cannot exist without them) and address them accordingly. With some it may be possible to co-opt them by recognizing their informal leadership capabilities and delegating special projects and tasks accordingly, but with others it may be necessary to deal with them through coaching and counseling and perhaps, in a few instances, through disciplinary action.

Another avenue open to Helen to break up the camps is to utilize ad hoc or project teams for various assignments, deliberately staffing these teams across the boundaries of the camps and thus making it necessary for the groups to mix and to form different working relationships.

Helen also should ensure that she is dealing with her staff as though they were indeed a team rather than a collection of individuals. Therefore, she should involve all group members in developing and addressing departmental goals, provide as much positive feedback to the group as a whole rather than to specific individuals (recognize them, of course, but first recognize the team), and treat each individual the same as all others.

If she makes the right moves, Helen has every chance of forging an effective team out of the enemy camps; however, doing so will be a lengthy process.

---

## REVIEW QUESTIONS

1. Describe what is wrong with this statement: *"Let's give this problem to a hand-picked group of employees to see what they can come up with. There's no danger, because all they can do is recommend. As management we're free to accept or reject what they suggest."*

2. Briefly describe the issues that should never be offered for consideration by a team composed primarily of rank-and-file employees.

3. In reference to the employees of a department as a "team," what is the *team effect?*

4. Once formed and fully functioning, is an effective department team self-perpetuating thereafter? Why or why not?

5. For an effective departmental team, to what extent must the individual employee become submerged in a team identity?

6. In many present day organizations, why has it proven difficult to appropriately reward and recognize team performance?

---

## CASE: THE SILENT MAJORITY

As the newly placed manager of the admitting department, it didn't take long to discover that morale in the department had been low for quite some time. As you worked to become acquainted with employees by meeting with each of them alone, you were rapidly inundated with complaints and other evidence of discontent. Most complaints involved problems with administration and the business office and with the loose admitting practices of a few physicians. There also were complaints from the admitting staff about other department members and some thinly veiled charges about admitting personnel who "carry tales to administration."

In listening to the problems you detected a number of common themes. You decided that most misunderstandings could be cleared up by airing the gripes openly with the entire group. You then scheduled a staff meeting and asked all employees to prepare to air their complaints (except those involving specific other staff members) at the meeting. Most employees thought this was a good idea, and several assured you they would speak up. You were encouraged by what you heard; it seemed as though most employees were of a similar mind, indicating something of a team outlook. However, your first staff meeting was extremely brief; when offered the opportunity to air their complaints, nobody spoke.

The results were the same at the next staff meeting two weeks later, although in the intervening period you were bombarded with complaints from individuals. This experience left you frustrated because many of the complaints you heard were problems of the group rather than problems of individuals.

### Questions

1. What can you do to get this group to open up about what is bothering them?

2. What should you consider doing to get this department on track toward becoming an effective team? Identify at least two significant actions and explain why they should be considered.

3. How would you approach the specific problem of the employees who supposedly "carry tales to administration"?

## NOTES

1. "Special Report: Employee Representation Committees at Electromation Are Illegal: NLRB," *Management Policies and Personnel Law*, January 15, 1993; 1–2.
2. B.S. Murphy et al., "Manager's Newsfront: NLRB Decides Labor-Management Committees Case," *Personnel Journal* 72, no. 2 (1993): 20.
3. "NLRB Charges Polaroid with Forming New Employer-Dominated Labor Group," *Labor Relations Week* 7, no. 23 (1993): 560.
4. J.R. Redeker and D.P. O'Meara, "Safe Methods of Employee Participation," *HR Magazine* 38, no. 4 (1993): 101–104.
5. J. Swan, Jr., "The Most Effective Employee Committees Are Probably Illegal," *Personnel* 63, no. 11 (1984): 91.
6. R.J. Doyle, "Caution: Self-Directed Work Teams," *HR Magazine* 37, no. 6 (1992): 153–155.
7. L. Blake, "Reduce Employees' Resistance to Change," *Personnel Journal* 71, no. 9 (1992): 72–76.

## CHAPTER 24

# Methods Improvement: Making Work—and Life—Easier

*There's a way to do it better—find it.*
*—Thomas A. Edison*

## CHAPTER OBJECTIVES

☛ Convey the belief that there is usually room for improvement in the way most tasks are performed.

☛ Outline a simple but logical approach to the improvement of work methods.

☛ Introduce some of the more common tools and techniques of methods improvement and provide guidelines for their application.

☛ Outline an organized approach to methods improvement that is applicable institutionwide.

☛ Identify the role of the supervisor in encouraging a "methods-minded attitude" on the part of the department's employees.

## SITUATION: IS THERE A BETTER WAY TO ACCOMPLISH THIS TASK?

You manage a health information management (HIM) department (formerly, and still to some, medical records). You are being forced by circumstances to seek ways of accomplishing more work with no increase in staff. In looking for improvement opportunity you are finding it necessary to examine every distinctly identifiable task in the department.

One task that concerns you is the fulfillment of legitimate information requests. These usually require locating patient charts and making and mailing copies of appropriate documents. You believe that the individual ordinarily assigned to fulfilling information requests is applying reasonable effort to the job, but the process strikes you as inefficient. For one thing, there appears to be a great deal of walking—clearly a nonproductive activity—in the fulfillment of each request.

In thinking about the problem of the information requests and other departmental tasks, you believe you can see a number of ways to improve task performance. However, you are stymied in your efforts to determine how much improvement any particular change would accomplish. It occurs to you that any proposed new method would need to be tested against the present method; to that end you begin to look for ways to measure what is being done at present.

*Instructions*

As you proceed through this chapter, keep the information request in mind and consider the potential applicability of the material to the improvement of that process. The information request will be addressed in example form following the introduction of some tools and techniques of methods improvement.

## EDISON-PLUS

You will notice there is no hedging in Thomas Edison's statement quoted previously, no qualifier that might keep the door to improvement closed. Edison did not say there is sometimes, often, or even usually a better way. Often there are several better ways.

Some of the pioneers of industrial engineering, the branch of engineering dealing with work methods, insisted on the need to seek something they called the one best way. In recent years, however, the notion of a single best way to do something has come to be regarded as something of a theoretical ideal. Rather, we now recognize that there are usually several better ways of accomplishing a given task and that we must seek one of these better ways that reasonably meets our needs and fulfills our objectives.

We can describe methods improvement as the organized approach to determining how to accomplish a task with less effort, in less time, or at a lower cost, while maintaining or improving the quality of the outcome. You may find this process referred to in different organizations by various other labels, among them methods engineering, job improvement, and work simplification. Regardless of label, however, the intent remains the same: to alter the performance of a task in such a way that the results represent a desired improvement over the way it was formerly accomplished.

Methods improvement is understandably a subject that is not near and dear to a great many supervisors. Rarely is the need for change in a specific work procedure so pressing that it takes priority over the day-to-day, hour-to-hour operating problems of a department. However, methods improvement is another of those management activities that puts us in something of a bind— rarely is it critical and it is usually readily postponable, but unless it is made part of today's effort we will never realize its near-future benefits. Much like delegation, it is one of those activities we promise to get serious about after the rush is over. Somehow, however, we never quite get around to it.

A modest but active methods improvement program can be a valuable part of any supervisor's pattern of management. There are economic benefits to be gained: when you manage to accomplish a job in less time, with less effort, or with fewer material resources, you are improving your department's efficiency by bettering the relationship between output and input. There are a few intangible benefits to consider as well. When methods improvement is approached with a spirit of participative management, making use of the contributions of the people who actually do the work, there are positive returns in employee attitude.

## ROOM FOR IMPROVEMENT

Methods improvement may exist as a formal program in the organization, coordinated by a department such as management engineering or industrial engineering. Or it may exist at the department level, at the discretion of the supervisor, as an informal, ongoing effort to "tune up" and otherwise improve work procedures. At the very least, methods improvement should exist in the department as an attitude. Such a "methods-minded" attitude, a practiced belief in the possibility of continuing improvement, will encourage employees to utilize time and other resources more effectively.

Methods improvement applies largely to tasks, to problems of things—such as procedures, processes, forms, equipment, and physical layout—as opposed to problems of people. We generally recognize that the overall task of getting things done through people puts the supervisor in a position of being largely a solver of people problems. However, we must also recognize that work procedures and other essentially nonhuman factors are nevertheless shaped or influenced by the people who do the work. A certain procedure may lose efficiency over months or years because of the changing environment in which the job is performed, but efficiency may also be lost because people bring their own habits, attitudes, and preferences onto the job, which influence the way they work. Dig deeply enough into causes and you will often find that many apparent nonpeople problems have human origins.

Each person coming to work in your department is a unique individual and as such exerts a unique influence on the workplace. Thus a work procedure, especially one that was perhaps not particularly well defined in the first place, becomes at least in part a reflection of the worker. Run several consecutive individuals through a specific task and the result is a composite "procedure" that incorporates the subtle and perhaps not so subtle influences of these several people. Since we train many employees on the job using the example of the person actually doing the job, we pass along not only essential job knowledge but also the influences of other workers.

It is not unusual for the procedure for performing a given task to exist in the department in three distinctly different ways. It can exist in one form in the mind of the supervisor who, perhaps having done the job at one time, thinks of a specific (and quite likely outdated) collection of steps. The procedure can also exist in the mind of the worker in the form of all the steps this person actually performs to accomplish the task. It may also exist in written form in the department's procedure manual in a form different from either the supervisor's concept or the worker's practice. How often are such manuals referred to when people believe that the same old task is being done in the same old way?

In some organizations the concern for methods improvement techniques is left to a specific function such as management engineering. However, the power to improve procedures and make work easier need not be limited to some special staff. A simple philosophy of methods improvement might suggest the following:

- There are few, if any, existing tasks that cannot be improved.

- The people who actually do the work are potentially valuable contributors to improvement.

- The power of participative management can bring out the best in each employee.

From a healthy, participative management point of view, methods improvement may be simply described as applied common sense.

## AT THE CENTER OF TOTAL QUALITY MANAGEMENT

With variations in terminology and occasional differences in emphasis owing to the organizational environment in which it is applied, the process described in the remainder of this chapter is largely the process that drives work improvement within a total quality management (TQM) program. You may find this process referred to as team-oriented problem solving (TOPS) or as the mission of "self-directed work teams." It has also been called "team-oriented process improvement" and "work simplification," the latter label identifying an organized approach to work improvement dating back to 1932.[1]

The overall process has also been known by the most broadly generic label of "methods improvement." Regardless of label, however, the following two critical characteristics run through all of these approaches:

1. A multidisciplinary approach is taken to problem solving, involving all departments that have a relationship to the problem.
2. Solutions are generated—and implemented—at the level of the people who actually do the work.

## THE METHODS IMPROVEMENT APPROACH

The generalized several-step approach to methods improvement presented in this section will be followed by a review of some of the simpler tools and techniques of methods analysis. Successful methods improvement ordinarily begins with concentration on a single, specific task. A supervisor has far too much to do to attempt to improve everything at once; a shotgun approach will lead to the start of many projects but the likely completion of few or none. Simply select one task or isolate one problem—one that is causing trouble or simply one that some members of the department feel could be done more efficiently—and go to work.

### Select a Task or Isolate a Problem

You must, of course, become aware of a problem before it can be solved. The need for methods improvement often becomes apparent on a number of fronts if you examine in detail the several areas in which the department's problems usually arise. The significant signs that often suggest a particular task deserves analysis and improvement follow:

- An activity is costing you more than you know or believe it should cost.
- Bottlenecks occur as work backs up at various stages of a process, or there are chronic backlogs of incomplete work.
- Confusion is evident as employees appear uncertain as to what happens next, how it happens, and why.
- Poor morale prevails in the work group.

- Walking, handling, transportation, and other nonproductive activities appear to occur in excess.

In locating and defining problems that may highlight the need for improvement, it is important to distinguish between symptoms of problems and true problems. For example, what may appear to be a bottleneck of work caused by poor work methods might seem correctable through a small amount of overtime, a bit of extra effort, or a rearrangement of task assignments. However, if the true causal problem happens to lie in ineffective scheduling practices, the bottleneck, supposedly fixed, is highly likely to return once conditions revert to "normal." When the area addressed head-on is really only a symptom of the problem, the difficulty will probably return within a short time or resurface in a somewhat altered form. Thus it is necessary to look beyond the apparent immediate problem and identify the force or forces that lie behind a manifestation of difficulty.

## Gather the Facts

The next step is to learn thoroughly how the task is done now—everything one could possibly learn about the way the job is being performed. The total process involved in the task under consideration must be described through sketches, flow charts, or whatever other techniques are available. Sketching out "the system" often increases understanding of the relationships among system components, since you can often observe a logical order or reasonable interrelationship among the pieces once they are all captured on paper. Recording the present method in full also allows others who may be able to provide insight into the problem to examine the problem and compare it with their understanding of the situation.

In getting the facts—in applying the information-gathering tools and techniques of methods improvement—one may gather information from

- written procedures, if they exist
- architectural and layout drawings, if the problem concerns layout or physical space in any way
- work schedules
- samples of pertinent forms and records
- accounting data, payroll data, purchasing information, and other financial records
- statistical reports and other records of operating results

Rest assured, however, that what you collect from any of the foregoing sources will often be insufficient. You must usually expend additional effort in the one major area of concern that you cannot learn from existing information: How the task is currently being performed.

## Reduce the Problem to Subproblems as Necessary

Often a single apparent methods improvement problem may seem too large or complex to tackle as a whole. Such a problem can often be broken down into a number of smaller, separately identifiable problems that can be solved independently. Once the problems have been separately addressed and tentative solutions developed, the subsolutions may be combined and integrated into a solution to the total problem.

## Challenge Everything

All of the information gathered to this point must be subjected to searching study. Take nothing for granted. At every step along the way, ask: What is actually being done? Where is it done? By whom is it done? How is it done? Always, for every step, ask: Why?

Examine every step and challenge every detail in an effort to

- Eliminate activities whenever possible. Just because something is being done is no reason it must be done. Ask of each step: If this were not done at all, what would be the result?
- Combine steps whenever possible.
- Improve the manner of performing various steps.
- Change sequence of activities, location of workstations, assignments of people involved, and any other factors that might have a bearing on efficient task performance.

The process of challenging every last detail lies at the heart of methods improvement. At this point methods improvement, while appearing to many to be a logical "scientific approach," must become a wide-open, no-holds-barred creative process. It is here that participation and teamwork have far-reaching implications. A number of factors come together to challenge every detail of the problem thoroughly and carry the problem solvers toward the results of the next step: brainstorming and other creative idea-generating techniques; optimism, other "up" attitudes, and genuine belief in the necessity for improvement; willingness to experiment, innovate, fail occasionally as part of the learning process, and try the untried; knowledge of the tools and techniques of information gathering and analysis; the complete involvement of all parties who have a stake in the problem, regardless of their level in the organization; and a healthy positive attitude toward the need for constructive change.

## Develop an Improved Method

Having learned thoroughly about the task and uncovered its weaknesses and strengths, you can use the results of your analysis to develop a proposed new method. However, the process is not as simple as replacing the old method with the new method with no further preparation. Rather, it is necessary to

- Check out the proposed method thoroughly using flow charts and other analytical techniques, subjecting it to the same kind of detailed examination that you applied to the present method, to provide reasonable assurance that the difficulties leading to the consideration of this task have been corrected.

- Analyze the impact of the proposed method in terms of human involvement, since the effective application of the new method will fall to people who actually do the work each day. The best methods-engineered procedure ever to hit the department is bound for eventual failure if it includes elements that the worker—the critical human factor—considers demeaning or dissatisfying. When combining the "perfect" solution—perfect in a technical sense—with the human element, you sometimes need to back off from technical perfection to accommodate the needs of employees.

- If at all possible, make some trial runs of experimental applications to test proposed methods. In this way you can also test variations in methods to determine which might work better in practice or be more palatable to the employees who do the work.

- In general, assess the practicability of the proposed method in light of any possible constraints. It is one thing to idealize a method; it is quite another matter to make that method work in the face of constraints of cost, time, and quality considerations.

## Implement and Follow Up

Action is a must. The best work method ever devised is useless as long as it remains solely on paper.

Be prepared to accept a certain amount of "tuning up" and "debugging." Steps that appear to work well on paper often require modification in actual practice. Also, conditions are constantly changing, and needs and circumstances present at the time of implementation may be different from those existing when the analysis was started. Rarely is a plan of any consequence implemented 100 percent as planned in every detail, so it is necessary to stay on top of implementation until all the hitches have been worked out of the method.

Always be aware of potential human relations problems and of the value of employee participation in methods improvement. Often you will find that the extent of participation that may have preceded implementation will have already determined the success or failure of a proposed new method.

The human problems encountered in the implementation of new work procedures are often the classic problems of resistance to change. As for employee participation, there is usually an identifiable relationship between employee involvement and resistance to change: the more intimately involved employees are in determining the form and substance of a change, the more likely they are to accept that change and thus be less resistant.

When it comes to implementing new methods or procedures or in general instituting any change, as supervisor you have three available avenues of approach: you can tell the employees what to do, you can convince them of what must be done, or you can involve them in determining what must be done. Employee involvement in determining new and revised methods is advisable for a number of important reasons:

- The employee who is involved will thoroughly know the details of the new method as it is created.

- The involved employee will "own a piece" of the new method and will thus be more likely to accept it.
- The employee is one of the most valuable sources, if not the single most valuable source, of information on how the task is performed now and how it might be performed better. The supervisor, who might have the superior perspective of departmental operations, may be able to stand back and observe what pieces do not fit together well and that a number of things need to be improved. However, when it comes to specific tasks it is the employee performing these tasks day in and day out who knows best of all people in the organization the inner working details of those tasks. Employees are a source of information that should not be allowed to go untapped in methods improvement.

Close follow-up on implementation is essential, and for many tasks it must be maintained for a considerable length of time. Time is necessary for new habits to form and replace old habits completely, and for new methods to dominate employees' actions fully and negate any fond remembrances of "the way we used to do it." Also, any method installed today is immediately subject to unforeseen problems and "creeping changes" that can affect performance. Thus supervisors must follow up a new method until it has completely taken its place among the department's normal processes. Even then the new method—as all of a department's procedures—should be subjected to a periodic audit of effectiveness and appropriateness.

## THE TOOLS AND TECHNIQUES OF METHODS IMPROVEMENT

A number of analytical tools and techniques are available to a person pursuing methods improvement. We introduce only a few such techniques in this chapter, but these are easy to use and broadly applicable to many situations.

One of the most valuable tools available for examining an activity is the flow process chart, used for tracking and recording the steps of an activity and assessing the nature of each step. Flow process charts appear in many forms, but most make use of the five basic activity symbols shown in Figure 24–1. For proper analysis all work activity should be divided into at least these five basic categories:

An operation is any activity that advances the completion of the task. It is the actual doing of work, whether writing on a form, dialing a telephone, giving an injection, making a photocopy, tightening a bolt, or whatever.

A transportation represents any movement encountered in the process. It may be the movement of a patient from here to there, the delivery of a memo from you to your supervisor, the carrying of a record from here to the copy machine, or any other activity that has movement as its primary characteristic.

An inspection is an activity in which the primary emphasis is on verification of the results of prior operations. For instance, a housekeeping supervisor may periodically check areas that have recently been cleaned; an admitting supervisor may check an admission form to ensure it is appropriately completed; a business office supervisor may assign an employee the task of verifying statements before they are sent out.

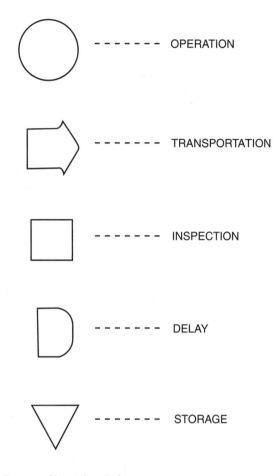

**Figure 24–1** Flow Process Chart Symbols

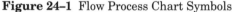

A delay is an unplanned interruption in the flow of necessary steps. A pencil breaks and must be replaced; a copier jams and must be cleared; a beverage spills, necessitating cleanup and replacement; a waiting line is encountered at the central supply window; the person who must sign your hand-carried requisition is on the telephone—all of these are examples of delays that might be encountered in flow process analysis.

A storage is indicated whenever a step results in an anticipated interruption of the process, or it may represent the end of the process. More in-depth analysis than we are dealing with sometimes calls for distinguishing between temporary and permanent storage. For example, that completed bill just dropped in the mailroom out-basket is in temporary storage; the process will be resumed after some period of time. However, although the completed medical record just filed on the shelf may be retrieved some time in the future, it is for all practical purposes in permanent storage.

Although the activity symbols of Figure 24–1 can be used in charting activity in freehand fashion, they are usually incorporated into prepared forms. A simplified version of a portion of a flow process chart form appears in Exhibit 24–1. If this form is used, it is necessary only to describe each activity, preferably in no more than two or three words; indicate the appropriate symbol for that activity; and, as you wish, connect the symbols to indicate sequential flow of activities.

An important indicator of the proper use of the flow process chart is embodied in the need for the user to note whether the chart follows the activities of a person or the flow of material. This decision must be made before beginning the analysis. For instance, if you are observing a clerk preparing and processing a three-part form, you may reach a point in the activity where the form is

**Exhibit 24–1** Flow Process Chart (Form)

| SUMMARY | PRESENT NO | PRESENT HRS | PROPOSED NO | PROPOSED HRS | SAVINGS NO | SAVINGS HRS |
|---|---|---|---|---|---|---|
| ○ OPERATION | | | | | | |
| ⇨ TRANSPORT | | | | | | |
| □ INSPECTION | | | | | | |
| D DELAY | | | | | | |
| ▽ STORAGE | | | | | | |
| DISTANCE TRAVELED | | | | | | |

| | |
|---|---|
| PROCEDURE CHARTED | |
| PERSON □ MATERIAL □ | |
| CHART BEGINS | CHART ENDS |
| CHARTED BY | DATE |
| □ PRESENT | □ PROPOSED |

| | STEPS IN PROCEDURE | OPERATIONS (OPER. TRAV. INSP. DELAY STOR.) | DISTANCE IN FEET | TIME IN HOURS | REMARKS |
|---|---|---|---|---|---|
| 1 | | ○ ⇨ □ D ▽ | | | |
| 2 | | ○ ⇨ □ D ▽ | | | |
| 3 | | ○ ⇨ □ D ▽ | | | |
| 4 | | ○ ⇨ □ D ▽ | | | |
| 5 | | ○ ⇨ □ D ▽ | | | |
| 6 | | ○ ⇨ □ D ▽ | | | |
| 7 | | ○ ⇨ □ D ▽ | | | |
| 8 | | ○ ⇨ □ D ▽ | | | |
| 9 | | ○ ⇨ □ D ▽ | | | |
| 10 | | ○ ⇨ □ D ▽ | | | |
| 11 | | ○ ⇨ □ D ▽ | | | |
| 12 | | ○ ⇨ □ D ▽ | | | |
| 13 | | ○ ⇨ □ D ▽ | | | |
| 14 | | ○ ⇨ □ D ▽ | | | |
| 15 | | ○ ⇨ □ D ▽ | | | |
| 16 | | ○ ⇨ □ D ▽ | | | |
| 17 | | ○ ⇨ □ D ▽ | | | |
| 18 | | ○ ⇨ □ D ▽ | | | |
| 19 | | ○ ⇨ □ D ▽ | | | |
| | APPROVED BY | TOTALS | | | PAGE OF PAGES |

taken apart and goes in three directions while the clerk either remains working with one part of the form or perhaps goes off in a fourth direction. It is necessary for the user to make an early decision on the focus of the analysis (e.g., either "purchasing requisition" or "purchasing clerk") and stick with it.

Note also the space on the chart form where you can summarize total number of work activities and total distance traveled in transportation steps. You can use this part of the form for comparing possible changes with present methods.

Another simple but helpful tool is the flow diagram, a sample of which appears in Figure 24–2. A flow diagram is simply a layout drawing, drawn to approximate scale, on which lines are placed to indicate paths of personnel movement or material flow. This can be especially helpful in determining how to rearrange equipment, furnishings, and workstations for improved effectiveness. This technique may be used to assess the approximate amount of movement necessitated by a particular layout, and any potential new layout may thus be tested on paper to see if it represents improvement over the present layout.

Numerous additional techniques are available for analyzing work activities of various kinds. Some of these are as follows:

**Figure 24–2** Flow Diagram Charting Route of X-Ray Technician Travel

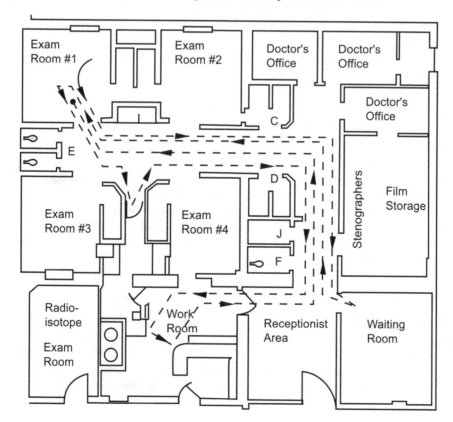

- *The operation process chart.* While a flow process chart captures an entire sequence of all operations, transportations, delays, inspections, and storages during a process or activity, an operation process chart typically focuses only on operations (the circular symbol) and inspections (the square symbol). It is most conveniently used to examine all the separate small activities or suboperations that may take place within a given larger task.

- *The multiple activity flow process chart.* This tool is most useful if you wish to examine, for example, a multipart form that is processed over a period of days. Using the standard charting symbols, this chart would perhaps display the multiple parts of the subject form in a vertical column at the left and a time scale of perhaps several days of the week across the horizontal dimension. Using this technique you can illustrate, usually on a single sheet of paper, what happens to each part of the multipart form on each day of the processing cycle.

- *The multiple activity chart.* Formerly referred to as a man-and-machine chart, this form is used to chart the activities of an employee in conjunction with one or more pieces of equipment. The heart of this particular chart is a vertical time scale calibrated in either minutes or decimal parts of an hour. The activities of the worker and the utilization of the equipment are indicated parallel with this time scale. This technique makes it possible to identify times when worker or equipment is waiting or being productively applied and thus to consider rearrangements of activity that may reduce idle (nonproductive) time for workers, equipment, or both.

- *The gang process chart* is a flow process chart applied to the analysis of the activities of a crew of two or more persons who must work together to accomplish a given task. The steps taken by each member of the crew are charted relative to each other on a time scale; that is, what worker A is doing at any particular time appears directly beside the activity that worker B is performing at the same time.

The foregoing overview of methods improvement barely scratches the surface of management engineering technology. For the supervisor who wishes to pursue methods analysis in considerably more detail, helpful published references are available. Three of the best such references are *Motion and Time Study,* by Ralph M. Barnes; *Maynard's Industrial Engineering Handbook,* edited by Kjell B. Zandin and H.B. Maynard; and *Hospital Management Engineering,* by Harold E. Smalley. These are described in more detail in the Annotated Bibliography.

## EXAMPLE: THE INFORMATION REQUEST

Returning to the "Situation" cited at the beginning of the chapter, we now have the means available to determine whether there is indeed a better way to accomplish the task in question. We first apply some of the simpler tools of methods improvement to documenting the present method, thus establishing a solid baseline with which to compare any potential improvements.

Exhibit 24–2 is a flow process chart documenting 17 steps involved in the processing of a single information request in the health information management department. The activity begins when a request for information is pulled from the incoming mail; it ends when the fulfilled request is "filed," which means it may be inserted into an actual file or put away in a desk drawer or other storage container. The nature of the steps between receiving and filing should be evident from their brief descriptions.

With the complete task of answering an information request recorded on a flow process chart, we can begin to question the individual steps involved to determine whether there might be room for improvement. For example, observation has revealed that considerable travel is involved in what would seem to

---

**Exhibit 24–2** Flow Process Chart: Information Request (Single)

| SUMMARY | PRESENT NO/HRS | PROPOSED NO/HRS | SAVINGS NO/HRS |
|---|---|---|---|
| ○ OPERATION | 10 | | |
| ⇨ TRANSPORT | 3 | | |
| □ INSPECTION | 1 | | |
| D DELAY | 1 | | |
| ▽ STORAGE | 2 | | |

PROCEDURE CHARTED: Information Request (Single)
PERSON □  MATERIAL ☒
CHART BEGINS: Get Request  CHART ENDS: File
CHARTED BY: CRM  DATE: 3/9/91
DISTANCE TRAVELED: 100 ft (for 1)
☒ PRESENT  □ PROPOSED

| # | STEPS IN PROCEDURE | OPERATIONS | DISTANCE IN FEET | TIME IN HOURS | REMARKS |
|---|---|---|---|---|---|
| 1 | Get, Open, & Read | ⊗⇨□D▽ | | | |
| 2 | Verify, Authorization | ○⇨☒D▽ | | | |
| 3 | Get Chart | ⊗⇨□D▽ | 15 | | |
| 4 | Chart to Desk | ○⊠□D▽ | 15 | | |
| 5 | Locate & Remove Pages | ⊗⇨□D▽ | | | |
| 6 | To Copier | ○⊠□D▽ | 20 | | |
| 7 | Start Copier | ⊗⇨□D▽ | | | |
| 8 | Wait for Warm-Up | ○⇨□⊠▽ | | | |
| 9 | Make Copies | ⊗⇨□D▽ | | | |
| 10 | Return to Desk | ○⊠□D▽ | 20 | | |
| 11 | Re-Assemble Chart | ⊗⇨□D▽ | | | |
| 12 | Re-File Chart | ⊗⇨□D▽ | 30 | | |
| 13 | Type Bill & Envelope | ⊗⇨□D▽ | | | |
| 14 | Assemble to Mail | ⊗⇨□D▽ | | | |
| 15 | Into Outgoing Mail | ○⇨□D▼ | | | |
| 16 | Enter into Log | ⊗⇨□D▽ | | | |
| 17 | File Request | ○⇨□D▼ | | | |
| 18 | | ○⇨□D▽ | | | |
| 19 | | ○⇨□D▽ | | | |

APPROVED BY          TOTALS          PAGE     OF     PAGES

be a small task—in all, about 100 feet of walking. This should raise questions as to whether any furniture or nonpermanent fixtures could be relocated to reduce personnel travel.

The delay recorded on line 8, waiting for the copy machine to warm up, should raise some questions. It may be perfectly legitimate—there are some copy machines that should be shut down between infrequent uses—but you will never discover this without probing to determine why.

In this example it is also reasonable to consider whether certain steps could be eliminated or combined. For instance, is it possible to obtain the chart as in step 3, then go directly to the copy machine and perform the next several activities there and thus eliminate a pair of transportations? Or if the copy machine warm-up should indeed be required, would it be productive for the employee to turn the copy machine on before getting the chart so the machine can be used without delay when needed?

Other pertinent questions should occur to you as you study the chart. However, we have not yet raised the most important question relative to this example: How many information requests are involved? If requests arrive at the clerk's in-basket in batches, then several additional questions become important:

- Can these requests be processed in batches, doing each step for several requests at a time?
- Can all necessary charts be obtained at once?
- Would it be practical to save all bill preparation for one time of day?
- Should all filing be done at the end of the day?
- Should you consider physical changes, such as moving a desk, to reduce transportation?

In the actual situation this example was taken from, mail arrived in the department once in the morning and once in the afternoon. The clerk was in the habit of running information requests twice a day, usually within an hour or so of the arrival of the mail, whether the batch consisted of a single request or several requests. A few simple changes in procedure were indicated as follows:

- The copy machine was turned on at the beginning of the day and left on (a little investigation showed this to be the manufacturer's recommendation).
- It was decided to run the requests in batches, with little change in the steps indicated (trial runs involving a clerk doing several steps at the copy machine produced a situation that was sufficiently awkward as to be counterproductive).
- An ideal batch size of 10 to 12 requests was established, thus providing that no request went unanswered longer than 2 days (the decision was simply to run 10 to 12 at once or a maximum of 2 days' requests, whichever accumulated first).
- A simple change in layout—turning the clerk's desk around and moving it about 8 feet—reduced total travel from 100 feet to about 70 feet. (A flow chart of the resulting activity appears as Exhibit 24–3.)

**Exhibit 24–3** Flow Process Chart: Information Request (Batch)

| SUMMARY | PRESENT NO / HRS | PROPOSED NO / HRS | SAVINGS NO / HRS |
|---|---|---|---|
| ○ OPERATION | 9 | | |
| ⇨ TRANSPORT | 3 | | |
| ☐ INSPECTION | 1 | | |
| D DELAY | 0 | | |
| ▽ STORAGE | 2 | | |

PROCEDURE CHARTED: Information Request (Batch)
PERSON ☐   MATERIAL ☒
CHART BEGINS: Get Request   CHART ENDS: File
CHARTED BY: CRM   DATE: 3/9/91
DISTANCE TRAVELED: 70 ft (for 10-12)   ☒ PRESENT   ☐ PROPOSED

| # | STEPS IN PROCEDURE | OPER. | TRAN. | INSP. | DELAY | STOR. | DISTANCE IN FEET | TIME IN HOURS | REMARKS |
|---|---|---|---|---|---|---|---|---|---|
| 1 | Get, Open, Read, & Sort by # | ⊗ | ⇨ | ☐ | D | ▽ | | | |
| 2 | Verify, Authorizations | ○ | ⇨ | ☒ | D | ▽ | | | |
| 3 | Get Charts | ⊗ | ⇨ | ☐ | D | ▽ | 10 | | |
| 4 | Charts to Desk | ○ | ⇨ | ☐ | D | ▽ | 10 | | |
| 5 | Locate & Remove Pages | ⊗ | ⇨ | ☐ | D | ▽ | | | |
| 6 | To Copier | ○ | ⇨ | ☐ | D | ▽ | 15 | | |
| 7 | Make Copies | ⊗ | ⇨ | ☐ | D | ▽ | | | |
| 8 | Return to Desk | ○ | ⇨ | ☐ | D | ▽ | 15 | | |
| 9 | Re-Assemble Charts | ⊗ | ⇨ | ☐ | D | ▽ | | | |
| 10 | Re-File Charts | ⊗ | ⇨ | ☐ | D | ▽ | 20 | | |
| 11 | Type Bills & Envelopes | ⊗ | ⇨ | ☐ | D | ▽ | | | |
| 12 | Assemble to Mail | ⊗ | ⇨ | ☐ | D | ▽ | | | |
| 13 | Into Outgoing Mail | ○ | ⇨ | ☐ | D | ▽ | | | |
| 14 | Enter into Log | ⊗ | ⇨ | ☐ | D | ▽ | | | |
| 15 | File Request | ○ | ⇨ | ☐ | D | ▽ | | | |
| 16 | | ○ | ⇨ | ☐ | D | ▽ | | | |
| 17 | | ○ | ⇨ | ☐ | D | ▽ | | | |
| 18 | | ○ | ⇨ | ☐ | D | ▽ | | | |
| 19 | | ○ | ⇨ | ☐ | D | ▽ | | | |

APPROVED BY   TOTALS   PAGE   OF   PAGES

The amount of effort put into such an analysis will depend largely on the total workload involved. In the situation just described, for instance, if information requests amounted to only one or two a day, as might be the case in a very small hospital, there is little to be gained by shaving a minute or so from each repetition of the task. The time of the supervisor or other analyst is fully as valuable as the time of the employee, and hours of effort can be wasted to produce obviously minuscule returns. Under conditions of high volume, however, there may be significant gains to be made through a few hours' effort. If, for instance, the institution was of sufficient size that processing such requests required a full-time person or more, analysis could make a difference as to whether one person could or could not do the job alone. As early as possible in the methods improvement process, assess the potential savings in time and resources. Let your best efforts be directed toward improvements having the greatest potential for savings in time or other resources.

## AN ORGANIZED APPROACH TO METHODS IMPROVEMENT

A formal, institution-wide methods improvement program should ordinarily consist of three phases: philosophy, education, and application.

### Philosophy

The belief in continual methods improvement effort and in the need for a methods improvement program should exist at the top of the organization. For a program to achieve long-run success, top management support should be active and visible. Regardless of where the idea begins, all employees must see top management as 100 percent supportive of an organized effort to maintain constant cost-containment pressure through regular, positive questioning of work methods. This commitment must be reflected in a shared belief that few if any activities cannot be improved.

Granted, the dissemination of the methods improvement philosophy throughout the organization may require a great deal of promotional effort, and the business of promoting the benefits of the continuous oversight of work methods is necessarily a selling job that is never truly complete. However, once a program is underway and some positive results have been generated, these results will in turn help to sell the philosophy.

Through meetings and printed matter, everyone in the organization should be encouraged to retain the basic message that cost containment is here to stay. All employees should realize that continuing attention to making each hour of labor and each dollar's worth of material input go further, do better, and produce higher-quality results is one of the important ways they can all help keep the institution solvent and thus continue to serve patients and protect their employment.

### Education

Education in the tools and techniques of methods improvement should begin some weeks after the introduction of the philosophy. This activity should bring supervisors and middle managers together and begin to acquaint them with the ways and means of work analysis. Ideally, the educational process should include some pilot methods improvement projects taken from the jobs of the participants.

Once a number of supervisors and managers have been at least partly oriented to a working knowledge of methods improvement tools and techniques, selected nonsupervisory employees—especially those having skills applicable to potential projects—should be brought into the education process.

## Application

Ideally, an ongoing methods improvement program should be guided and monitored by either an administrative steering committee or a methods improvement coordinator who is a member of administration, a management engineer, or both. In addition to assisting actively and coordinating necessary skills and resources, the primary task of the steering committee or coordinator is to keep the methods improvement projects moving. Methods improvement will necessarily not always be particularly high on the average supervisor's priority list; there is usually more than enough to do without it. In constantly monitoring the program, the committee or coordinator serves as an ever-present reminder that keeping methods improvement alive requires periodic activity. This monitoring also makes the process easier for supervisors who are involved in active projects.

Common sense suggests that it is best initially to pursue those projects that hold the greatest potential for returns or that are most readily completed. Although this may seem like "skimming" or going after just the "easy stuff," there is a distinct advantage in proceeding in this fashion: some early, visible successes often serve as a much-needed boost to the momentum of the entire program.

Individual project teams may take two forms: the ad hoc group assembled for a single project, or the ongoing group formed to deal with a particular department or specific function.

The ideal ad hoc project team might consist of the following individuals:

- the supervisor responsible for the task being studied
- the assistant to the supervisor (if there is one)
- one or two of the persons who regularly perform the task
- one "expert" knowledgeable in the most prominent technical specialty related to the task (for example, an accountant to deal with aspects of a billing problem, a materiel management specialist to deal with a transportation problem, a personnel professional to deal with personnel policy issues)

An ongoing project team formed to deal with a series of projects relating to a specific department or function might consist of the following individuals:

- the department head or assistant
- a representative of administration
- a finance representative
- a management engineer or systems analyst
- one or more "experts," persons from particular technical specialties that might be involved in most projects
- one or two nonsupervisory employees of the department

Given the history of many methods improvement undertakings, and recognizing that in many organizations much has been started that has died of its own weight or gradually dwindled to nothing, much of the foregoing may appear idealistic. Regardless of the organization's overall attitude toward methods improvement, there remains the opportunity for individual supervisors to pursue methods improvement strictly within the confines of their own departments.

Granted some projects can never be undertaken or successfully completed without interdepartmental cooperation. However, such projects aside, in each department are countless ways in which a conscientious supervisor and a few positively motivated employees can improve work methods and contain costs. In the average department of any health care institution a great deal of improvement is there for the making; the supervisor has only to recognize the possibilities for improvement and provide the example of leadership required to bring the employees into the improvement process.

### Total Quality Management in Action

The preceding few paragraphs have largely described the TQM process. Certainly the major phases of the process—philosophy, education, and application—are identical, as is the critical need for solid top management commitment. Much of the organization for TQM is the same, with a high-level "steering committee" providing guidance, and a methods improvement coordinator who may be referred to as "quality coordinator" or "quality director" or the like.

A true total quality management approach rightly calls upon the organization as a whole and each function or activity therein to identify its mission—the essential reasons for its existence—and further identify its customers, both internal and external, and to pursue quality, described in one of many of its current variations as meeting or exceeding customers' expectations.

Regardless of label or variation in application, however, the ultimate goals of TQM and methods improvement are identical: ensure that the organization is doing the right things, and doing them right the first time.

### THE METHODS-MINDED ATTITUDE

The "methods-minded" attitude referred to earlier has its foundation in each employee's belief that improvement is always possible, and that, left to themselves for prolonged periods, work activities will experience "creeping changes," that are usually not changes for the better. Methods-mindedness will often be reflected in the person who develops efficient work habits and always approaches a task in such a way as to achieve satisfactory results with minimum effort. Methods-mindedness, then, might seem to be a talent. Rather, however, it is a habit, or, more appropriately, a collection of habits. And as a habit, methods-mindedness can be learned.

Your attitude toward methods improvement will do the most to encourage your employees to become methods-minded. You need not plunge into methods improvement in a full-scale manner; rather, limit your attention to one or two troublesome tasks at a time—or simply to one activity or process that you feel includes room for improvement. Even if you simply keep one such project open at a time, working on it as time allows or as you make time, you are bound to make noticeable progress and stimulate the interest of some of your employees.

Your employees, of course, are once again counted among the keys to your success as a supervisor. You may be able to stand back at an objective distance and see problems your employees cannot see, but when you get into specific procedural details the situation is reversed: Nobody knows most of the inner workings of a task better than the employees who do it day in and day out. Your employees can see much that is hidden from you.

Effective methods improvement in a department requires a merger of structural and human considerations. Referring to the organization types discussed in Chapter 2, methods improvement is able to produce an effective blend of the job organization system and the cooperative motivation system by tapping the individual enthusiasm and motivation of your employees to organize and refine the task they must perform.

---

## REVIEW QUESTIONS

1. Do you ascribe to the existence of *one best way* to perform a task? Why or why not?

2. In your own words, explain what you believe is meant by the *methods-minded attitude.*

3. Providing quality is not an issue in a particular instance, what should be the key factor in determining how much effort goes into achieving an improved process?

4. Why, in so many instances, will a new method incorporating greatly improved efficiency and productivity be resisted by the employees who perform the work?

5. Why is it often extremely difficult to obtain funding and other resources for educating employees in methods improvement?

6. What do you believe to be the stage of the methods improvement process at which resistance or reversion to former ways is most likely to occur? Why?

---

## EXERCISE: "THE PENCIL"

Using the basic flow charting symbols, chart the following simple activity.

Get a wooden pencil from your desk, sharpen it at a sharpener located near the door of this room, and return to your place. Also, account for the following:

- somebody else got to the sharpener a step ahead of you, so you had to wait

- the sharpener gave you a poor job; you found it packed with shavings that you had to clean out before you got an acceptable point

- Assuming "pencil sharpening" to be of sufficient importance to deserve a few minutes further study, sketch a flow diagram showing your relationship to the sharpener (use your actual surroundings). If you had to sharpen at least ten pencils each day, what could you do to reduce the time and effort spent on this task?

---

**NOTE**

1. Kjell B. Zandin and H.B. Maynard, eds., *Maynard's Industrial Engineering Handbook*, 5th ed. (New York: The McGraw-Hill Companies, Inc., 2001).

## CHAPTER 25

# Reengineering and Reduction in Force

*The future never just happens; it is created.*
—*V. Clayton Sherman*

## CHAPTER OBJECTIVES

☞ Provide a basic understanding of the process referred to as "reengineering."

☞ Relate reengineering to the concepts of methods improvement and total quality management (TQM).

☞ Provide a perspective on reduction-in-force as an undesirable but sometimes necessary adjustment for the sake of organizational viability.

☞ Outline the individual supervisor's likely involvement in a staff reduction.

☞ Stress the essential nature of all forms of communication with the survivors of a staff reduction.

## SITUATION: EXPANDING RESPONSIBILITIES

You are the nurse manager (or head nurse) of a 22-bed medical-surgical unit known as 3 West. There is also a medical-surgical unit known as 3 East. Unit 3 East is a mirror-image of 3 West, and the two are laid out such that their nursing stations are back-to-back in a center core although not fully open to each other. Over the recent 12-month period each unit has averaged approximately 60 percent occupancy.

For several weeks your employees asked you questions concerning rumors of impending layoffs at the hospital. You did all that you could to answer their questions but you were able to say very little of substance. Finally, after two months of speculation, a reduction-in-force occurred.

The third floor lost two part-time nurse aides and one part-time housekeeper. The only nurse affected was the manager of 3 East, your counterpart in the adjoining unit. One week following the layoff you were told that you were now the manager of both 3 West and 3 East.

*Instructions*

As you proceed through this chapter, consider how you would address the following questions:

- What would be the likely impact on your individual span of control as a supervisor?

- Conceding that you were always constructively occupied managing 3 West, how can you merge the responsibilities of the two units and successfully run both?

- What kinds of tasks you once engaged in will now be performed less often than when you ran 3 West alone?
- What skills will increase in importance because of your new role in running the combined units, and how might your management style have to change?

## REENGINEERING: PERCEPTION, INTENT, AND REALITY

As a term frequently used in business, reengineering has replaced a number of other "-ings" over the years, including repositioning, rightsizing, downsizing, reorganizing, revitalizing, and modernizing. Regardless of label, however, there has always been one critical factor these terms have in common by the way they have been perceived by the majority of employees. In one way or another they all convey an extremely unsettling message: Some people are going to lose their jobs.

One can argue about differences in perceived meaning of all of the "-ings." For instance, "reorganizing" can be perceived as "simply moving things around;" perhaps "downsizing" is seen as no more than "cutting back." One of the oldest of the "-ings," "modernizing," at one time inspired fear of technology as it was perceived as people being displaced by machinery. But there remains a common thread holding all of the "-ings" together: change in the way we do business.

The term "reengineering" has evolved just as the basic intent of the process has itself evolved. Reduction in numbers of employees has never been the primary intent. Rather, reduction-in-force has frequently been a byproduct of a process intended to improve operations overall. This improvement might result from decreasing costs, increasing revenues, or improving operating efficiency by getting greater results from the same or less resources.

### A Working Definition

Reengineering may be defined *as the systematic redesign of a business's core processes, starting with desired outcomes and establishing the most efficient possible processes to achieve those outcomes.* One begins the process with a desired result in mind. Whether the envisioned result is a physical product or other specifically desired outcome, basic engineering involves designing and developing the product or outcome and the means of producing it. Reengineering literally means engineering something again, looking at the same product or outcome again and determining how it is to be produced or attained. What may seem simple in concept, however, can be extremely difficult to achieve in practice.

An original engineering effort begins cleanly: nothing exists in the way of a process, so there is nothing in place to channel our thoughts or efforts in any particular direction. Once a process is in place, however, especially a process that has been considered by some to be reasonable and workable, it serves to draw us back to this previously traveled path.

Note that at the heart of all classical methods improvement or problem-solving processes (see Chapter 24) is how something is presently done. Reengineering, on the other hand, ignores—or at least tries to ignore—the manner in which something is done, focusing instead on the desired outcome and independently establishing a new way to achieve that outcome. This new way might or might not look like the old way. What is important is that it be developed without undue influence from the present process and that it represent the most effective means of achieving an essential outcome. And *essential* is the key. Methods improvement and problem-solving processes focus on doing things the right way. The concept translates to reengineering when the focus becomes one of doing the right things in the right way.

Why reengineering? Because nothing remains unchanging, because conditions, circumstances, and needs change. The rationale for reengineering was well stated in the October 5, 1995, cover story in *Hospitals and Health Networks:* "Day-to-day activities change dramatically, and you *eliminate things that do not add value for customers—for patients and the people paying for health care* (emphasis added)."[1]

## Obstacles to Reengineering

The appropriate path to reengineering includes the following steps:

- identification of the organization's mission
- identification of the outcomes necessary to fulfill the organization's mission
- establishment of the processes needed to achieve the necessary outcomes

Existing processes, traditional divisions of work, and the assumptions and expectations fostered by the environment in which we are accustomed to working all conspire to frustrate our reach for innovation. Thus the principal barriers to reengineering continue to be:

- present processes that distract us from an essential focus on desired outcomes
- existing rules and regulations that place boundaries around our thinking from the outset
- departmental boundaries that reinforce perceived limitations on the scope of our responsibility and authority
- functional and occupational boundaries that cause us to enter each problem with preconceived notions of who can do what and when
- normal resistance to change that is experienced as we are forced into unfamiliar and thus discomforting territory
- individual paradigms and perspectives, through which our perceptions are narrowed—we see no more than what we have been conditioned to see, and in some instances we are actually closed off from certain kinds of information

## Using Outside Help

Many organizations use outside consultants to assist in reengineering. Although consultants are dramatically overused and misused in many organizations, reengineering is one area of need in which consultants can be highly effective precisely because they are outsiders. The outsider's perspective is likely to be broader and more open than that of the insider, and the person from outside does not have the emotional or intellectual stake in present processes that the insider is likely to have. Frequently the external perspective can perceive that to which the internal perspective is blind.

Another important reason for the outsider's involvement in reengineering lies in the need for a view that is as unbiased as possible of the organizational changes that appear to be needed. Employees who may become involved in a reengineering effort can hardly be expected to recommend themselves out of a job. The insider who becomes involved in a serious reengineering effort potentially affecting his or her own position is ill prepared to participate constructively.

## REDUCTION-IN-FORCE AND BEYOND

Reducing labor cost is probably the most common goal of organizational restructuring. Reduced labor cost comes about occasionally from reduced salaries, sometimes by way of reduced hours for employees, and most often in the form of reduced numbers of staff.

It goes without saying that a considerable amount of thought and effort are required in structuring and implementing a reduction in a manner that will be as fair as possible to all concerned while supporting the primary responsibility for delivering quality health care. However, the effort associated with this significant undertaking cannot stop simply when the staff members who have been appropriately identified for separation have been released. For those at all levels who remain with the organization—and in the vast majority of work force cutbacks the people who remain are far more numerous than those who leave—the implementation of the reduction-in-force (RIF) is the beginning of a completely new work situation in what will, and what in fact must, become a dramatically different organization culture. Although many will tend to seek a "business as usual" state of affairs following a staff reduction, they will find that this is not possible.

## What Follows Reduction in Force?

A major RIF will forever alter many employees' beliefs and attitudes concerning their employment. Consider the following:

- For many years health care workers saw reductions occurring in manufacturing and commercial industry in their communities while feeling relatively safe against the likelihood of ever having to share the experience. For a long time we felt certain that, as an absolutely essential service, health care would remain untouched by the severe economic concerns that plagued other industries.

- Many health care organizations long enjoyed a sense of employment security that has been severely—and for all practical purposes permanently—damaged.
- Health care workers have been forever awakened to the hard fact that health care is subject to many of the external forces from which we believed it was relatively protected. That is, we now see that forces beyond our control can cause permanent changes to health care whether we do or do not seek these changes ourselves.

The immediate responses to a health care organization's RIF can include the following:

- Many employees may at first—and permanently, if positive steps are not taken—feel more like a cost of doing business than valued members of a work organization; they view themselves as simply another purchased commodity of which the organization will henceforth purchase less.
- Employee commitment to the organization will tend to erode as perceived employment security is diminished.
- Employee morale will be automatically reduced.
- Some key staff the organization desires to retain may resign to seek employment in environments they may perceive as more stable, further impacting the morale and outlook of those who remain.
- Managers and supervisors, with their thinking still bound by former ways of doing things, may attempt to compensate for lost staff by increasing the use of overtime and temporary help. They will experience additional frustration as controls are placed on hiring and on the use of overtime and temporaries.

In the time immediately following a RIF, there is a severe risk of cost reduction becoming universally perceived as a higher priority than people. It is true that successful cost control is an essential element of survival; the health care organization that cannot adapt to financial reality will not survive to employ anyone. People, however, still remain the driving force. It is people working together who must bring the organization into line with financial reality, yet the same organization's continued existence then and forever will depend on serving people.

What should necessarily follow any RIF is a revitalization of the remaining work force. An organization cannot and should never attempt to simply "lay off" a number of employees and call upon those who remain to close ranks and continue as before. All who remain have a more difficult and more responsible task looming before them, and the organization's top management should endeavor to give all of the support and assistance that can reasonably be provided in making the transition to a leaner, more purposefully directed organization.

## The Necessity of Reducing the Work Force

Although the scenarios have differed to some extent from state to state, health care provider organizations across the nation have been experiencing reductions in revenue from most payment sources. Further significant revenue shortfalls will likely be occurring because of additional limitations placed on reimbursement levels by most payers, the commercial insurers and major not-for-profit insurers as well as Medicare and Medicaid. This should come as no surprise to those who have been aware of the budget and health care debates continually raging at all levels of government. The simple fact of the matter is that the health care system is being forced by external circumstances to continually deliver the best of care while holding down increases in cost. Because the demand for service remains as high as ever and, in many respects continues to grow, the system is called upon to accomplish more results with fewer resources.

Consider the circumstances of one particular teaching hospital. This hospital's modest financial circumstances and generally good fiscal health sustained operations for several years during which costs rose at more than twice the rate that its income increased. This hospital employed a delaying tactic used by many not-for-profit organizations by annually reallocating modest reserves of various sorts to bring the current year into line, while avoiding any attempt at serious cost cutting—until the reserves ran dry during the same year that serious cuts in Medicare and Medicaid occurred.

Thus following literally decades of fiscal performance that was at a break-even or better level, the hospital faced a projected loss of such significance that two or three such years together could render the organization insolvent. Not the least of top management's concerns was the task of communicating the facts of their situation truthfully and believably to a work force that had never experienced layoffs, had never felt more than token pressure to contain costs, and had been conditioned by years of experience to believe that costs and revenue would somehow always be made to balance.

One should hope that realistic cost-containment activities, pursued as a normal course of business, might help an organization avoid or at least lessen a massive financial crunch of the kind just described. However, the problem remains the same regardless of its immediate magnitude and it must be dealt with. The communication issues are difficult enough when faced squarely with realistic data on a year-to-year basis; they become all the more difficult when the work force has been conditioned to believe that nothing serious is amiss.

In brief, when a RIF is planned and before the cuts occur, the work force must be given every opportunity to understand why this is going to happen. The more openly the employees have been treated all along and the more frankly they have been advised of the organization's real circumstances on a continuing basis, the easier it will be to communicate why.

Any RIF, while preferably designed and recommended by senior management and the medical staff leadership and approved by the board of directors, should proceed after all other reasonable efforts to reduce costs have been explored as follows:

- All realistic short-term savings opportunities should be identified and implemented.

- Maximum effort should be expended to reduce staff through attrition before the actual reduction is done by freezing hiring in most positions and, as much as possible, transferring current employees into areas of greatest need.

- Overtime should be severely curtailed, essentially reserved for true emergencies only and approvable by only a select few. Also the use of temporary help should be curtailed (along with overtime, agency temporary help can tend to increase under staff reduction pressure if not closely monitored).

- Supply inventories should be reduced to levels conforming to the true needs indicated by reduced levels of activity.

It must be stressed that no matter how much cost control effort precedes a RIF, the reduction itself is never the end of the process. For the organization's continued financial viability and effectiveness, it becomes the job of all employees to pursue continuous cost control in concert with continuous quality improvement if the organization is to prevail as a quality provider of health care.

### The Employees Who Remain

A RIF instantly establishes two entirely different groups of employees: those who leave and those who remain. Except in rare instances, those who remain far outnumber those who leave. Judging from many of the health care staff reductions that have occurred in recent years, it is not unusual for the "survivors" to outnumber those leaving by eight, nine, or ten to one.

Management must recognize that the manner in which it deals with the reduction's survivors has a considerably greater bearing on the organization's future than how the terminations related to the RIF have been addressed. Those who have departed are gone, probably forever, but the survivors are there and are critical to the organization's future.

Stress and stress-related fear among those who remain following a RIF is natural, predictable, and essentially universal throughout the organization. A fully understandable feeling among survivors is the fear that they may be the next to go.

It becomes necessary to unite the survivors into a forward-moving team and to motivate them to work harder in a leaner, more efficient, and yet initially a completely alien, situation. Through a concentrated and continuing communication program, the survivors of the reduction need to learn several things:

- why they remain and what will be expected of them, why the old organization is gone forever, and how they can help shape the new organizational culture that will be emerging

- that as the survivors of the reduction they are among the best in their occupations, and that is essentially why they are still in place

- that a future in which continually doing more with less will remain critical to organizational survival and continued employment

## Immediate and Natural Reactions to Staff Reduction

The issues emerging in the wake of a RIF are all essentially people issues. The major issues that surface usually include the following:

- The short-term loss of good talent in the form of productive employees that the organization would wish to retain. At special risk are valuable "free-agent" employees, those professional and technical employees whose primary loyalty is to an occupation and whose movement between and among organizations may be governed more by labor market circumstances than by ties to a specific organization or group.

- An immediate drop in productivity, precisely at a time when productivity increases are needed for the sake of long-term survival. This occurs because morale has dropped and employees are preoccupied with issues of security and concern for their future.

- Increases in the use of sick time, health care benefits, on-the-job accidents, medication errors, and other lapses in quality. These are often experienced during and after a RIF, again owing to employees' concern for their employment.

During and after a reduction there may be a fully understandable tendency to cut all financial corners and curtail all possible expenditures in an effort to save jobs and achieve an acceptable financial position. However, this may be precisely the time for the organization to be devoting money and effort to developing new sources of income and to ensuring the increased flexibility, adaptability, and effectiveness of the remaining work force.

## Employee Motivation Following Reduction

Under normal circumstances—without the direct prospect of a reduction in the work force and with each employee's reasonable expectation of continued employment—job security and wages are not particularly active motivating forces. Rather, they are potential dissatisfiers; as long as wages and job security are perceived as "reasonable," the concern for them is secondary. However, when they are disturbed—when raises are eliminated, for instance, or when security is perceived as threatened—these become factors in heightening employee dissatisfaction, which in turn negatively impacts motivation.

It becomes necessary to help the surviving employees reestablish a sense of equilibrium with their altered surroundings and achieve a relative sense of security. An employee who may come to work each day wondering "Will I be next?" will be neither effective nor productive. As long as an employee is preoccupied with personal survival, individual productivity will decline at the time its improvement is needed more than ever.

It is necessary to communicate with employees fully, completely, and repeatedly until they understand the following:

- Nobody—neither the organization nor a labor union—can absolutely guarantee continued employment, which frequently plays upon fears and uncertainties attendant to downsizing.

- A certain amount of stress is inevitable regardless of what management does following a RIF, but stress can be energizing as well as debilitating and can serve as a spur to improvement.
- A future emphasis on improved productivity is essential to survival as an organization.
- Employees' aggregate job performance is the organization's best survival guarantee, and as far as individual employees are concerned, their performance is their own best job security.

The most potent motivating forces—perhaps the only true long-run motivating forces—are inherent in people's work. These forces are largely opportunities: the opportunity to learn and grow, to do interesting work, to contribute, and to feel a sense of accomplishment and worth. However, these motivators can work only when employees are able to feel relatively secure and reasonably compensated. Management needs to provide conditions under which all employees can become self-motivated and then act on that belief.

Attendant to employees' motivational needs, the organization might also consider the creation of incentive programs and other flexible rewards to encourage and acknowledge innovation, commitment, and enhanced productivity. Overall, top management should at all times let employees know what is expected of them and tell them exactly how this desired behavior will be rewarded.

### Changes in Supervisors' Roles

Any significant RIF includes the elimination of some positions and the combination of positions responsible for managing the work of others. In the presence of a generally flatter management structure—overall fewer levels from top to bottom—supervisors and managers are likely to find their roles enhanced. They will essentially assume new roles, roles that are more challenging and that require more direct decision making.

The individual who directly supervises others will be the organization's primary conduit for communication with staff. At each management level, the supervisor is always a critical link in the movement of information up and down the chain of command. The supervisor is the primary communicating link between each direct reporting employee and the rest of the organization. It is through the supervisor that the individual employee receives assignments, evaluations and performance feedback, praise and criticism, information about the organization's fate and future, and information about nearly all other aspects of employment.

The supervisor's role is critical. As the one member of management who the employee knows best and the one whose role it is to be the employee's communicating link, the supervisor influences the attitudes and outlooks of a significant portion of the organization. Thus as the individual employee views the supervisor, so too is he or she likely to view the organization. In other words, if a supervisor of 15 people is seen as distant, uncommunicative, and uncaring, so are 15 people likely to see the total organization as distant, uncommunicative, and uncaring. Because the size of direct reporting work groups generally increases following a RIF and flattening of the organization, the influence of the individual supervisor becomes even more significant.

Some of the supervisor's key concerns after a RIF are as follows:

- the need to be conscious of the employee's motivational needs and to work to control turnover both immediately and over the long term
- the need to function as a strong advocate for the staff, to achieve the best for those who must leave as well as for those who remain
- the need to begin preparing to work with the survivors, helping them to internalize the dramatic change well before the reduction is fully implemented
- the need to actively encourage employee participation more than ever before, stressing involvement and drawing all possible employees into the decision-making processes. More than ever the supervisor's focus needs to be "we," never "I" or "you"
- the need to develop and utilize employee teams to the maximum possible extent
- the need at all times to communicate, communicate, communicate, remaining in touch with employees' fears and concerns even when some of the answers have to be, "We simply don't know yet, but we'll keep you informed"

Assistance in responding to these and other concerns can be provided to supervisors and middle managers in part through enhanced educational opportunities.

## Education and Training after Staff Reduction

It has been almost a foregone conclusion that an organization's education function is among the first to be cut back during lean times. The traditional treatment of the education function, at least as far as non-clinical education such as management development and supervisory training are concerned, implies that such education is seen as a frill, that it is dispensable often to a greater degree than most other functions. Clinical education, much of which is continuing nursing education, is another matter; the largest part of such continuing education is required by state regulations and Joint Commission standards, so it is largely reduction-proof. Because education departments are usually small and a cutback usually removes one or more full-time positions, in terms of percentage of staff reduction non-clinical education is frequently harder hit than many other activities.

No staff reduction rationale is more counterproductive than the across-the-board cut in which every department is expected to surrender an equal percentage of staff. Yet this rationale is frequently applied out of a misguided sense of "fairness" that suggests the pain must be equally borne by all.

Some functions are simply more valuable at certain times than are others. In a manufacturing company that is reorganizing in response to a declining market share, for example, it could be folly to reduce staff in marketing and new product development because this may be precisely the time to be enhancing and reemphasizing these functions. Likewise in many health care organizations, it can be short-sighted to reduce the resources allocated to education as part of a RIF that leaves in its wake a dramatically increased need for education.

Following a RIF, it is necessary to assist all remaining employees to become more flexible and adaptable. To that end, an enhanced program of continuing education is strongly recommended for all employee levels, that is, for supervisors and managers as well as nonmanagerial employees.

## COPING WITH YOUR EXPANDING RESPONSIBILITIES

In the position in which you were asked to imagine yourself in the "Situation" at the beginning of the chapter, you will of course find that your responsibilities have expanded considerably. It may even seem to you, at least until you begin to bring the combined position under control, that your workload has grown to unmanageable proportions.

Your span of control has essentially doubled with the addition of 3 East to your responsibilities. The physical territory has doubled, and the number of staff has almost doubled (the original total staff of 3 West and 3 East, less the few losses through layoff).

You must take an approach that combines similar tasks in the most efficient possible manner. For example, you would not do the schedule for 3 West and later do the schedule for 3 East; rather, you would schedule at one time using one process or perhaps schedule as a single unit. Also, you must understand that there will probably never be enough time for everything you believe must be done, so it will be more important than ever to be conscious of priorities to ensure that you are always at work on the most important task facing you.

When running 3 West alone you might have tended to do much of your own support work, such as memos, schedules, audits, filling in as a direct caregiver, or other tasks that do not require a manager's authority. Running the combined unit you will discover that you have less and less time to devote to tasks that are not true management duties, so you should look to using support services where and when available.

High among the skills that will become more important to you are: delegation, because you will experience a need to get more done by others; planning, because you now have a greater area and larger staff to worry about; time management, because you have more to do and more to keep track of; decision making, because there will be more decisions to make; and employee relations because a larger staff invariably raises more personnel concerns. Generally, your style will necessarily become more open and participative than it might once have been if you are to cope with the increased demands placed on you. You will have to make the best use of the talents and capabilities of staff. Your concern cannot be "How can I possibly run this new unit by myself?" Rather, your concern, directly reflected in your management approach, should be "How can we make this new unit run as efficiently as possible?"

## RESISTANCE TO CHANGE: COPING WITH DRAMATIC PARADIGM SHIFTS

A RIF in a health care organization involves a forced paradigm shift that affects workers in a dramatic and considerably disturbing fashion. For many years health care providers have been locked into a particular paradigm, clinging especially to a number of assumptions about the manner in which care must be delivered in a hospital setting. As a reduction approaches and the visible signs such as deliberate slowdowns in filling open positions or hiring freezes begin to emerge, much of the resistance of supervisors and managers to delays in filling positions will center on the contention that quality of care will suffer without the one-for-one replacement of departing personnel. The extremely strong paradigm at work here is that which assumes that our present way of delivering care is the best and most efficient way, that cost and quality exist in a direct relationship so if we take cost out (in this instance remove staff), quality will automatically decline, and, therefore, because we would never willingly or knowingly deliver poor quality care, we believe we have to have the staff whether the money to pay them exists or not. (Implicit in this argument is the belief that the answer lies in more money for the system or, at the very least, money diverted from other parts of the system: "Cut their program, not mine.")

For a number of complex reasons the cost of health care has grown far more rapidly than any other significant societal cost for a considerable number of years. Steps are now being taken to stem that alarming growth by simply reducing the amount of money allowed to flow into health care. In doing so, the government and other third-party payers are forcing health care out of its age-old paradigms, quite literally making health care providers look for ways of accomplishing the same ends at much less cost. Yet the strength of the old way of doing things hampers the ability to quickly find a new way.

When we are forced into unwanted change, we typically respond through a grieving process. (Actually, it is not change itself we resist so much as *being changed*.) Loss and uncertainty prevail. Those who survive a staff reduction may even experience guilt over having done so. There is considerable trauma experienced by those who leave the organization involuntarily, but the trauma is just as great for those who remain. Those who remain have to make the painful adjustments that organizational survival requires.

The survivors of a RIF typically perceive dwindling control over their work circumstances. Therefore, every effort should be made to keep employees advised of the organization's circumstances. Employee communication and involvement are critical in establishing the future direction of the work force that remains following a reduction. To ensure maximum possible communication and involvement, management should

- hold regular employee meetings to answer questions and to explain where the organization is going
- make necessary changes rationally, whenever possible calling upon the participation of affected employees
- seek regular employee feedback by way of surveys and other means so as to be continually aware of employee concerns

- continually explore new business strategies and other potential means of enhancing the organization's value to the community and its financial viability as an organization

For some who leave, a staff reduction seems like the end of the world, at least for a while. Many who remain also tend to see the dramatic changes forced upon them as marking the end of the world as they knew it. Because none who survive, neither line managers nor rank-and-file, can control what happens to the organization, it is indeed the end of the world as many knew it. But for the survivors it can also be the beginning of a challenging new world.

---

## REVIEW QUESTIONS

1. Describe what you believe is the common employee perception of "reengineering," and state how you would suggest working to change this perception if possible.
2. Cite at least three significant elements of the supervisor's essential role in reduction in force and its aftermath.
3. What do you believe is the principal contradiction generally perceived between the concepts *total quality management* and *reengineering.*
4. What do you believe are the immediate major needs and concerns of the "survivors" of a reduction in force?
5. What are the implications for the role of the individual supervisor following a reduction in force (that is, in what ways might the supervisor's job be altered?)

---

## CASE: IDENTIFYING FOR LAYOFF

Dan Carey, director of facility operations, was meeting with Arthur Brooks, engineering supervisor, about the possible need to soon identify one or two employees from engineering for possible layoff. Layoffs were not new to the hospital, having occurred twice over the previous 3 years.

Dan said, "I'm new to this place. What did you do the last time there were layoffs?"

Arthur answered, "We were given a sort of scale to use for comparing people. It gave roughly equal weight to four factors—basic job qualifications, seniority, performance evaluations, and what I'd guess you'd call conduct."

"What's that?"

"It involves warnings and suspensions and such for violating hospital policy," Arthur said. "You know, like a written warning for being late too many times."

Dan said, "I don't see how we're going to escape losing at least one person in this next cutback. I want you to make sure the one we lose is Fredericks."

"He's been here a long time," Arthur said, "lots longer than most. Offhand I don't see how to make him fit the criteria."

"You make him fit," Dan said. "You and I both know he's one of the biggest goof-offs in the hospital and our least productive worker. We can't help it that past management didn't do what they should have done."

"Should have," Arthur said, "but didn't."

Dan shook his head vigorously. "We've got tons of work-order history that proves he's our least productive person."

"But not a negative word in his file," said Arthur.

Dan Carey and Arthur Brooks discussed Fredericks and his situation for a quarter of an hour. Their positions are summarized as follows:

Dan: "We shouldn't have to keep the worst employee of the whole lot over all the others. We have no union here so there's no contract to make us observe seniority. If I have to then I can prove he's the least productive person. It's a legitimate layoff—the hospital has got to reduce staff—and this is a lot easier and cleaner way of dealing with Fredericks than going through a whole long, drawn-out process that someone else should have followed long ago."

Arthur: "Laying off Fredericks is risky. Seniority has always been a major factor in determining who gets laid off here; it's an established policy. You might be able to prove he's our least productive person, but there's no file we can open up and use to prove that he ever knew how he was doing. There's only a bunch of average evaluations. He might be the one who really deserves to go, but this isn't the way to get him out of here."

### Instructions

1. Consider the summaries of Dan's and Arthur's positions as alternatives for addressing the potential impact on Fredericks. Which alternative are you more willing to support, and why?

2. Fredericks reports to Arthur Brooks who in turn reports to Dan Carey. Imagine that Arthur has recommended against laying off Fredericks, instead recommending the department's newest member for the reduction. Dan Carey, however, chooses to reject Arthur's recommendation and directs him to lay off Fredericks. If you found yourself in Arthur's position, how would you proceed?

---

**NOTE**

1. K. Lumsdon, "Mean Streets," *Hospitals and Health Networks* 69, no. 19 (1995): 44–52.

## CHAPTER 26

# Continuing Education: Your Employees and You

*Your education begins when what is called your education is over.*
*—Oliver Wendell Holmes*

## CHAPTER OBJECTIVES

☞ Establish the importance of continuing education as a legitimate concern of every supervisor.

☞ Stress the necessity for management commitment to continuing education.

☞ Describe various approaches to continuing education.

☞ Establish the role of the supervisor in providing and guiding the department's continuing education program.

☞ Examine the special emphasis on education necessitated by reengineering, reduction in force, and other dramatic organizational changes.

☞ Identify avenues of continuing education available to the supervisor for self-development.

## SITUATION: CROSS-TRAINING AND THE SUPERVISOR

You supervise a sizable group of people, perhaps 20 or more employees, including a number of individuals who do different jobs but are in the same labor grade or on the same pay scale.

For example, maybe you work in food service where you have a general category that could be called food service aide, but within that category there are three or four different jobs (e.g., food preparation aide, cafeteria aide, dining room aide, or tray line worker).

Or perhaps you supervise in the patient billing division of accounting where your employees have three job titles—outpatient biller, inpatient biller, Medicare biller—that are all on the same pay scale.

You have been directed by your immediate supervisor to develop a cross-training plan by which you will be able to prepare all of your employees working in the same general labor grade to perform all jobs in the department in that labor grade.

*Instructions*

As you proceed through this chapter, try to determine what information you need to assemble concerning the affected employees and their jobs.

Also, be prepared to sell the idea of cross-training with sound reasons why it is to the advantage of both the organization and the employees.

Consider also what your approach might be to the occasional employee who seems completely unwilling or unable to cross-train.

## WHY CONTINUING EDUCATION?

It can be difficult and at times nearly impossible for people working in the delivery of health care to keep up with all of the changes affecting their work. Some health care workers, subject to continually evolving techniques, procedures, and equipment, must feel as though the more they learn the more there remains to be learned.

The rate of technological change was discussed in Chapter 18 and it was concluded, in part, that what we know and how we must apply it does not, in fact cannot, remain stable. Today's knowledge is not sufficient for the needs of tomorrow, so without the presence of a learning attitude we seem doomed to remain forever behind the times. Although the rate of technological change will not have equal impact on all skills and all professions, there is sufficient reason to suggest that standing still relative to developments in one's field—however slowly these developments may seem to accrue—is to guarantee falling short of the ability to meet some future job needs. In some areas of work activity, including nursing, radiology, administration, medical records, and health finance, to name only a few, it is often necessary to absorb and react to change at a rapid pace simply to remain abreast of the times.

Continuing education affords a significant means of bringing change under control, of making change work for you rather than against you. Properly focused, continuing education provides the ability to increase knowledge, improve skills, and change attitudes as job performance needs change.

In addition to providing a means of keeping up with new developments, continuing education also serves at least two other major functions. One of these is the provision of reinforcement through refresher education. Knowledge that lies unused or infrequently used can get rusty from lack of application, but relearning what one has learned before can revitalize knowledge and sharpen skills.

The other major function of continuing education is to increase individual capabilities and thus to improve the potential effectiveness of all members of a work group. Later in this chapter we will highlight the benefits of cross-training which is the practice of ensuring that employees become proficient in the performance of jobs other than those to which they are regularly assigned.

All of the foregoing benefits of continuing education aside, there is also one compelling reason driving a great deal of continuing education in the hospital setting: much of it is required, or at least strongly encouraged, by accreditation and regulatory bodies. For example, in the current *Accreditation Manual for Hospitals*, accreditation survey criteria for the continuing education of hospital staff appear in more than 50 places.[1] For the department of nursing, for a considerable number of years the education criteria of the Joint Commission on Accreditation of Healthcare Organizations (Joint Commission) has had the status of an accreditation standard, meaning that a number of criteria must be satisfied for the hospital to receive accreditation.

The health departments of some of the states also require continuing education (as well as new-employee orientation) in a number of topics. In 1985, for example, the New York State Department of Health issued regulations to the effect that "Hospital policies must require that all staff receive orientation training and annual in-service training in the following areas."[2(p.5)] A list of seven topic areas followed in which education of all employees was required. Among the topics were the patients' bill of rights, the hospital's incident reporting program, and the safety practices of both the hospital at large and its specific departments.

Just as the Joint Commission has long applied standards to nursing in-service education, many state governments have long applied regulatory requirements to nursing in-service education by way of individual state hospital codes. With the regulatory requirements of various governmental bodies increasing steadily, more legally mandated continuing education is certain during the coming several years.

Thus some continuing education takes place—and grudgingly, at that—simply because it is required. However, much essential education—and specifically the education of supervisors and managers and the cross-training of employees—remains voluntary. It must therefore be accomplished through desire and commitment.

## COMMITMENT

Education receives a great deal of verbal tribute in our organizations; not many managers will deny the supposed value of continuing education for working people. In practice, however, education in the work organization is often little more than a bit of surface motion that produces little or no behavioral change.

It is true that education presents some problems in the functioning health care organization. There are numerous activities of necessarily higher priority than education. It remains something that "we ought to do when we have time," but because it is eminently postponable it is usually put off until "after the current crunch is over." Also, some forms of continuing education require noticeable added cost, and many in health care know that money is a fundamental resource that is often in short supply. It is natural that various activities are seen as competing for available funds; it is just as natural that limited funds are channeled toward points of urgent need—uses possessing the potential for generating readily measurable returns.

Quite often—we might even say too often—continuing education loses out in direct competition for management's time and the organization's resources. There is certainly not a sense of immediate need for most proposed education endeavors, nor is the return on an investment in education necessarily immediate or measurable in any direct sense.

Much continuing education is undertaken without a great deal of out-of-pocket spending, so the principal avenues of commitment become time and effort. However, it becomes difficult for you as an individual supervisor to devote sufficient time and effort to education if such a posture is not encouraged by higher management.

Regardless of the resources going into a program of education (the time you have available to apply and the materials and assistance at your disposal) there is one critical element without which no educational undertaking can long succeed, an element that cannot be mandated. This is the personal and organizational commitment to continuing education as a necessary and desirable activity. This commitment must be present and visible at a level and scope sufficient to support the training effort. That is, management training for department heads must have the support of administration; supervisory development for nursing supervisors must have the support of the director of nursing service; skill training for housekeeping workers must have the support of the housekeeping supervisor; and so on. Some measure of commitment is behind every successful education endeavor, whether personal, departmental, or organizational.

## MANY OPTIONS

Approaches to continuing education can range from the formal and highly structured to the informal and almost totally unstructured. Continuing education need not always be a structured program of formal classes on specific topics. It may indeed be this, but it may also be, for example:

- a simple demonstration of manual skills or work methods for a small group of employees, or perhaps one-on-one for a single employee
- employee orientation and guided on-the-job training in which an employee learns while doing
- self-study, perhaps job-related reading, correspondence courses, or outside classes

Thoughts of continuing education tend to inspire visions of classes, teachers, and classrooms; indeed much of continuing education is approached in schoolroom fashion. Such programs and classes, however, can vary considerably in type according to their purposes.

### Informational Programs

Informational programs are intended to implant specific information for later recall and application. This is "going to school" in the fundamental sense, with students receiving information that they will be expected to absorb as received, recall when necessary, and apply as appropriate in the future.

Informational programs are subject to evaluation by direct testing or examination. You are familiar with the pattern: you attend classes and participate in a number of assignments, following which you deal with a number of questions designed to test your recall of the information you received.

### Skill Programs

Skill programs are intended to impart specific skills: perhaps how to operate a computer, how to start an intravenous drip, how to abstract a patient record, or how to clean a patient room. To some extent, the results of skill programs can also be measured by test or examination, especially if these require the learner to demonstrate the skill.

**Concept Programs**

This type of program deals with concepts and concept-based patterns of behavior that, when translated into action and refined through application in specific situations, result in the development of "skills" of a sort. Most management education falls under this heading. Although we frequently speak of skills, as in "supervisory skills development program," we are really dealing with something much more fundamental. Consider as an example one topic drawn from the manager's bag of skills: delegation. You may sit through a class or a series of classes on delegation and learn about the concept of delegation. You may also consider cases and exercises in delegation, reinforcing your knowledge of the concept, but the program does not allow you to benefit from real-world applications. The applications, when you get to them, usually vary to some extent from the class examples and from each other so that each situation itself becomes a learning process in which you must continually adjust the elements of the concept to suit reality. If you do this successfully a sufficient number of times, then you will have incorporated the delegation concept into your pattern of behavior. Thus you will have absorbed a concept in the classroom, carried it onto the job and put it into practice in a number of situations, and developed the hazily defined skill called delegation.

The problem with most concept programs, and thus with most management, supervisory, or leadership programs, is that they are treated by many learners and teachers alike as informational programs. As a result, concepts are absorbed but are not applied. Many supervisors can tell you about proper delegation, but not nearly as many practice delegation wisely and well.

For a concept program you can test for retained knowledge as you would with an informational program. However, the true success of a concept program depends largely on changes in behavior and attitude.

## YOUR EMPLOYEES

Regardless of how small the group you supervise may be, you will often find it difficult to meet all the educational needs of all your employees. Thus continuing education becomes an ongoing job—with the focus truly on continuing—made necessary by promotions, transfers, and replacements. Unless all your employees do precisely the same things, which is a condition encountered by very few supervisors, any of the foregoing actions can create gaps in the capability of your work group. Even if your group remains stable in terms of personnel transactions, there are always gaps created by illness, vacation, and other time off.

A recommended objective for continuing education in any employee group is the achievement of the maximum possible amount of cross-training among employees working at comparable skill levels. For example, put yourself in the position of a supervisor in health information management who has three clerical employees assigned to three distinctly separate functions. Although all three may be classified as record assistants or technicians, one is assigned to chart completion and assembly, another to filing and retrieval, and the third to correspondence and information requests. The absence of any one of these workers could mean the development of a disruptive backlog if no one else is able to step into that person's job for a day or two. However, if all three individuals were trained in all three functions, the two on the job could be shifted around to serve the greatest needs. If all three were present, similar positive action could be taken if one activity was backlogged but the other two were current.

Cross-training of employees is of value to the supervisor because of the versatility of coverage just described. It can also be of appreciable benefit to employees. Many employees welcome the opportunity to learn different tasks and undertake activities new to them, and enjoy breaking away from prolonged periods spent performing the same tasks. The stimulation and thus the motivation provided by task variety is often sufficient to encourage the supervisor to rotate employees through several different assignments at regular intervals. (Take care, however, to assure that cross-training and job rotation are limited to employees and jobs in the same general job classification or pay range.)

Your immediate goal in approaching continuing education with your employees is to impart knowledge or skill. However, your long-range goal should be to create a learning attitude among your employees. Not all employees can be encouraged along these lines, so the creation of a learning attitude remains an ever-present goal that is never completely fulfilled. However, you will know that this goal is being served when some of your employees begin to seek out additional knowledge on their own, without further supervisory urging.

## Getting Started

Because this discussion is no more than an overview, the initial suggestion offered for pursuing continuing education in your department is to obtain a comprehensive book on the subject and screen it for information.

The second suggestion is to look around your institution for advice and assistance from other managers who are already involved in continuing education. If your institution is large enough or sufficiently committed to continuing education, you may have an education department or staff development department. Lacking these, you are at least likely to find an in-service education function in the nursing department. The extent and effectiveness of nursing in-service education are fully as sensitive to commitment as are other departments' programs, but in nursing the function will exist because, as mentioned earlier in this chapter, nursing in-service education has long been required by the standards of the Joint Commission and by most state hospital codes. The director of in-service education can help with program structure and general approach; more likely, however, the in-service director can provide plenty of advice, information, and assistance to another supervisor preparing to begin a continuing education program.

Before launching any program of education, however, examine the apparent needs of the work group and select some potentially fruitful starting points. In other words, it is best to begin with some form of learning-needs analysis.

## Determining Needs

A portion of a skills inventory matrix created for the employees in a food service department is shown in Exhibit 26–1. All of the employees in the food service aide job classification are listed in the column on the left side of the form. The remaining columns contain the supervisor's assessment of each employee's capabilities in the jobs identified at the top of each column. Note the simplicity of the breakdown. A number 1 indicates that the employee needs complete training in this activity; a number 2 designates the need for some degree of refresher training; and a number 3 indicates that the employee now performs that particular job satisfactorily. Do not be misled by the simplicity of the matrix. To be sure, each number is a judgment call on your part. In creating the matrix, especially in determining the 2s and 3s, because a 1 is automatically indicated for an employee who has not done a particular job, it is necessary for you to speak with each employee and observe each at work. When you have completed such an exercise you will have a fairly good idea of where to focus your early training efforts.

Another form of the skills inventory, a variation applicable to the assessment of the learning needs of all employees' capabilities relative to all jobs in the department, is shown in Exhibit 26–2. For each employee and each job you are really asking two questions: (1) Is training on this job applicable to this employee? and (2) Can this employee, working under normal supervision and direction, perform this job satisfactorily?

A not applicable answer may be called for because a job is totally unrelated to an employee's general line of work or is of a different labor grade or pay classification. Be careful, however, of how freely you apply the "N/A" indicator;

---

**Exhibit 26–1** Skills Inventory: Food Service Aides

| Employees | Tray Preassembly | Tray Line | Transport | Clean Up |
|---|---|---|---|---|
| P. Abel | 2 | 3 | 3 | 3 |
| C. Brown | 3 | 3 | 1 | 2 |
| N. Carter | 1 | 1 | 3 | 3 |
| J. Davis | 3 | 3 | 1 | 2 |
| D. Evans | 2 | 1 | 3 | 3 |

> 1. Needs complete training
> 2. Needs refresher
> 3. Satisfactory

**Exhibit 26–2** Skills Inventory: Medical Records Department

| Employees | Transcription | Information Request | Completion Review | Assembly and Analysis |
|---|---|---|---|---|
| R. Baker | Yes | No | Yes | Yes |
| P. Fredericks | N/A | Yes | Yes | No |
| M. George | Yes | Yes | Yes | Yes |
| N. Lori | N/A | No | No | Yes |
| D. Quincy | N/A | No | Yes | No |

Yes—Fully qualified
No—Training (or refresher) required
N/A—Not applicable to pay grade

it may be advantageous to both you and the employee to consider training in completely different areas of activity as long as the jobs are consistent in classification and pay grade.

For the major question regarding the employee's capability of performing the job with normal supervision and direction, your task, again accomplished through individual observation and judgment, is simply to answer yes or no. All of your no answers indicate potentially productive starting points for staff education.

## The Supervisor as a Teacher

You will likely do some, although not all, of the teaching in a continuing education program for your department. For some of the topics and skills you must deal with you will be the most qualified, most readily available instructor, but chances are that at least a few topics will be better handled by others. For instance, if you are the manager the health information management department and you are interested in cross-training several record assistants in chart completion review, it might be wise to use the employee who is regularly assigned to this task as an instructor. With proper encouragement and assistance, the person who best knows how to perform the details of a given task can become the best possible resource for teaching that task to others. You should not presume to do all the teaching all the time. However, your department's continuing education program will remain your responsibility, and you will be fulfilling part of this responsibility by helping others develop as instructors.

Teaching a class can loom as a formidable task to a newcomer. If the idea of teaching a small class of employees frightens you, you can rest assured that you are not alone in that feeling: just about everyone involved in teaching or public speaking has experienced similar qualms. It helps to regard your early ventures into teaching as learning experiences in themselves, remembering also that you are not a professional teacher, that your employees are familiar to you and not a group of unknown students, and that instruction in this environment is best accomplished in an informal, friendly atmosphere.

The keys to building your effectiveness as an instructor are preparation and practice. As long as you are reasonably comfortable with your knowledge of the subject and take care to organize your material for logical presentation, you can overcome your apprehensions about teaching. The more you teach a given subject, the better you will be able to teach it in the future. The more often you face a class of learners, the less bothersome your uneasiness about teaching will become.

## The Process

Speaking now primarily of the process of imparting skill or knowledge to nonsupervisory employees, in teaching you should be trying to do the following for your trainees:

- Motivate them. Attempt to reach them with reasons why they should want to learn. Let them know what is in it for them—new skills; something interesting for its own sake; or an opportunity for more interesting, challenging, or varied work. Let them know what they stand to gain, and what the department stands to gain by taking advantage of what is to follow.
- Tell and demonstrate. Present your subject in logical order, and when teaching skill-related topics (for instance, how a particular task is performed) actually show them how it is done.
- Check for their understanding. Ask for questions and discussion and generally encourage feedback. If you can hear what you have been saying coming back to you to your satisfaction in someone else's words, chances are you are moving along lines of effective communication.
- Let them try it. Again related primarily to skill training, having told them how it is done, shown them how to do it, and received reasonable assurance that they understand, have them actually perform the task. Encourage feedback and work with them until they are able to perform the task to your satisfaction.

## Some Points to Remember

We have already mentioned the importance of preparation. However, preparation is only a part of what is necessary to get your message across. The balance of the task lies in dynamic instruction. Entertaining instruction can at least partially salvage thin material, but dry, lackluster presentation can render the best-prepared material useless. Consider the following presentation approaches:

- Combine your instructional methods whenever possible. Telling, showing, or doing alone is not nearly as effective as combining approaches (for instance, telling and showing, or ideally, telling, showing, and doing).
- Use multiple modes of presentation. Avoid reliance on pure lecture, 100 percent transparencies, complete tape-recorded presentations, or the predominant use of any other single medium of presentation. Mix up your media, perhaps lecturing for a while, supporting your comments with transparencies, showing a brief film now and then, or using short segments of tape-recorded material. Also, use interactive techniques whenever possible—discussion, exercises, case studies, and in general anything that will draw your employees into the learning process.
- Always be aware that your learners are workers, not students. You are meeting with them in the middle of or perhaps after a regular workday, and chances are they have not come to your class fresh and relaxed. Never forget that they are full-time workers who probably have job problems on their minds.
- Accept the high likelihood that you will rarely reach everyone in every way. People are different; some are receptive to new information and new skills and some are not. But you must always try. Failure to reach everyone is not necessarily an indication of a teacher's shortcomings, but failure to try to do so is such an indication.
- Remember that for the instructor the process of teaching is itself a valuable form of learning. Most supervisors who have done some teaching have discovered that there is no better way to expand one's knowledge of a subject than to teach that subject.

## AN URGENT AND EXPANDING NEED

Continuing education in health care organizations has become increasingly important in recent years, and this trend promises to continue for quite some time. The primary driver of this need is change.

One might be tempted to suggest that change has always been with us and that learning and relearning and adapting have always been necessary. This is entirely true. However, the difference creating the present urgency is the rapidity of change. Change has always been present in our working circumstances, but in this era of health care mergers and acquisitions, of hospital closings, of reengineering, and of the creation of new forms of health care delivery, rapid change is altering roles at such a pace that employees at all levels are hard put to keep up.

### Supervisory Education

In particular circumstances like major reengineering and especially following a reduction-in-force (RIF), the organization needs to provide assistance to supervisors who may find their scope of responsibility increased. Subsequent management education should include two types of programs:

1. An orientation for new supervisors, both for those new to management within the organization as well as those entering management for the first time. This program may also serve as a refresher in basics for those for whom a need is expressed or indicated.

2. Management development programs, with either individual classes or multisession offerings as appropriate, addressing a number of important "how-to" subjects. Possible "how-to" programs are listed in Exhibit 26–3.

An area of constant emphasis in supervisory and management training, running through most of the programs presented for these people, should be the importance of the individual supervisor being visible and available to staff, constantly reinforcing the supervisor's key role in each employee's relationship with the organization.

## Employee Education and Training

Individual department orientation and on-the-job training that have long been facts of organizational life should continue in full force following a staff reduction. In addition, a number of practices involving education and training

---

**Exhibit 26–3** Management Development: Possible "How-To" Programs

HOW TO
- improve personal effectiveness as a supervisor
- delegate work and appropriately empower staff
- utilize corrective processes in dealing with problems of employee performance and conduct
- enhance employees' ability to adapt to the demands and requirements of a changing environment (largely motivational concerns)
- deal with certain employee issues that arise from time to time (problem employees as well as employee problems)
- maintain effective communications, upward, downward, and laterally
- conduct interviews and make the best possible legal employee selection decisions when necessary
- effectively manage day to day in spite of an ever-expanding body of law affecting the employment relationship
- develop and work with a departmental budget and effectively control costs at the department level
- protect your employees' and your organization's best interests during union organizing
- make effective decisions in a realistic manner
- organize, develop, and run effective employee teams—while keeping them legal
- enhance productivity at the department level
- guide employees through change
- effectively manage time
- make the transition from traditional management to effective leadership
- write effective letters and memos
- organize and conduct productive meetings
- develop and deliver effective presentations

should be considered for their potential to assist the reinvigoration of the remaining work force.

With appropriate orientation and on-the-job training, some employees who might have been offered transfer as an alternative to layoff may be allowed a normal probationary period during which to attain standard performance (assuming the presence of the basic qualifications for the job). An employee who is offered a transfer should be strongly urged to accept the new assignment as it will likely be the sole alternative to layoff.

A program of cross-training should be undertaken between, among, and within certain departments as appropriate. Each cross-trained employee will enhance the work force's flexibility as well as increase the individual's potential value through improved flexibility and versatility.

Programs should be planned and developed for the education of multiskill specialists, those usually technical employees who are qualified to work in more than one area (e.g., a phlebotomist who is also a specimen processor, a licensed practical nurse who is also an electrocardiogram technician, or a secretary/receptionist who is also a medical office assistant). Multiskill specialists enhance their own potential job security while providing greater flexibility to the organization.

Enhanced tuition assistance benefits should be considered for employees who wish to advance themselves by pursuing education in occupations for which the organization has identified current and projected needs.

The organization might also make available remedial education in certain basic skills (e.g., reading and basic mathematics) to assist employees who have otherwise demonstrated the capacity to seek advancement through self-improvement.

Whenever possible, the organization should pursue a policy of promotion from within, providing all reasonable assistance and preparation for employees who wish to advance themselves.

## The Cross-Training Exercise

The activity posed in the "Situation" at the beginning of the chapter called on the reader to plan for the development of a program of cross-training. Some who perform this exercise will be working supervisors who can refer to their own departments and develop actual cross-training programs. The majority who peruse these pages will not presently supervise others, however. Therefore, to keep all participants in this exercise on an equal footing, an actual plan need not be provided; rather, participants should demonstrate an understanding of what needs to be done to accomplish cross-training.

The cross-training plan should include the following:

- identification of all of the jobs to be involved in the actual cross-training, and assurance that these jobs are all in the same labor grade or on equivalent pay scales
- identification of the employees to be involved, with assurance that they are all past the learning period and thus fully familiar with what is presently their own positions

- knowledge that the job descriptions of all involved positions are current and complete
- consideration of who will do the actual training (Hint: Utilize well-performing employees to the fullest extent possible in training each other)
- consideration of how long the training should require and what, if any, special training aids or processes may be required
- a decision concerning how training results will be measured; that is, how to recognize when an employee is ready to proceed on the job unaided
- identification of the motivational aspects of cross-training, so that employees may be "sold" on it as necessary

As with any other activity in which you ask employees to take on different tasks and vary their routines, most employees react more positively if they first understand why the change is being made and then have the opportunity to be involved (as in training each other as noted above). Certainly the department has increased flexibility when people are cross-trained; scheduling is facilitated, and covering for illnesses and vacations is much easier because each person can do more than one job. But advantages accrue to employees as well, because cross-training gives employees the following benefits:

- variety in work, because employees can count on rotating through different jobs
- challenge in the job, because there is more to learn and retain
- greater interest in the job overall
- growth that can make an employee more valuable for future consideration
- versatility that could conceivably protect one's employment when layoff decisions are made

Is cross-training for everyone? Probably not; some employees who have performed the same duties for a prolonged period may not wish to change their ways. If that is the case, it is probably best to "go around" such an employee and cross-train all who are willing. However, it could be to the department's benefit once it implements cross-training to henceforth recruit and fill the involved positions on the condition that the job requires rotating through these two, three, or four assignments on a regular basis.

## CONTINUING EDUCATION AND YOU

Formal continuing education programs for the supervisor often deal with matters of supervisory skill or management practice—usually the "concept programs" discussed earlier. Because of the inability to include practical applications in this kind of program, because even the best prepared exercise or case problem is at best only a model of reality, concept programs deal primarily with ideas and theories. As many people in management are constantly discovering, the gap between theory and practice can be broad and deep. The principal shortcoming of most management programs lies in their failure to provide any substantial means of bridging the gap between theory and practice; many managers learn things that they may retain in an information sense but never take the steps necessary to incorporate changes based on this information into their patterns of behavior.

Your opportunity to attend management programs usually comes about because administration, human resources, or staff development has made such training available. You may occasionally be given the option of attending such a program; this is the preferred method of obtaining your attendance. However, you may sometimes find you are asked to attend in such a way that you clearly cannot refuse without prejudice. Or you may simply be ordered to attend. Even if you feel your attendance is mandated or forced, however, do not allow this to influence you negatively toward the program.

Take advantage of the opportunity to attend supervisory and management programs whenever possible. You may feel inclined to bypass such opportunities because you are too busy, but if you approach management training with an open and receptive attitude you are practically guaranteed to come away with something that will help you do a better job.

Again, because of the concept-based nature of management education, management programs, at least many of the better ones, are oriented more toward attitude change than toward imparting specific skills. Because of this, a great deal of self-starting is required on your part if you are to get the maximum benefit from such education. Even the best of programs leave it largely up to you to translate what you learn in the classroom into action on the job.

Aside from management and supervisory programs provided by your organization, your continuing education can also include the following:

- books, journals, and professional bulletins and newsletters and other publications
- courses available outside of the institution, such as professional seminars, and workshops and management programs at local colleges
- audio- and videotape programs made available for individual self-study
- correspondence courses and conferences, seminars, and workshops made available by various professional organizations

The key difference between continuing education for you and continuing education for your employees lies in the matter of who makes such education available. It is up to you to make continuing education available to your employees. However, do not assume that it is up to your superiors to make continuing education available to you. Your institution, if prompted by you and other supervisors, may make an occasional management program available. However, your access to most other forms of supervisor-oriented continuing education is largely controlled by you. In the last analysis, the most lasting and effective form of continuing education is self-education.

## YOUR KEY ROLE

Briefly recalling the matter of commitment discussed in the early part of this chapter, it is your personal commitment to continuing education that will most influence how you and your employees develop educationally. If your commitment is verbal only—if, for instance, you simply launch a continuing education program for your employees and then back away—your employees are likely to follow your lead and participate only superficially. Your employees will take their cues from you. If they see you as truly "into education" they are much more likely to take your program seriously.

Continuing education for both you and your employees is one of your responsibilities as a supervisor. It is not unreasonable that you may be expected to stimulate and guide your employees' continuing education while actively pursuing your own.

## REVIEW QUESTIONS

1. Describe in a few words each, two examples of *skill programs*.
2. What is the essential difference between a *skill program* and a *concept program*?
3. What effects do reengineering, reduction in force, and other dramatic organizational changes have on continuing education?
4. Describe the benefits of cross training, placing them in what you believe to be their primary order of importance in most departments.
5. Provide two examples of multiskill specialists, with only one of these examples coming from the text.

## EXERCISE: THE SKILLS INVENTORY

Using the approach of either Exhibit 26–1 or Exhibit 26–2, prepare a preliminary skills inventory for your department or a portion of your department.

The technique of Exhibit 26–2 is adequate for a smaller department, for example, fewer than 10 employees and not more than 10 or 12 major tasks. If you supervise a larger department, concentrate on a single job classification or labor grade and apply the technique of Exhibit 26–1.

Do not simply render all judgments off the top of your head; when you have doubts concerning a person's ability to perform a certain task, spend a few minutes with the employee and ask some pertinent questions.

Use your skills inventory to develop a listing of learning needs for your employees: who must be trained in certain tasks and who could be of greater benefit to the department (by providing greater flexibility, improved task coverage, for example) by being trained in additional tasks?

**NOTES**

1. Joint Commission on Accreditation of Healthcare Organizations, *Hospital Accreditation Standards* (Oakbrook Terrace, Ill.: Joint Commission, 2001).
2. State of New York Department of Health Memorandum, Health Facility Series H-6, January 16, 1986.

## CHAPTER 27

# The Supervisor and the Law

*Laws should be like clothes. They should be made to fit the people they are meant to serve.*
—*Clarence Darrow*

## CHAPTER OBJECTIVES

☛ Provide a review of pertinent areas of legislation with which the supervisor should be generally familiar, with emphasis on the National Labor Relations Act, wage and hour laws, and laws dealing with affirmative action and equal employment opportunity.

## SITUATION: WHAT KIND OF EMPLOYEE?

Relatively new to department management within a health care organization, you have heard the terms *exempt employee* and *nonexempt employee* used with some regularity. Only recently your organization reissued its employee handbook to include two sections of supposed wage-and-hour rules identified only by the headings Exempt Employees and Nonexempt Employees. The handbook provides no defining distinction between the two, and as a result you find you have been the target of numerous clarification requests from your employees. Beyond a simple definition, a number of your employees are asking you, "Just what does this exempt and nonexempt stuff mean, anyway?"

In preparation for a staff meeting at which you will be expected to address this issue with your employees, review all of the apparent advantages and disadvantages of being classed as an exempt employee or a nonexempt employee. This should include knowing the difference between those employees who must, under law, be treated as nonexempt and those employees who, although they might qualify as exempt, may be treated as nonexempt for payroll purposes at the organization's option.

*Instructions*

In proceeding through this chapter, be aware of your need to be knowledgeable of the risks of incorrectly classifying employees and of treating the same employees as exempt or nonexempt at different times.

## LEGAL GUIDES FOR SUPERVISORY BEHAVIOR

This chapter will cover some major areas of legislation that place requirements on our organizations and thus influence supervisory behavior. In particular we will discuss the following topics:

- The National Labor Relations Act, highlighting its applicability to health institutions. Comments will be limited to appropriate highlights of the act; the supervisor's role in dealing with union organizers and labor organizations will be discussed in Chapter 29.

- Wage and hour laws, for the benefit of the supervisor's familiarity in dealing with rates of pay, hours of work, and related matters.
- Affirmative action and equal employment opportunity, encompassing consideration of several laws that proscribe organizational behavior in regard to interviewing (see Chapter 8), hiring, and making certain work assignments.

It is not intended that you read a small amount about law and undertake to decide legal issues for yourself. Rather, this material is meant to increase your awareness of some of the things you should or should not do as a supervisor because of the existence of various forms of legislation. When a true legal question arises, seek the answer through administration, through human resources, or through in-house legal counsel if this function is available in your organization.

## THE NATIONAL LABOR RELATIONS ACT

The National Labor Relations Act (NLRA) of 1935, known as the Wagner Act, provided the basis for most labor law in the United States. The way was paved for the 1935 Wagner Act by the lesser-known Norris-LaGuardia Act passed in 1932. The Norris-LaGuardia Act marked a significant change in public policy from suppression of union activity to significant encouragement of such activity. However, it did little to restrain employers in their conduct toward collective bargaining.

The NLRA was amended significantly in 1947 by the Labor Management Relations Act, known otherwise as Taft-Hartley. It is Taft-Hartley to which we are primarily referring when speaking of aspects of union organizing. One can find numerous references to the NLRA that are actually references to this law as amended by Taft-Hartley. The Taft-Hartley Act provides the framework for modern labor law.

Prior to 1975, not-for-profit hospitals were exempt from all provisions of Taft-Hartley. In 1975, the act was amended to remove the not-for-profit hospital exemption; before that time, hospital employees were covered only in special subsections of the labor relations laws of various states. The Taft-Hartley amendments were passed over the objections of numerous hospitals and the organized opposition of the American Hospital Association. Generally, hospitals wanted to see the inclusion of a mandated "cooling off" period after the expiration of a contract and before a strike could occur; however, what they received was mandated fact-finding prior to the end of contract negotiations.

Employees of public hospitals, those institutions operated by cities, counties, and other arms of government, continue to be exempt from Taft-Hartley.

Contrary to the misgivings of many, coverage of not-for-profit hospitals under the act did not mean automatic unionization. It does not make unionization inevitable, provided the individual hospital has or institutes "thoughtfully conceived personnel programs, realistic and attractive compensation policies, and provided there are first-line supervisors who are well trained in supervisory and employee relations skills."

### The 1975 Amendments

The Taft-Hartley amendments affecting not-for-profit hospitals are summarized as follows:

- As stated above, these amendments remove the exemption of not-for-profit hospitals from the act. This specific exemption had been in effect since 1947.
- The term health care institution is broadly defined to include "any hospital, convalescent hospital, health maintenance organization, health clinic, nursing home, extended care facility, or other institution devoted to the care of sick, infirm, or aged people."
- The legal notification period for negotiations on collective bargaining contracts is set at 90 days. That is, a 90-day notice by either the employer or labor organization is required for renewals or modifications of contracts, rather than the 60-day notice required for all other industries covered by the act.
- The Federal Mediation and Conciliation Service must be notified 60 days prior to the termination or expiration of an existing contract, as opposed to the 30-day notification required for other industries covered under the act.
- The labor organization will be required to participate in the mediation process in both renewal and initial contract situations. No such requirement exists for other industries covered by the act. (This requirement is not to be taken as suggesting compulsory arbitration in any form.)
- Written notice must be provided by the labor organization to the health care institution and the Federal Mediation and Conciliation Service 10 days prior to engaging in any picketing, strike, or other concerted refusal to work. There are no strike or picketing notice provisions in the act for other industries.
- Prior to the expiration of the notification periods on renewal and initial contracts, and at the discretion of the director of the Federal Mediation and Conciliation Service, an impartial board of inquiry could be established to investigate any labor-management dispute and make a written report of its findings of fact. This process is applied only when the Federal Mediation and Conciliation Service judges that an actual or threatened work stoppage could substantially interrupt the delivery of health care to the community involved. Again, there is no such provision for other industries covered under the act.
- An employee of the health care institution who is a member of a recognized religion, body, or sect that has historically held conscientious objections to participation in or support of labor organizations will not be required to join or support financially such an organization as a condition of employment. This position applies to health care institutions only as defined within the act.

- The 1975 amendments preempt all state labor laws previously applicable to nongovernmental hospitals. Also, the amendments apply to health care institutions previously covered by the act (such as proprietary hospitals and nursing homes) as well as to all those institutions brought under federal law by the amendments to the act.

### Congressional Intent

The congressional intent of the amendments is summarized as follows:

- Congress wished to avoid fragmentation of bargaining units in health care institutions, with numerous small units working with and bargaining with the same institution.
- Congress wished to establish special priority attention in handling by the National Labor Relations Board of cases involving unfair labor practice charges and labor-management disputes in health care institutions.
- Congress intended that it be possible to transfer patients from a struck or threatened institution to another institution and obtain limited assistance from another institution without risking secondary strikes or boycotts against the assisting institution.
- Congress wished to reaffirm existing National Labor Relations Board definitions of supervisors among professional employees in health care institutions.

### Fragmentation of Bargaining Units

A major point in the congressional intent of the 1975 amendments was the wish to avoid fragmentation of bargaining units in health care institutions. However, in spite of this wish, in the late 1980s the National Labor Relations Board (NLRB) moved decidedly in the direction of proliferation of bargaining units.

In mid-1988 the NLRB issued proposed new rules for determining bargaining unit boundaries in hospitals. To be applied in nongovernmental acute-care hospitals (nursing homes and psychiatric hospitals excluded), these rules would leave hospitals very limited flexibility with which to challenge proposed units.

During late 1988 and throughout 1989 and beyond, the proposed rules underwent some modest modifications but continued to call for a multiplicity of bargaining units. The proposed rules were vigorously opposed by the American Hospital Association and other interests. The rulemaking authority of the NLRB came under legal challenge, culminating in an April 1991 decision by the United States Supreme Court favoring the NLRB.

The decision of April 1991 officially established eight separate bargaining units as appropriate in acute-care hospitals:

1. registered nurses
2. physicians
3. all other professionals

4. technical employees
5. skilled maintenance employees
6. business office clericals
7. security guards
8. all other nonprofessionals (service, etc.)

Previously units were determined on a case-by-case basis, and a hospital, especially one of less than 100 beds, stood a good chance of having to deal with only two or three unions at most. Present rules, however, mean that a hospital of any size could conceivably have to deal with eight or more separate unions. Concerning bargaining unit proliferation the NLRB has gone far afield from the congressional intent of the 1975 amendments.

Although petitions filed for NLRB-supervised elections increased in the months following the Supreme Court ruling, there was not the flood of petitions that some had predicted. The groups that were initially most affected of the eight designated units were registered nurses, all other professionals, and skilled maintenance employees.[1] This came as no surprise. The previous long-standing combination of nurses and other professionals had inhibited organizers for a number of years; for example, the individual state units of the American Nurses Association sought units of professional nurses only. And the skilled trades have long been associated with union membership; in separating them from all others, the NLRB essentially encouraged them to organize. In past years when bargaining unit determinations were made on a case-by-case basis, skilled maintenance employees had been grouped with the larger body of service employees.

## WAGE AND HOUR LAWS

Of primary interest is the 1938 Fair Labor Standards Act (FLSA), which is the federal wage and hour law and as such the model for the wage and hour laws of many states. Occasional points that might not be covered by federal law may be covered by pertinent state laws. Generally, if the same points are covered by both state and federal laws but differences exist between the two, the more stringent legislation will apply.

### Exempt Employees

Prior to 1967, hospitals were exempt from the minimum wage and overtime requirements of the Fair Labor Standards Act. Since the amendments of 1967, however, minimum wage and overtime requirements have applied equally in hospitals as in other industries. Three types of employees remain exempt and are identified as follows:

1. *Executives.* An executive employee must generally spend 50 percent or more of the time in direct management of an enterprise or an organizational subunit such as a department. In addition, an executive employee must direct the activities of two or more persons. The executive definition may also require that a person possess the authority to hire and fire

or so recommend; possess discretionary powers rather than being assigned largely routine work; and from work week to work week spend no more than 40 percent of the time on nonmanagerial work.

2. *Administrative.* An administrative employee must spend 50 percent or more of the time on office or nonmanual work related in some way to policy, general business, patient care, or people in general and must be required to exercise discretion and independent judgment. Other tests of the administrative classification may be assisting executive or administrative personnel; handling special assignments with only general supervision; working in a position requiring special training, experience, or knowledge; and spending not more than 40 percent of the time on nonadministrative work.

3. *Professional.* Professionals in health care institutions (e.g., chemists, registered nurses, pharmacists, physicians) are so classified by virtue of spending 50 percent or more of the time in work that requires advanced specialized knowledge or is original or creative in nature. The definition may also require that the professional be consistently required to exercise discretion and independent judgment, be employed at intellectual and varied work, and be engaged in nonprofessional activities not more than 20 percent of the time.

The FLSA specifies the minimum salary that executive, administrative, and professional personnel must be paid. The single exception applies to licensed medical practitioners and interns and residents; they are subject to no minimum salary requirements.

Arguments based on the applicability of a particular nonexempt definition are generally decided on the basis of the percentage of time spent on various activities. The time test applies on a workweek to workweek basis.

## Nonexempt Employees

All employees who do not fall under the executive, administrative, or professional category are considered nonexempt employees. They must be paid at least the prevailing legal minimum wage for each hour worked in a workweek, and they must be paid at a rate of one and one-half times the regular rate for all overtime hours. In addition, they must be given equal pay for equal work unless there are legitimate factors that justify the establishment of different rates. (Sex is not a legitimate factor.) The organization is required to keep detailed records of hours worked and wages paid.

There are a few well-defined exceptions to the payment of the legal minimum wage. Special regulations allow the payment of lower rates to students, learners, and apprentices. Employment of such persons is also subject to additional requirements and restrictions.

## What Kind of Employee?

In reference to the "Situation" presented at the beginning of the chapter, exempt and nonexempt are common organizational terms that are used essentially synonymously with salaried (exempt) and hourly (nonexempt). In simplest possible terms, "exempt" means exempt from the overtime provisions of the FLSA. A nonexempt employee must be paid overtime for hours worked in excess of 40 in a week; an exempt employee need not be paid overtime.

The preceding section concerning exempt employees describes, in summary fashion, the conditions that must be satisfied in order to designate a particular position exempt. Any position that meets the requirements for classification as executive, administrative, or professional may be designated exempt, and all positions not qualifying under these requirements must be designated nonexempt. Being nonexempt is advantageous to the employee because overtime must be paid for all hours in excess of 40 in a week. Being exempt may be seen by some as advantageous to the employee because of the associated rate of pay and flexibility of hours. It is advantageous to the employer because of stability of labor cost and the ability to get additional work accomplished (beyond 40 hours in a week) without additional payment.

It is important to recognize the difference between the uses of *may* and *must* in the preceding paragraph. The law clearly states that any position that does not meet the exempt criteria must be considered nonexempt and be paid overtime. However, a position that meets the exempt criteria is not legally required to be treated as exempt. It is true that many such positions are classified and treated as exempt; consider, for example, health care administrators; department heads; and others such as accountants, engineers, and the like. It is equally true that some positions that qualify as exempt are treated as nonexempt in that overtime is paid; for example, most registered nurse positions qualify as exempt under the professional criteria, yet they are ordinarily paid overtime for extra hours and extra shifts.

There is some risk in incorrectly classifying employees as exempt when they should in fact be nonexempt. In some organizations certain positions have been treated as exempt simply because they were compensated at or above the minimum exempt salary requirement. For example, a position as "secretary" might be retitled "administrative assistant" and made an exempt "administrative" position simply because of satisfying the salary requirement. However, because the position may not involve a sufficient percentage of true administrative work it may, upon audit by the Labor Department, be ruled nonexempt. If this occurs, the organization will be called on to pay imputed overtime costs for positions incorrectly classified. For a position to be treated as exempt, it must meet the requirement for work content as well as for salary.

## Overtime Compensation

### The Workweek

The FLSA defines the workweek as a fixed, recurring period of 168 hours; that is, seven consecutive 24-hour periods. These 24-hour periods need not be calendar days, and the seven periods together need not be a calendar week. For instance, work weeks beginning and ending at midnight Friday or midnight Sunday are not uncommon. The workweek may be changed, and many organizations have done so to facilitate payroll accounting, but it cannot be changed in such a way as to avoid payment of overtime.

*Time and One-Half*

The FLSA requires payment of one-and-one-half times a worker's regular rate for all overtime hours. Overtime hours are defined as those hours in excess of

- 40 hours in a 7-day workweek, where the usual 7-day workweek is used
- 8 hours per day or 80 hours per 14-day period, when the use of the 14-day period has been approved and posted

The institution may use either or both methods for certain of its employees but may use only one method at a time for a specific employee group. If the so-called 8-and-80 provision is used, overtime must be paid for all hours worked in excess of 8 in each day or in excess of 80 in the 14-day period, whichever results in the greater number of overtime hours.

In the example appearing in Exhibit 27–1, the employee worked a total of 80 hours. The employee is owed 3 hours of overtime that is derived from the fourth day, when 10 hours were worked, and the eighth day when 9 hours were worked (although on one day the employee worked only 5 hours).

Next look at Exhibit 27–2. In this case the employee worked more than 8 hours on one or more days and more than 80 hours for the 14-day period. This example assumes that the employee worked 8 hours in each of nine days and 10 hours on the tenth day and thus is due 2 hours of overtime. Note that the employee has worked 2 hours in excess of both the 8 hours per day and 80 hours per work period provisions. However, this does not mean that the employee is owed overtime for 4 hours (based on 2 hours in excess of 8 and 2

---

**Exhibit 27–1** "8 and 80" Illustration 1

| Day | Hours |
|---|---|
| 1 | 8 |
| 2 | 8 |
| 3 | 5 |
| 4 | 10 |
| 5 | 8 |
| 6 | 0 |
| 7 | 0 |
| 8 | 9 |
| 9 | 8 |
| 10 | 8 |
| 11 | 8 |
| 12 | 8 |
| 13 | 0 |
| 14 | 0 |
| 14 days | 80 hours |

Overtime owed—3 hours (2 from day 4; 1 from day 8)

**Exhibit 27–2** "8 and 80" Illustration 2

| Day | Hours |
|:---:|:---:|
| 1 | 8 |
| 2 | 8 |
| 3 | 8 |
| 4 | 8 |
| 5 | 8 |
| 6 | 0 |
| 7 | 0 |
| 8 | 8 |
| 9 | 8 |
| 10 | 8 |
| 11 | 8 |
| 12 | 10 |
| 13 | 0 |
| 14 | 0 |
| 14 days | 82 hours |

Overtime owed—2 hours (from day 12)

hours in excess of 80). The employee is owed 2 hours of overtime pay. Hours are not double counted; rather, when the totals of daily overtime and over-80 differ it is the higher that must apply.

The FLSA also specifies that only hours actually worked need to be counted toward determining overtime. That is, the institution is not required to count nonworked time such as vacation days, sick leave, holidays, and personal time as part of the 80 hours.

*The "Regular Rate"*

The so-called regular rate referred to in the FLSA includes the scheduled hourly rate plus on-call pay, call-in pay, and shift differential. Exhibit 27–3 presents an example of the effects of these additions on the rate.

Assume the employee in the example is paid overtime under the 7-day, 40-hour workweek. The employee receives the following amounts: an hourly rate of $9.00, a flat rate of $15.00 for on-call time, $50.00 for 4 hours work on call-in, and 60 cents per hour shift differential. Assume the employee actually worked a total of 50 hours including the 4 hours of call-in time, and that shift differential was not used for the 4 hours of call-in time.

Because the employee worked a total of 50 hours, divide $506.60 by 50 to arrive at a "regular rate" of $10.132 per hour. Therefore, for the 10 hours of excess time the employee must be paid time and one-half this regular rate, or 10 hours at $15.198 per hour. Having already been paid the regular rate for each of the 50 hours, the employee is owed only the difference between that and $15.198 for the 10 excess hours, that is, $5.066 × 10 hours or $50.66. The total owed the employee in this example is $557.26.

**Exhibit 27–3** Illustration of "Regular Rate"

---

Overtime period: 7 days, 40 hours

Employee worked 50 hours, including 4 hours of call-in time

Rates paid:    Basic: $9.00/hour
                  Shift differential: $0.60/hour
                  Call-in: $50.00 (4 hours)
                  On-call: $15.00 (flat)

| Calculation: | | | |
|---|---|---|---|
| $9.00 3 46 hours | $\times$ | $414.00 |
| 0.60 3 46 hours | $\times$ | 27.60 |
| 50.00 call-in | $\times$ | 50.00 |
| 15.00 on-call | $\times$ | 15.00 |
| | | $506.60 |

$\dfrac{\$506.60}{50} \times \$10.132$/hour "regular rate"

$10.132 31/2 \times $5.066/hour overtime premium

| Basic Earnings (above) | $506.60 |
|---|---|
| Premium ($5.066 $\times$ 10 hours) | 50.66 |
| Total Earned | $557.26 |

---

Generally, hours spent at home "on call" are not counted as hours worked. This treatment depends on the employee's freedom of movement while on call. Pay received for such time, however, is counted in determining the regular rate. Note also, however, that when an employee who is "on call" is actually called to perform work, the hours actually worked are counted in the total hours worked. In determining whether on-call time must be counted as hours worked, the government will generally look to determine whether the employee must remain on the employer's premises or be sufficiently close that the time cannot be used as the individual chooses. If this is the case, the hours will be treated as working time for purposes of both minimum wage and overtime requirements.

**Equal Pay**

A section of the FLSA prohibits discrimination among employees on the basis of sex when the employees are doing equal work on jobs requiring equal skill, effort, and responsibility and performed under similar working conditions. In correcting unlawful differences in rates of pay, the act requires that the lower rate be increased; it is not permissible to decrease the higher rate. The act does make provision, however, for unequal pay if the inequality is directly attributable to a bona fide seniority system, merit system, incentive compensation system, or any other plan calling for a differential in pay based on any factor other than sex.

## AFFIRMATIVE ACTION AND EQUAL EMPLOYMENT OPPORTUNITY

### Title VII of the Civil Rights Act of 1964

As amended by the Equal Employment Opportunity Act of 1972, this legislation prohibits discrimination because of race, color, religion, sex, or national origin in any term, condition, or privilege of employment. The Equal Employment Opportunity Act of 1972 greatly strengthened the powers and expanded the jurisdiction of the Equal Employment Opportunity Commission (EEOC) in enforcement of this law.

Title VII was amended to cover:

- all private employers of 15 or more persons
- all educational institutions, public as well as private
- state and local governments
- public and private employment agencies
- labor unions with 15 or more members
- joint labor-management committees for apprenticeship and training

The EEOC investigates job discrimination complaints, and when it finds reasonable cause that the charges are justified, it attempts, through conciliation, to reach agreement by eliminating all aspects of discrimination revealed by the investigation. If conciliation fails, the 1972 amendments give the EEOC the power to go directly to court to enforce the law. Among other important provisions, the 1972 act also provides that discrimination charges may be filed by organizations on behalf of aggrieved individuals, as well as by employees and job applicants themselves. Applicants may also go to court directly to sue employers for alleged discrimination.

### The Equal Pay Act of 1963

The Equal Pay Act of 1963 requires all employers subject to the FLSA to provide equal pay for men and women performing similar work. In 1972, coverage of this act was extended beyond employees covered by FLSA to an estimated 15 million additional executive, administrative, and professional employees (including academic, administrative personnel and teachers in elementary and secondary schools) and to outside salespeople.

### The Age Discrimination in Employment Act of 1967

The Age Discrimination in Employment Act (ADEA), addressing age discrimination in essentially all aspects of employment, was first passed in 1967. Amended a number of times since its initial passage, the ADEA applies to private employers and state and local governments having 20 or more employees and to labor unions having at least 25 members. The original act prohibited such employers from discriminating against persons in the 40- to 70-year-old age range in any area of employment because of age.

The Age Discrimination in Employment Amendments Act of 1986, effective for most employers on January 1, 1987, removed the age 70 limitation on ADEA protection. An employer can neither place an age limit on candidates for employment (except for those occupations for which it has been established that age is a *bona fide occupational qualification*) nor establish a mandatory retirement age for most employees.

The amended ADEA has also necessitated the amendment of numerous insurance plans and other employee benefits plans to permit their continued provision to all active employees regardless of their age. Essentially, ADEA in its present state requires employers to provide the same terms, conditions, and privileges of employment to all employees regardless of age.

The protections of the ADEA notwithstanding, many members of the so-called baby-boomer generation (74 million people were born between 1946 and 1965, the largest generation in the country's history) have been discovering the harsh reality of age discrimination. As the economy ebbs and flows and occasionally lags, older boomers being displaced from what has often been long-term employment are encountering significant age bias in the job market. A dramatic increase in age discrimination lawsuits and greatly increased visibility of the problem have done little to alleviate the effects of the perceived "silver ceiling." The situation is truly ironic in view of what have been described as increasing worker shortages in many occupations and in various part of the country.

### The Older Workers Benefit Protection Act of 1990

The Older Workers Benefit Protection Act (OWBPA) is essentially another amendment to the ADEA, clarifying the authority of the ADEA relative to employee benefits. Although it required equal benefits for all workers, following a number of legal decisions the ADEA allowed reductions in benefits for older workers in instances where added costs were involved. The OWPBA removed the option for the employer to justify lower benefits for older workers and required that any waivers or releases of age discrimination must be voluntary, part of a written agreement between employer and employee. In effect, this law says that an employer cannot unilaterally provide a reduced benefit to an employee on the basis of age.

### Title VI of the Civil Rights Act of 1964

Title VI of the Civil Rights Act of 1964 prohibits discrimination based on race, color, or national origin in all programs or activities receiving federal financial aid. Employment discrimination is prohibited because a primary purpose of federal assistance is the provision of employment, such as apprenticeship, training, work-study, or similar programs. Revised guidelines adopted in 1973 by 25 federal agencies prohibit discriminatory employment practices in all programs if such practices cause discrimination in services provided to program beneficiaries.

### The Americans with Disabilities Act

Passed in 1990 and largely effective in 1992, the Americans with Disabilities Act (ADA) affirmed the rights of persons with disabilities to equal access to employment, services and facilities available to the public (whether under public or private auspices), transportation, and telecommunications. Covered disabilities are defined in the law. This legislation provides a comprehensive mandate for barring discrimination against persons with disabilities and provides enforceable standards addressing such discrimination.

The ADA requires employers to provide reasonable accommodation for disabled individuals who are capable of performing the essential functions of the positions for which they apply. This may include altering physical facilities to make them usable by individuals with disabilities, restructuring jobs around their essential functions, and altering or eliminating nonessential activities so that disabled persons can perform the work.

Regulations implementing ADA were issued by the EEOC, the agency responsible for dealing with complaints of discrimination under all major federal antidiscrimination laws.

The ADA has been in the news frequently since it was passed. Fully 10 years after its passage it was argued before the Supreme Court that the ADA went too far in allowing disabled public employees to sue state and local governments in federal court.[2] States and localities generally enjoy immunity against such lawsuits unless Congress has documented sufficient discrimination to deny them that immunity and to invoke its power under the 14th Amendment to ensure that people have equal protection under the law.

In a decision rendered in January 2002, the Supreme Court unanimously narrowed the number of people covered by the ADA. The opinion held that ". . . merely having an impairment does not make one disabled for purposes of the ADA;" that a person's ailment must extend beyond the workplace and affect everyday life; and that the ability to perform tasks that are of central importance to most people's daily lives must be "substantially limited" before an individual can qualify for coverage under the 1990 law.[3] In another opinion that some regard as a defeat for disabled workers, the Supreme Court ruled that disabled workers are not always entitled to premium assignments intended for more senior workers.[4] Continuing its clarifications and rulings limiting rights under the ADA, in June 2002 the Supreme Court ruled that disabled workers cannot demand jobs that would threaten their lives and health.[5]

Cases continue to arise, and it is likely that the ADA will continue to be refined through Supreme Court decisions for a few years to come.

### Civil Rights Act of 1991

The Civil Rights Act of 1991 was essentially passed to reverse several Supreme Court decisions that had the effect of weakening existing law. It provided for the most extensive modification of Title VII (of the Civil Rights Act of 1964) in more than 20 years. This newer law relies on jury trials, along with statutorily limited compensatory and punitive damages, as the basic litigation scenario under Title VII of the Civil Rights Act of 1964 and the Americans with Disabilities Act.

This act introduces jury trials into employment law to determine liability and compensatory and punitive damages for violations that are found to constitute intentional discrimination. The net effect of this legislation on employers is to increase the likelihood of legal action and increase legal costs associated with trials because potential plaintiffs and their attorneys are attracted by the prospect of damage awards and attorneys' fees (rather than simply compensation for losses, as under Title VII).

## Family and Medical Leave Act

The Family and Medical Leave Act (FMLA) of 1993 makes it possible for an eligible employee (one who has been employed at least 1 year and has worked at least 1,250 hours) to take up to 12 weeks of unpaid leave in a 12-month period for certain specific reasons without loss of employment. The qualifying reasons are: for the birth of the employee's child or the care of that child up to 12 months of age; for the placement of a child with the employee for adoption or foster care; for the employee to care for spouse, child, or parent having a serious health condition; and for the employee's own serious health condition involving the employee's inability to perform the essential functions of the job. An employee returning to work within the 12-week limit must be returned to his or her original position or to a fully equivalent position in terms of pay and benefits and overall working conditions.

Leave taken under the FMLA must often be coordinated with short-term disability and other time-off plans. Also, because certain forms of leave may be taken intermittently or on a reduced day or hours schedule and because there are rules governing the treatment of employee benefits while on such leave, this act has created additional work for department management and human resources.

Millions of employed individuals have used FMLA to take up to 12 weeks of unpaid leave because of a serious illness or to care for a new infant or sick family member. As of early 2001, the U.S. Congress and a number of individual states were considering whether to cover more people under FMLA and grant partial pay for such leaves. Applying as it does to organizations of 50 or more employees, the FMLA covers close to 60 percent of the work force. It has been proposed to expand applicability to employers of 25 or more, which would increase coverage to more than 70 percent of the work force. Partial pay for such leave, resisted by employer groups and others and at this stage by no means certain to become law, would most likely be financed by state unemployment funds or other payroll taxes.[6]

The FMLA has created a number of problems relative to other laws governing employment. There is overlap in the treatment of sick leave between FMLA and the ADA, and rarely is it clear which law's provisions take precedence. Also, portions of the FLSA and various state workers' compensation laws conflict with provisions of both ADA and FMLA.

When confronted with any but the simplest questions raised by FMLA, the individual supervisor is advised to seek answers through human resources or in-house legal counsel if available.

## State and Local Laws

Many state and local government laws prohibit employment discrimination. When the EEOC receives discrimination charges, it defers them for a limited time to various state and local agencies having comparable jurisdiction and enforcement status. Determination of which agencies meet this deferral standard is a continuing process. These agencies' procedures and their requirements for affirmative action vary, but if satisfactory remedies are not achieved the charges will revert to the EEOC for resolution.

## The National Labor Relations Act and Related Laws

Discrimination on the basis of race, religion, or national origin may violate rights arising under these laws. It may be unlawful for employers to participate with unions in the commission of discriminatory practices unlawful under these acts, or to practice discrimination in a way that gives rise to racial or other divisions among employees to the detriment of organized union activity. It may also be unlawful for unions to exclude individuals from union membership, thereby causing them to lose job opportunities; to discriminate in the representation of members or nonmembers in collective bargaining or in the processing of grievances; or to cause or attempt to cause employers to enter into discriminatory agreements or otherwise discriminate against union members or nonmembers.

## Title IX, Education Amendments Act of 1972

In addition to extending coverage of the Equal Pay Act, this law prohibits discrimination on the basis of sex against employees or students of any educational institution receiving federal financial aid. Provisions covering students are similar to those of Title VI of the Civil Rights Act of 1964.

## The Rehabilitation Act of 1973

The Rehabilitation Act of 1973, as amended the following year, requires affected employers to maintain affirmative action programs to ensure the hiring and promotion of qualified handicapped persons. The Rehabilitation Act is significant as a precursor to the Americans with Disabilities Act of 1990.

## The Vietnam Era Veterans Readjustment Assistance Act of 1974

The Vietnam Era Veterans Readjustment Assistance Act of 1974 extends the protection of affirmative action to disabled veterans and veterans of the Vietnam period employed by contractors holding federal contracts of $10,000 or more.

## Other Laws

Employment discrimination has also been ruled by the courts to be prohibited by the Civil Rights Acts of 1866 and 1870 and the Equal Protection Clause of the Fourteenth Amendment to the Constitution. Action under these laws on behalf of individuals or groups may be taken by individuals, private organizations, trade unions, and other groups.

## The Health Insurance Portability and Accountability Act of 1996 (HIPAA)

The Health Insurance Portability and Accountability Act of 1996 has had and continues to have significant effects on a great many health care provider organizations. Ironically, this law's more far reaching effects have little or nothing to do with the "health insurance portability and accountability" of the title. This law is of such significance to many who work and manage in health care that it rates its own chapter (see Chapter 28—"Living With HIPAA").

## SPECIAL CONCERN: SEXUAL HARASSMENT

Because of its prominence in today's society, a few comments on the subject of sexual harassment are in order. The number of sexual harassment complaints filed with the EEOC and various state agencies continues to increase, as does the number of employers involved and the extent of monetary penalties. In recent years sexual harassment has been one of the two leading causes of legal complaints against employers (the other being age discrimination).

The legal basis for defining and addressing sexual harassment has been in place for some time; sexual harassment is in fact a form of sex discrimination under Title VII of the Civil Rights Act of 1964.

Sexual harassment consists of unwelcome sexual advances, requests for sexual favors, or other conduct of a sexual nature if submission is either an actual or implied condition of employment, submission or rejection is used as a basis for making employment-related decisions, or the conduct interferes with work performance or creates an offensive work environment. A key concern in the foregoing lies in the word unwelcome; conduct is considered unwelcome if the employee neither solicited nor invited it and regarded it as undesirable or offensive. To a considerable extent, whether a particular occurrence is or is not sexual harassment may depend largely on the perception of the victim.

Sexual harassment can take a number of forms. Sexually explicit pictures, calendars, or other materials; offensive sexually related language (including sexual humor) or other sexual conduct that creates a hostile environment; sexually explicit behavior; indecent exposure; sexual propositions or intimidation; offensive touching; and participation in or observation of sexual activity are all examples of sexual harassment. So also is something as seemingly innocent (to some) as repeatedly asking a coworker or subordinate for a date after having been turned down. This latter situation adds the dimension of repetition to some harassing behavior; asking a time or two might be considered reasonable, but asking repeatedly—especially after having been turned down—may be considered harassing.

Sexual harassment is not limited strictly to the workplace. Much does of course occur in the workplace, but it is also sexual harassment if it occurs off premises at employer-sponsored social events and even off-premises at private sites if it involves people who have an employment relationship with each other. In addition to involving employees, sexual harassment can involve visitors, vendors, patients, and others as potential perpetrators or victims.

To limit or avoid liability for sexual harassment it is necessary for the employer to promptly and confidentially investigate all complaints, take appropriate remedial action, and create and retain complete and accurate documentation.

The importance of a sound prevention program cannot be overstated as far as sexual harassment is concerned. At a minimum such a program should include a published sexual harassment policy and a detailed procedure for investigating complaints. Ideally, all employees—and most certainly all managers—should be educated in the recognition and prevention of sexual harassment.

## WHO NEEDS MORE RULES?

We have barely scratched the surface of the collection of laws, rules, and regulations with which health care institutions must comply, looking only at the major areas that are likely to be of concern to health care supervisors throughout the country. There are many additional regulations bearing on finance and reimbursement, quality of care, provision of services, medical practice, nursing practice, and many other aspects of organized health care activity.

The recent two to three decades have seen a dramatic increase in the amount of new and expanded federal legislation affecting employee benefits. Primarily among the day-to-day concerns of the human resource department, many of these changes will generally not be immediately visible to the individual supervisor. However, you are likely to see many of the effects of this legislation as regularly occurring change in the features and facets of employee benefits programs.

Many regulatory requirements vary from state to state, but overall they add up to a measure of external control that makes health care the most heavily regulated industry in the country.

Who needs more rules? Certainly not us. Remember, however, that as supervisors we are also employees and that the protection afforded our employees under legislation such as equal pay and affirmative action also extends to us. As supervisors we should be willing to recognize that certain laws represent a well-defined part of our boundaries—those outside limits within which we must learn to work in fulfilling our responsibilities.

---

## REVIEW QUESTIONS

1. How is the hospital industry different from non-health industries as far as a union's right to initiate a strike is concerned?

2. From a hospital manager's point of view, what are the most troublesome implications of the ruling allowing as many as eight separate bargaining units in a hospital?

3. What are the two means available of counting hours for overtime purposes available to hospitals, and what are the significant differences between them?

4. Explain as briefly as practical the determination of the "regular rate" for overtime payment purposes.

5. What are your primary sources of answers and assistance on legal issues, and how can you access these?

## EXERCISE: RATES, HOURS, AND OVERTIME

Your institution operates on the "8 and 80" basis for overtime.

One of your employees worked the following days and hours (mostly on the 11:00 P.M. to 7:00 A.M. shift):

| Day | Hours |
|-----|-------|
| 1 | 8 |
| 2 | 8 |
| 3 | 6 |
| 4 | 9 |
| 5 | 7 |
| 6 | 0 |
| 7 | 0 |
| 8 | 10 |
| 9 | 10 |
| 10 | 12 |
| 11 | 6 |
| 12 | 8 |
| 13 | 0 |
| 14 | 0 |

The employee's base rate is $8.60 per hour. The shift differential is $0.65 per hour. Day 10 included 4 hours of call-in, paid at a flat $40.00. (The employee was asked to come in at 7:00 P.M., 4 hours early.)

Determine the following:

1. the hours of overtime due the employee
2. the "regular rate" for determining overtime premium
3. the employee's total earnings for the two-week period

## NOTES

1. Legislative and Labor Committee, American Society for Healthcare Human Resources Administration of the American Hospital Association, and The Omni Group, Inc., ASHHRA/OMNI *Semi-Annual Labor Activity Report* (Chicago: ASHHRA, 1992): 10–11.

2. Hearst News Service, "High Court Scrutinizes Disabilities Act," *Democrat and Chronicle* (Rochester, NY), 12 October 2000.

3. Newsday, "High Court Limits Disability Law," *Democrat and Chronicle* (Rochester, NY), 9 January 2002.

4. The Associated Press, "Seniority Outweighs Disability," *Democrat and Chronicle* (Rochester, NY), 30 April 2002.

5. The Associated Press, "Top Court Disallows Dangerous Jobs for Disabled," *Democrat and Chronicle* (Rochester, NY), 11 June 2002.

6. Hearst News Service, "Family-Leave Program Could Expand," *Democrat and Chronicle* (Rochester, NY), 5 February 2001.

## CHAPTER 28

# Living with HIPAA

*The purpose of government is to serve, never to dominate.*
*— Dwight D. Eisenhower*

*It is difficult to make our material condition better by the best laws,*
*but it is easy enough to ruin it by bad laws.*
*— Theodore Roosevelt*

## CHAPTER OBJECTIVES

☞ Introduce the Health Insurance Portability and Accountability Act of 1996 (HIPAA) and overview its structure.

☞ Consider the expressed intent of HIPAA and examine some of the diverging views concerning intent versus effects experienced upon implementation.

☞ Identify the principal contentious portions of HIPAA and consider why they have generated resistance and discontent.

☞ Address the role and responsibilities of the individual supervisor in the ongoing implementation and observance of HIPAA.

## SITUATION: A LOOK AT PRIVACY

A gentleman walked into the reception area of a specialty medical practice a few minutes before his scheduled appointment. The waiting area was extremely congested and seemed far too small to properly hold the patients of the half-dozen specialists in the practice and the family members and others who might accompany the patients. The layout of the room was so tight that two or three people who were seated in the waiting area could have touched the receptionist's desk without leaning too far out of their seats, and these people were clearly near enough to the desk to hear everything said there.

The patient gave his name to the receptionist, named the physician he was there to see, and mentioned his appointment time. The receptionist nodded, located him in the appointment calendar, and asked, "What seems to be the problem today?"

The patient, fully aware that two or three people nearby were attuned to every word uttered at the desk, said simply, "This is a follow-up visit," although it was anything but that. He was not about to air his current health complaint in public and would probably not even have told a non-medical individual—a clerical receptionist—what his concern was even if no strangers could hear.

Before the receptionist could speak again she was approached by an individual in a white lab coat who laid what was apparently a lab report in front of her and said, "We need to get in touch with Mr. Johnson; his test results say he's probably diabetic. And remind me that I need to phone in Mrs. Wilson's prescription for (name of drug) before noon." The receptionist nodded and the person in the white coat moved on.

The waiting patient was about to seek a seat in the crowded room when the receptionist said, "We need to update some of your information." The following interchange followed:

Patient: "Update what? I was here not long ago, and nothing's changed."

Receptionist: "Bear with us just a moment. Now, do you still live at (address), is your phone number still (number), and has your insurance changed?"

Patient: "Again, nothing has changed."

Receptionist: "Do you have an answering machine at home?"

Patient: "Yes."

Receptionist: "May we leave appointment reminders on your machine if we can't reach you directly?"

Patient: "Yes."

Receptionist: "May we leave messages such as lab test results on your answering machine?"

Patient: "Yes, I suppose so."

Receptionist: "Is there anyone else with whom we can leave personal messages for you if we can't reach you personally?"

Patient: "I suppose you can leave word with my wife."

Receptionist (consulting a computer screen): "And that would be (spouse's name)?"

Patient: "Yes."

Receptionist: "Thank you. Have a seat and we'll call you when Dr. (name) is ready to see you."

*Instructions*

As you go through this chapter, prepare to comment on the foregoing scenario relative to what you understand about the privacy requirements of HIPAA. Consider all apparent privacy issues involved, as you interpret them from the "Situation" and as you glean from the chapter. While doing so, be sensitive to what one might be led to do out of common sense or common courtesy, and what changes in the described circumstances might be driven by HIPAA.

## INTRODUCING HIPAA

The Health Insurance Portability and Accountability Act of 1996, known commonly by the acronym HIPAA, came into being as PL 104-191 (Public Law Number 104 of the 191st Congress). This law is made up of five sections. Titles I, III, IV, and V address regulation of the continuity and renewability of employee health insurance, promote the establishment and use of medical savings accounts, and set standards for the coverage of long-term care. Title II, described hereafter, provides the basis for most of this chapter.

### An Inconspicuous Beginning

As far as many persons working in health care were concerned, when it was passed in 1996 HIPAA more or less crept quietly upon the scene. At that time the most visible portion of HIPAA, the portion broadly described by the name of the law and the portion that went into effect in 1996, addressed "portability and accountability" in reference to employee health insurance. The intent was to enable American workers to change jobs, whether voluntarily or involuntarily, without fear of losing health care coverage. The portion of HIPAA implemented in 1996 enabled workers to move from one employer's plan to another's without gaps in coverage (no waiting periods) and without encountering restrictions based on pre-existing conditions. Simply, a worker could move from plan to plan without disruption of coverage.

Not a great many managers in health care concerned themselves with HIPAA in 1996. It is likely that human resource managers were the ones who became most aware of the new law because of the involvement of their benefit plans. However, even many human resource managers had little to concern them about HIPAA. In most instances the required notifications were handled by the employers' health insurance carriers, so there was little to do other than answering employee questions as they arose.

In the minds of many who did not look beyond the simple implications of the law's title, the organization had little more to do than ensuring the portability of health insurance so therefore they would have few concerns about HIPAA overall. However, the real impact of HIPAA was yet to come, and its arrival was a considerable surprise to many.

### The Contentious Title II

The portion of HIPAA having the most far-reaching effects on patients and health care providers and related organizations is Title II. This section is identified as "Preventing Health Care Fraud and Abuse, Administrative Simplification, and Medical Liability Reform." It is often referred to as just "Administrative Simplification," a name fraught with irony for those who feel that its effects, at least upon many organizations that must comply with it, have been quite the opposite of "simplification."

"Administrative Simplification" includes a number of significant requirements that were designated for implementation at differing times. All affected entities were to be in compliance with the Privacy Rule, by far the most contentious portion of HIPAA, by April 14, 2003. Following this, compliance with the Transactions and Code Sets (TCS) Rule was required by October 16, 2003, and the Security Rule was scheduled for complete implementation in April 2005.

### THE INTENT AND THE REALITY

There is continuing controversy over whether HIPAA is in fact doing what its framers intended it to do. As its name suggests, it was intended in part to ensure the continuity and renewability of employee health insurance. There is little disagreement on this point. The controversy over the intent versus the reality of HIPAA primarily concerns the Privacy Rule and the requirements supporting this rule.

The essential intent of this portion of HIPAA may be described as an effort to strike a balance between ensuring that personal health information is accessible only to those who truly need it and permitting the health care industry to pursue medical research and improve the overall quality of care. In the effort to do so, the pertinent portions of HIPAA have created considerable work and expense for health care providers and organizations that do business with them, plus inconvenience and often frustration for patients and their families and representatives.

## TITLE II AND BEYOND

The implementation of HIPAA is overseen by the Department of Health and Human Services (DHHS).

"Standardization," the first of HIPPA's several Administrative Simplification rules, was published in August 2000. Compliance was ordered for October 2002, 24 months after publication.

On December 20, 2000, DHHS released the "final" health information Privacy Rule, the requirements of which were met with mixed reactions from various elements of the health care system. Much of the health care industry, and particularly health maintenance organizations (HMOs) and other managed care plans, saw this collection of new rules and requirements as a hindrance to the fulfillment of their objectives of service. On the other hand, patient advocates believed that the new rules did not go far enough in protecting patients' medical information. There were sufficient objections raised to suggest that the Bush administration might concede to health care industry demands and abandon the new rules in favor of a less rigorous version; however, although the rules governing privacy were disputed they were re-released by DHHS in March 2001 without the changes that many people expected. Compliance with the nearly 1,500 pages of the Privacy Rule, bringing about the most frustration with HIPAA, was ordered for April 2003. Most health care organizations were in reasonable compliance by that date or at least well on their way to being so.

First proposed in May 1998, the first version of the Transactions and Code Sets (TCS) Rule was published in August 2000 with a compliance deadline of October 2002. In January 2001, the compliance deadline was extended to October 16, 2003. Affected organizations were to file TCS compliance plans with the Centers for Medicare and Medicaid Services by October 16, 2002, to qualify for the extension. Affected organizations had a TCS testing deadline of April 16, 2003, while the compliance date remained October 16, 2003.

The Security Rule was published in its final form on February 20, 2003. Two dates were set for its effectiveness: April 21, 2005 for larger organizations (think hospitals, nursing homes, etc.) and April 21, 2006 for smaller organizations (such as physician practices). Specifically, a "small" organization is a provider of services having fewer than 25 full-time equivalent employees (FTEs) or an involved supplier (other than a provider of health services) having fewer than 10 FTEs. The Security Rule addresses the confidentiality, integrity, and availability of electronic patient data. To differentiate Security from Privacy: the Privacy Rule covers paper-based, oral, and electronic patient health information, while Security applies only to electronic health data stored or transmitted electronically. Electronic information, for example, does not include paper-to-paper faxes, video conferencing, or voice mail messages because the information being exchanged did not exist in electronic form before transmission.

Other rule sets concerned in HIPAA implementation are the National Provider Identifier, the National Employer Identifier, the National Health Plan Identifier, Claims Attachments, and Enforcement.

## THE PRIVACY CONTROVERSY

Reactions to the Privacy Rule, ordered for compliance by April 16, 2003, were many and varied. Patients and patient advocates claimed that these new requirements were forcing Americans to choose between access to medical care and control of their personal medical information. Federal officials, however, were claiming that the rules would effectively balance patient privacy against the needs of the health care industry to provide Americans with "efficient and effective" access to health care. Expressed another way, the Privacy Rule would ensure that personal health information was available only to those who need it while allowing the health care industry to pursue research, promote public health objectives, and improve the quality of care.

As already suggested, HIPAA has many and varied things to say in its several sections, but to a great many people who have been exposed to the Privacy Rule from either the organizational position or the position of the patient, "Privacy" *is* HIPAA.

In early 2001 when many of HIPAA's regulations were first receiving widespread exposure, hospitals, insurers, health maintenance organizations, and others claimed that the Privacy Rule would impose costly new burdens on the industry. They lobbied to have the proposed regulations killed, while at the same time Congress was claiming that HIPAA's proposed protections were immensely popular with consumers. Consumer advocates generally hailed the proposed rules as the first comprehensive federal standards for medical privacy, while at the same time suggesting that they did not go far enough.

The comprehensive Privacy Rule was finally effective April 14, 2003 following two years of debates and numerous hearings.

To achieve compliance with the Privacy Rule affected organizations were required to:

- Revise, or develop as necessary, policies and procedures addressing the handling of patient medical information ("Use and Disclosure of Protected Health Information").
- Ensure that employees are trained in the handling of protected health information, this training to include the proper orientation of new employees in all confidentiality requirements.
- Provide for the active management of administrative issues arising from or associated with the handling of protected health information.
- Monitor compliance with all requirements for handling protected health information.

- Create and maintain documentation as proof that all pertinent information-handling requirements are being fulfilled.

**Privacy and the Individual**

It would be difficult to deny that patient privacy is at the center of most interest in HIPAA. It is for the provider's compliance with the Privacy Rule that all patients who begin a relationship with a provider are asked to sign a statement acknowledging receipt of the provider's privacy notice. A typical privacy notice is shown in Appendix A. This is a lengthy document, as are most privacy notices, and we might perhaps reasonably ask ourselves whether very many patients who have signed an acknowledgement and received a provider's privacy notice have taken the time to actually read the notice in its entirety. The form and format of the privacy notice may vary from one organization to another, but it must provide all of the information required by HIPAA.

Generally, the rights of patients under HIPAA encompass the following.

- Patients are entitled to know how their personal medical information will be used or disclosed.
- Patients may request and receive copies of their health records. (This is a dramatic change from past practice, when a patient record was considered the provider's property to be shared only with another legitimately concerned provider.)
- Patients may ask for corrections, amendments, or restrictions to their personal medical information.
- Patients may request a full accounting of disclosures of their personal medical information; all persons are entitled to know who is in receipt of their information.
- Patients may file complaints if they believe their privacy rights have been violated by improper or unauthorized disclosure.
- Employers and marketers are prevented from obtaining patient medical information without the patient's express written authorization.
- Any hospital inpatient may direct the facility to refrain from releasing information on his or her medical condition to anyone, whether relatives or the public, and may even forbid the facility to even acknowledge one's presence as a patient.

In many instances the new privacy requirements are causing frustration for patients and others. Consider, for example, one's spouse or other family member, who might be expected to help in obtaining a referral or following up on a test result, or perhaps a benefits representative at one's place of employment attempting to resolve a simple billing problem. In brief, nothing in any way related to a patient's medical condition can be addressed by anyone other than the patient unless the designated party has the signed authorization of the patient (except, of course, when the patient is a minor).

There are, however, instances in which personal medical information can be used without patient consent. This can be done in the following situations.

- Information can be provided for certain purposes, for example, for research or study, when no patient is directly identified and there is no way to infer any patient's identity.
- Information can be given to someone else in the provider's practice who has a legitimate need for it, for example, a billing service.
- Personal medical information can be given to a representative who has legal authority to represent a patient (parent or guardian of a minor, designated health care proxy, a medical power-of-attorney, a patient's written permission, or such).
- Medical information can be gathered by a legal public health authority to be used to prevent or control disease, injury, or disability.
- Information can be supplied to the Food and Drug Administration (FDA) in the form of reports of adverse events, for product recalls, or to track health care product problems.

### Effects on the Organization

Essentially all health care plans and health care providers must comply with HIPAA. Provider organizations include physicians' and dentists' offices; hospitals, nursing homes, and hospices; home health providers; clinical laboratories, imaging (radiologic) services; pharmacies, clinics and free-standing surgical centers and urgent care centers; and any other providers of health-related services to individuals. Also required to comply are other organizations that serve the direct providers of health care, such as billing services and medical equipment dealers. All affected entities are required to:

- Protect patient information in all forms from unauthorized use or distribution;
- Protect patient information from malfeasance and misuse;
- Implement specific data formats and code sets for consistency of information processing and preservation; and
- Establish audit mechanisms to safeguard against fraud and abuse.

All subcontractors, suppliers, or other involved entities coming into contact with any protected patient information must also comply with the HIPAA Privacy Rule. In addition, all arrangements with such entities must define the acceptable uses of patient information. Overall, contracts with involved organizations must:

- Define the proper uses of all patient data;
- Specify necessary audit mechanisms and other safeguards;
- Require disclosure when and if patient information is improperly used or disclosed; and
- Call for the destruction or return of all remnants of protected patient information once it is no longer needed.

Depending on organization size and structure, compliance with the HIPAA Privacy Rule could involve several departments (e.g., in a mid-size to large hospital), a few people (e.g., in a small hospital or nursing home), or a single person (e.g., in a small medical office). Whether accomplished by separate departments, a person or two, or an office manager, compliance involves a number of functions including:

- Information technology;
- Health information management (medical records);
- Social services;
- Finance;
- Administration; and
- Various ancillary or supporting services.

There was little doubt from initial exposure to the new regulations that every provider organization would have to make some changes in procedures and adopt some practices that would add to their workload. The most visible new requirement was the "notice of privacy practices" that would have to be provided to each individual beginning a relationship with the provider (refer again to Appendix A).

Providers must now obtain written consent from patients or their legal representatives for the use or disclosure of information in their medical records. Patients or their representatives grant this permission by signing to acknowledge receipt of the privacy notice. Further, in the privacy notice providers must define the acceptable use of patient information and forbid its use for all other purposes. Providers are also legally required to disclose when patient information has been improperly accessed or disclosed.

The HIPAA Privacy Rule created a widespread need for health care providers to reengineer their systems to protect their patient information infrastructures and combat misuse and abuse. Providers now must:

- Guarantee protection of patient information in both paper and electronic forms;
- Secure their information systems from unauthorized access;
- Implement specific data formats and code sets as specified in the law;
- Institute audit mechanisms to monitor systems to safeguard sensitive information to guard against fraud and abuse;
- Monitor compliance within their organizations by conducting periodic formal audits, investigating complaints and incidents, and generally overseeing internal compliance with the rules;
- Establish and maintain appropriate polices and procedures for the use and disclosure of protected information;
- Ensure that all employees are trained in HIPAA's privacy requirements; and
- Compel the organization's business partners—contractors, suppliers, consultants, business services, and such—to return or destroy protected health information once it is no longer needed.

And concerning the foregoing requirements on the organization, it is not enough to simply do everything that is supposed to be done. There are also requirements for the inevitable documentation; it is necessary to be able to produce documentation to verify compliance.

Also, a provider organization's telecommuting or home-based program must also be HIPAA compliant, so specific privacy guidelines for telecommuting employees must be implemented.

*Physical Layout Considerations*

The HIPAA Privacy Rule has necessitated changes in the physical arrangements in which various tasks and services are performed to ensure that no one other than the patient and involved caregiver or other legitimately involved person knows the nature of the patient's problem. For example, previously a physician's office nurse might have given a patient specific care instructions at a front desk where others—perhaps patients departing or waiting to be seen, or other persons—could hear what was said. This can no longer happen; any information about a patient's medical condition must be conveyed with a guarantee of privacy; no one other than those who are party to the conversation may hear what is being said. This applies in any instance in which information of a personal medical nature must pass between patient or representative and a legitimately concerned party.

One striking example of HIPAA's influence is readily noticeable on any given day when one walks into a retail pharmacy. Surely most persons have become aware of the changes at retail pharmacies—consultation and prescription pick-up counters arranged within privacy areas, waiting lines isolated such that persons waiting are unable to ascertain a customer's business, and even prescriptions packaged so that the name of any particular medication cannot be read on the outside of the package. These pharmacy changes have all been in response to the HIPPA Privacy Rule, in recognition of the fact that the name of one's medication is part of that individual's personal health information.

*The Privacy Officer*

Every health care provider organization must have an individual designated to oversee HIPAA compliance. In a large organization this could be a full-time HIPAA coordinator; in a small organization, say a medical office, the task will likely be an additional responsibility for whoever manages the office. In addition to monitoring all aspects of compliance on an ongoing basis, this individual must also ensure that appropriate policies and procedures are in place and maintained current.

*Signs of the Future*

It seems reasonably clear at this time that many of HIPAA's requirements point toward the promotion of standardized electronic transmission of health care transactions that are currently or were formerly set on paper by manual means. In other words, HIPAA is seen as encouraging the steady conversion of paper records to all-electronic patient records.

## Penalties

Just as documentation is inevitable in compliance with any law, penalties are also inevitable for non-compliance or deliberate violation. The smaller

penalties to be encountered relate to failure to comply with HIPAA's requirements, and more severe penalties are associated with wrongful disclosure of
protected information. Civil fines can range from $100 to $25,000 depending
on the nature and extent of violation, and individuals found to be deliberately
marketing protected information can be subject to criminal penalties.

## RESPECTING PRIVACY IN A PUBLIC SETTING

In the "Situation" described at the start of the chapter there were a number
of instances in which privacy considerations were ignored or overlooked. Certainly the congested waiting area, with its inappropriately placed reception
desk, would necessarily have to be rearranged for compliance with the HIPAA
Privacy Rule. No one in the waiting areas should be able to hear other persons' personal health information exchanged at the reception desk (or anywhere else). One might be able to argue that the patient could reasonably be
expected to identify his present medical problem for the reception person or
other non-medical provider employee, but the patient has the right to do so
without others overhearing. However, if the patient chooses not to tell the
receptionist even without others hearing, common sense suggests that the
receptionist should accept the "follow-up visit" statement.

It was, of course, fully inappropriate for the white-coated individual—probably a physician—to mention Mr. Johnson's likely problem and to name Mrs.
Wilson's medication in the presence of others.

The need to update some information may have been appropriate, but
again, doing so should not take place within the hearing of others. The inquiry
about the answering machine and the questions that follow were part of an
effort to obtain the patient's permission to leave personal health information
recorded so that it could conceivably be heard by persons other than the
patient. Ideally, in true conformance with HIPAA the provider's representative should have obtained signed permission.

It could also be argued that no one else in the waiting room should have
been able to hear the name of the physician the patient was waiting for,
because at times it may be possible to infer the kind of medical problem a
patient has by the identity of the medical specialist involved.

Consider much of today's privacy concerns as addressable using a combination of common sense and common courtesy. The sharing of personal health
information should always be subject to strict "need to know" criteria.

## HIPAA AND THE SUPERVISOR

Depending on the kind of activity supervised, the requirements of HIPAA
could significantly affect the supervisor's role. For example, in addition to
being concerned with the Privacy Rule, as are all supervisors to some extent,
an individual supervising within health information management (HIM, formerly known as medical records) must also be concerned with implementation
of the Transactions and Code Sets (TCS) Rule. As another example, a supervisor involved with information technology or information systems (still
referred to by some as data processing) will be significantly concerned with

the Security Rule because of its applicability to health data stored or transmitted electronically.

Like numerous other laws affecting the workplace, there is considerably more to compliance with HIPAA than simply putting the appropriate policies and procedures and systems in place and mandating their use. Some of the HIPAA regulations are relatively complex, and in the areas of an organization that are most affected a significant amount of training can be required. Also, HIPAA necessitates a certain amount of training for most staff regardless of department or function; anyone who comes into contact with protected patient information must receive privacy training. This suggests that most supervisors will be both trainees and trainers, learning HIPAA's privacy requirements and communicating them to and reinforcing them with employees.

It is necessary for the supervisor to be aware of HIPAA's requirements, especially as it affects his or her specific function, and to be knowledgeable of the contents of the organization's privacy notice and all applicable policies and procedures. Beyond this familiarity, however, each supervisor should harbor an attitude that reflects an abiding respect for every person's right to privacy. Concerning all personal health information of all persons, never has the phrase *need to know* been so completely applicable. An individual's health information must never be communicated to anyone who does not have a legitimate need for the information in the fulfillment of the individual's needs, and then only with agreement of the individual or that person's legal representative. Also, the supervisor has an obligation to safeguard all personal health information against accidental disclosure.

In addition to knowledge of HIPAA regulations, the supervisor's attitude concerning patients' personal health information should reflect both common sense and common courtesy.

## HERE TO STAY

Although a number of HIPAA requirements are still being shaken out and all the dust has yet to settle, it is clear that the law's basic privacy requirements are here to stay in one form or another. Although there may be changes in how some aspects of privacy are addressed, it remains likely that the privacy rules will continue to affect every physician, patient, hospital, pharmacy, other health care provider, and all other entities having contact with patient medical information in any form.

The Health Insurance Portability and Accountability Act is likely to remain controversial for some time to come. Some patient advocacy groups strongly believe that the rules do not go far enough in protecting patient medical information. On the other side of the controversy, much of the health care industry—and especially those providers in managed care—describe the new rules as mostly bureaucratic barriers to the provision of good patient care. In general, the health care industry's reaction to HIPAA seems to be that the government went overboard in pursuit of a worthy goal.

## REVIEW QUESTIONS

1. In reference to the partial name of Title II of HIPAA, "Administrative Simplification," what, if anything, appears most likely to be truly simplified?

2. If a state happens to have a privacy law—portions of which are different from the regulations of HIPAA's Privacy Rule, how is the conflict between the two laws to be reconciled?

3. Why do you suppose the framers of HIPAA made it necessary for even one's spouse or other immediate family members to have written permission to learn one's condition when hospitalized?

4. Explain how, if at all, the HIPAA Privacy Rule affects the long-standing practice in many small communities of publishing hospital discharges or notices of births.

5. In either the sample "Privacy Notice" (Appendix A) or the text of the chapter, identify at least three conditions or sets of circumstances that might be prompting privacy advocates to claim that the law does not go far enough. Explain.

## CASE: PRIVACY VERSUS THE "NEED TO KNOW"

Elaine Spring, an employment representative in the human resource department of Valley Memorial Hospital, was visited by Norma Michaels, a nurse manager who was actively recruiting to fill an open LPN (licensed practical nurse) position. Norma had already interviewed three candidates supplied by Elaine; all three happened to be current employees who were looking to transfer. Two were new LPNs still working in the entry-level jobs they held while going to school; the third, Janet Cook, was an experienced LPN who was looking to leave the hospital rehabilitation unit and return to a medical/surgical floor. Norma wanted someone with some experience, so she considered Janet to be the only real possibility she had before her. In part, the conversation between Norma and Elaine went as follows:

Norma: "The only real possibility you've found for me is Janet Cook. I can't go with a new, inexperienced LPN—our unit's just too hectic. Do you have anyone else for me to interview? Someone from outside?"

Elaine: "No, we haven't had a single outside applicant for this job. And you've seen all three transfer candidates."

Norma: "I was afraid of that, so I dug out Janet's personnel file to check her out."

Elaine (with something of a surprised look): "Oh? Who got the file for you? Cindy?"

Norma: "I got it myself."

Elaine: "You know you're not supposed to do that. You needed to ask Cindy."

Norma (shrugging): "I didn't see her, so I helped myself. Anyway, this tells me almost nothing."

Elaine: "Everything should be there—evaluations, attendance records, the works."

Norma: "I happen to know that Janet's had a stretch of disability time off and I heard she was once a Workers' Compensation case. I need her *entire* personnel file so I can judge whether she's fit to do the job."

Elaine: "You *have* her entire personnel file. Disability reports and other health-related documents are now kept in a separate file in the employee health office."

Norma: "All that stuff used to be in one file."

Elaine: "Not any more."

Norma (impatiently): "Then get me the file from employee health."

Elaine (shaking her head): "No can do."

Norma: "Part of that HIPAA nonsense?"

Elaine: "Yes and no. The separate files were established before HIPAA, but HIPAA rules apply to the files in employee health."

Norma (scornfully): "It makes no sense whatsoever to have parts of the same file kept in two different places. And I need to know whether this Janet Cook can keep up the pace on our unit."

Elaine: "You're not entitled to the other file. In fact, neither am I. You'll have to go ahead based on your interview and the file you can review here."

## Questions

1. Why do HIPAA regulations apply to the portions of the personnel file maintained in the employee health office?

2. Why would Norma be forbidden to see the record maintained in employee health?

3. Because she is not allowed to see Janet's employee health file, how can Norma judge whether Janet could or could not perform the job as required?

4. In just a few words, describe the fundamental distinction between the file kept in human resources and the one maintained in employee health.

# Typical Privacy Notice

(Organization Name)

This notice describes how your medical information may be used and disclosed and how you can obtain access to that information. Please review this information carefully.

## Our Commitment to Privacy

(Name or organization or practice) is committed to maintaining the privacy of your protected health information, which includes information about your medical condition and the care and treatment you receive. This notice describes how your information may be used and disclosed by (organization) and also describes your rights regarding your personal health information.

## How Your Medical Information May be Used and Disclosed

(Organization) may use and disclose your personal health information for purposes related to your care, payment for your care, and health care operations of (organization).

*Care:* Your personal health information will be provided to those health care professionals, whether on this organization's staff or not, directly involved in your care so that they may understand your medical condition and needs and provide advice and treatment to you. For example, a physician treating you for arthritis may need to know what medications have been prescribed for you by the medical providers from (organization).

*Payment:* To secure payment for the health care provided by (organization), your personal health information will be sent to the appropriate third-party payer, for example your insurance carrier.

*Health Care Operations:* In order for (organization) to provide quality and efficient care for you, it may be necessary to compile, use, and disclose your personal health information for health care operations purposes. For example, we may use your information to monitor the performance of the physicians providing your treatment.

## When an Authorization Is Not Required

(Organization) may use or disclose your personal health information, without your written authorization, under the following circumstances:

*Unidentified Information:* When your personal health information is amended so that it does not identify you directly and your identity cannot otherwise be inferred.

*Business Associates:* When it is submitted to a business associate, someone with whom (organization) contracts to provide a service necessary to operations, for example a billing service. All business associates will be required to appropriately safeguard your personal health information.

*Personal Representative:* When it is revealed to an individual who, under applicable law, has the authority to represent you in making decisions related to your care.

*Public Health Activities:* When information is collected by a public health authority for activities for the public good such as the prevention or control of disease, injury, or disability. This includes reporting of child abuse or neglect.

*Food and Drug Administration:* When required by the Food and Drug Administration (FDA) in the reporting of adverse events, product defects or problems or biological product deviations, or to track products, or to enable product recalls, repairs or replacements, or to conduct post-marketing surveillance.

*Abuse, Neglect, or Domestic Violence:* When (organization) is required by law to make such disclosure to a government authority. Upon such requirement, (organization) will do so if convinced that the disclosure is necessary to prevent harm or if (organization) believes that you have been the victim of abuse, neglect, or domestic violence. Such disclosure will be made in accordance with the requirements of law, which may also involve notifying you of the disclosure.

*Health Oversight Activities:* When certain activities required by law concern government agencies involved in oversight activities that relate to the health care system, government benefit programs, government regulatory programs, and civil rights law. Such activities include criminal investigations, audits, disciplinary actions, or general oversight activities relating to the community's health care system.

*Judicial and Administrative Proceedings:* When, for example, your personal health information must be supplied in response to a court order of subpoena.

*Law Enforcement Purposes:* Your personal health information may be disclosed to the appropriate persons for law enforcement purposes including:

- complying with a legal process such as a subpoena or as required by law;
- for identification and location purposes; for example suspect or missing person;
- provision of information concerning one who is or is suspected to be a crime victim;
- when the death of an individual may have resulted from criminal conduct;
- when a crime occurs on the premises of (organization); or
- when there is a medical emergency and it appears that a crime has been committed.

*Coroner or Medical Examiner:* Your personal health information may be disclosed to a coroner or medical examiner for the purpose of identifying you or determining your cause of death, or to a funeral director as permitted by law and as necessary to fulfill his or her duties.

*Organ, Eye, or Tissue Donation:* When you are a designated organ donor, (organization) may disclose your personal health information to the facility that is to receive the donated organs.

*Research:* When the practice is involved in research activities, your personal health information may be used subject to governmental requirements intended to protect the privacy of your personal health information, such as approval of the research by an institutional review board and the requirement that protocols be followed.

*Threat to Health or Safety:* Your personal health information may be disclosed if (organization) believes that disclosure is necessary to prevent or lessen a serious and imminent threat to the health or safety of a person or the public and the disclosure is to a party or parties who are reasonably able to prevent or lessen the threat.

*Specialized Government Functions:* When the appropriate conditions apply, (organization) may use the personal health information of individuals who are members of the armed forces:

- for activities deemed necessary by appropriate military command authorities;
- for determination by the Department of Veterans Affairs of eligibility for benefits; or,
- to a foreign military authority if you are a member of a foreign military service.

(Organization) may also disclose your personal health information to authorized federal officials for conducting national security and intelligence activities including the provision of protective services to the President or others legally authorized.

*Inmates:* The practice may disclose your personal health information to a correctional institution or law enforcement official if you are an inmate of that correctional facility and your information is necessary to provide care and treatment to you or is necessary for the health and safety of other individuals.

*Workers' Compensation:* If you are involved in a Workers' Compensation claim, (organization) may be required to disclose your personal health information to an appropriate person in the Workers' Compensation system.

*Disaster Relief Efforts:* (Organization) may use or disclose your personal health information to a public or private entity authorized to assist in disaster relief efforts.

*Required by Law:* If otherwise required by law, but such use or disclosure will be made in compliance with the law and limited to the specific requirements of the law.

### Authorization

Uses and disclosures other than those described above will be made only with your written authorization. You may revoke your authorization at any time.

### Sign-in Sheet

(Organization) may use a sign-in sheet at the registration desk. Your name may also be called in the waiting area when your caregiver is ready to see you.

### Appointment Reminder

(Organization) may contact you to remind you of scheduled appointments. The reminder may be in the form of a letter, postcard, or telephone call, or message. The amount of information included in the reminder will be kept to an absolutely essential minimum.

### Treatment Alternatives/Benefits

(Organization) may contact you about treatment alternatives or other health services or benefits that may be of interest to you.

### Marketing

(Organization) may use and disclose your personal health information for marketing purposes only if we obtain your prior written authorization. Marketing activities include communication to you that encourages you to purchase or use a product or service when such communication is not made for your care or treatment. However, marketing does not include, for example, sending you a newsletter about (organization). Marketing also includes receipt of remuneration, directly or indirectly, from a third party whose product or service is being marketed to you. You will be informed if (organization) engages in marketing and your written authorization will be requested.

### Fundraising

(Organization) may use and disclose some of your personal health information in order to contact you for fundraising activities supporting (organization). Any fundraising materials sent to you will describe how you may voluntarily choose not to receive further such communications.

### On-call Coverage

In order to provide you with on-call coverage, it is necessary for (organization) to establish relationships with other providers who will take your call if your regular caregivers are not available. Such on-call providers, when accessed, will provide (organization) with whatever personal health information they create and will keep your personal health information confidential.

### Family and Friends Involved in Your Care

(Organization) may disclose to your family member, other relative, close personal friend, or other person your personal health information relevant to such person's involvement with your care. We may also use or disclose your information to notify or assist in the notification of a family member, a personal representative, or another person responsible for your care, of your location, general condition, or death. However, the following conditions apply:

- You must agree to such uses or disclosures, or (organization) provides you the opportunity to object and you do not object, or we can reasonably infer from the circumstances, based on the exercise of our judgment, that you do not object to the use or disclosure.
- If you are not present, (organization) will exercise judgment in determining whether the use or disclosure is in your best interests and if so, disclose only the personal health information that is directly relevant to the person's involvement in your care.

## Your Health Information Rights

You have the right to:

- *Revoke any authorization* in writing at any time. To request a revocation you must submit a written request to (organization)'s designated privacy officer or coordinator.
- *Request restrictions* on the uses and disclosures of your personal health information. However, (organization) is not obligated to agree to requested restrictions. To request restrictions, submit a written request to the privacy officer or coordinator describing the information you wish to limit, whether you wish to limit (organization)'s use or disclosure or both, and to whom you want the limits to apply. If in agreement with your request, (organization) will comply unless the information is needed to provide you with emergency treatment.
- *Receive confidential communications* of personal health information by alternate means or at alternative locations. You must make your request in writing to the privacy officer or coordinator. All reasonable requests will be accommodated.
- *Inspect and copy your personal health information* as provided by law. To inspect and copy your information, submit a written request to the privacy officer or coordinator. In certain situations defined by law, your request may be denied, but you will have the right to request review of the denial. You can be charged a reasonable fee for the cost of copying, mailing, or other supplies associated with your request.
- *Request an amendment of your personal health information* as provided by law. To do so, submit a request to the privacy officer or coordinator and provide reasons supporting your request. Your request may be denied if the information to be amended was not created within (organization) (unless the individual or entity that created the information is no longer available), if the information is not part of your personal health information maintained by (organization), if the information is not part of the information you would be permitted to inspect and copy, or if the information is accurate and complete. If you disagree with denial of your request, you have the right to submit a written statement of disagreement.
- *Receive an accounting of disclosures* of your personal health information as provided by law. To request an accounting, submit a written request to the privacy officer or coordinator stating a time period not longer than six

(6) years and excluding dates prior to April 14, 2003. The request should indicate in what form you want the list (paper or electronic). The first list requested within a 12-month period is free, but you may be charged the cost of providing you with additional lists in the same 12-month period. You will be notified of costs involved, and you can decide whether to withdraw or modify your request before costs are incurred.

- *Receive a paper copy* of this Privacy Notice from (organization) upon request.
- *Complain to (Organization)* or to the Secretary of Health and Human Services, Office for Civil Rights, (address of office of appropriate state or region). You may locate a regional office at www.hhs.gov/ocr/regmail.html. To file a complaint directly with (organization), contact the privacy officer or coordinator. All complaints must be in writing.
- *To obtain more information* about your rights, or have questions about your rights answered, you may contact (organization)'s privacy officer (name and contact information).

## (Organization)'s Obligations

This health care provider organization:

- Is required by law to maintain the privacy of your personal health information and to provide you with this Privacy Notice.
- Reserves the right to change the terms of this Privacy Notice and to make new Privacy Notice provisions effective for all of your personal health information that it maintains.
- Will not retaliate against you for making a complaint.
- Must make a good faith effort to obtain from you an acknowledgment of receipt of this Notice.
- Will post this Privacy Notice on (organization)'s website.
- Will provide this Privacy Notice to you by e-mail if you so request; however, you also have a right to obtain a paper copy.

## Effective Date

This revised notice is in effect as of (date).
The original notice was effective April 14, 2003, as required by federal law.

## CHAPTER 29

# Organizational Communication: Looking Up, Down, and Laterally

*The trouble with this place is there's no communication.*
*—Anonymous*

## CHAPTER OBJECTIVES

☛ Compare and contrast the characteristics of upward communication and downward communication in the organizational setting, with special attention to the barriers to upward communication.

☛ Define and describe the supervisor's role in organizational communication.

☛ Provide suggestions for strengthening communications with other organizational elements including your immediate superior.

☛ Suggest ways of dealing with "the grapevine."

☛ Stress the importance of the supervisor's visibility to the department's employees.

## SITUATION: THE UNREQUESTED INFORMATION

One morning about 15 minutes before the normal starting time for the day shift, you are enjoying a solitary cup of coffee when you are joined by Mrs. Morris, one of your direct reporting employees. Mrs. Morris proceeds to advise you ("In strictest confidence, please don't say that I told you") that another employee, Mrs. Greely, has been actively talking with the department's staff, passing derogatory remarks about you and your leadership style and essentially undermining your management of the department.

Mrs. Morris proclaims that she ordinarily does not carry stories but she felt that you "had a right to know, for the good of the department."

The options that appear immediately open to you are as follows:

- Thank Mrs. Morris, and ask her to report anything else she might hear.
- Acknowledge her concern "for the good of the department," but tell her to bring you no more such stories.
- Thank her, ask her to say nothing to anyone else, and decide to keep an eye on Mrs. Greely.

*Instructions*

As you proceed through this chapter, think about whether you would opt for one of the three choices given above, or pursue some other course of action.

## WHAT GOES DOWN MAY NOT COME UP

It is safe to assume that in any organization, communication should, and in fact must, move both upward and downward through the structure. However, an informed management view of organizational communication will recog-

479

nize that much information does not flow both upward and downward with equal ease. Downward communication is facilitated largely by management's control of its own actions and by its control of most of the means of communication in the work setting, but much upward communication remains dependent on stimulation, encouragement, and the creation of a climate conducive to communication.

The essential differences between the accomplishment of upward communication and downward communication can be highlighted by consideration of a number of factors that inhibit upward communication.

## Organizational Concerns

Simple physical distance between supervisor and employee can inhibit upward communication. Simply put, the more time you spend physically separated from the location where most of your employees work, the tougher it is for them to communicate with you. This was suggested in the discussion on "span of control" in Chapter 4, where it was pointed out that supervisors with employees who have considerable on-the-job mobility or are scattered over an extended physical area need to take steps to keep in touch. The more time you spend physically removed from your employees, the more likely you are to miss something that might have otherwise been communicated to you.

The problems posed by physical distance are becoming more of a concern for an increasing number of supervisors. In this era of rapid and dramatic change in health care, as mergers and acquisitions and other affiliations create health systems from what were formerly individual organizations, some supervisors find themselves responsible for activities in multiple locations. Under these circumstances, when travel time and distance as well as the division of one's time become determinants of availability to employees, the supervisor must be highly conscientious concerning the need to stay in touch with all employees no matter how scattered they may be.

The number of levels in the organization structure can also inhibit upward communication. If a piece of information originating with a single hourly-rated employee truly deserves to reach the top, the chances of it being properly communicated up the line diminish as the number of levels it must go through increases. Each level that a message must pass through presents another set of opportunities for the message to be misinterpreted, sidetracked, or stopped entirely.

While some modern health care organizations are making upward communication inherently more difficult by splitting supervisors among multiple locations, many of these same organizations are also "flattening"—reducing the number of levels in the management hierarchy. Because the presence of fewer levels reduces the opportunity for miscommunication and also reduces resistance to the upward movement of information, this flattening may at least partially offset the problems caused by multiple locations.

The relative complexity of a given problem or situation can also hamper upward communication. Some employees are often unable to define complex problems fully, especially if these problems appear to involve jobs or departments other than their own. Also, some employees lack sufficient command of communication skills to enable them to translate their thoughts and observations into concise, understandable messages, so they simply do not bother to try.

## Problems Involving Managers

The attitude exhibited by a supervisor or manager can have a great deal to do with how well information flows upward. If your manner and attitude should seem to say, "No news is good news," or "Don't tell me anything I don't want to hear," then employees are likely to be discouraged from speaking up. Also, if the supervisor appears to behave defensively—perhaps seeming to regard opinions, problems, or requests as personal jabs—then employees are likewise discouraged from speaking up.

Some managers frequently exhibit apparent resistance to becoming involved with the personal problems of employees. This resistance, coming no doubt from the supervisor's understandable uneasiness with hearing things that might be considered "confessional" in nature, serves as a wall that unfortunately keeps out desired feedback as well as unwanted information. Recall the notion of the employee as a "whole person," and learn to accept the high likelihood that many supposedly personal problems have their work-related sides.

The manager's available time can also be a factor inhibiting the upward flow of information. True effective listening is a time-consuming process, and under the pressure of many high-priority tasks it is easy to find yourself dealing with some items lightly, briefly, or not at all.

Present-day problems generated by increasing spans of control and multi-location assignments threaten to limit your available time even further. It therefore becomes necessary to make yourself remain focused on true priorities—your employees and their needs—and not allow the apparently important to divert you from what is genuinely important.

Probably one of the greatest inhibitors of upward communication lies in actions of the recent past: management's failure to respond to some earlier communication. A question, problem, or observation coming from an employee remains one-way communication and thus not true communication at all unless you make an effort to "close the loop" by providing the required feedback. This is not to say that employees should always expect to receive the responses they desire. Rather, they need simply to receive something indicating that their messages have been considered and that management responses are offered. Your feedback, after proper investigation, consideration, or consultation as appropriate, may be a simple, "Thanks very much for pointing it out; it's being taken care of," or "I'm sorry, but it can't be done (for such and such a reason)." However, without feedback your employees are likely to regard their concerns as "swallowed up by the system" and will be discouraged from communicating at all.

## Problems Involving Employees

Employees will invariably see downward communication as occurring more freely and frequently than upward communication could possibly occur. Tradition, authority, and prestige are all on the side of the management hierarchy in the way they favor downward communication over upward contact. After all, you feel free to call on your employees at just about any time, just as your manager is likely to feel free to call on you at any time. However, rarely will nonsupervisory employees feel that same degree of freedom in their ability to call on the boss.

Most of the mechanics of organizational communication favor the downward flow of communication, and management controls most of the means. Bulletin boards, public address systems, employee newspapers and other printed matter, and duplicating services are largely controlled by elements of management. The individual employee with something to communicate must usually do so either by writing it out or relating it orally to another person. Some things never get communicated upward because some employees are unwilling to communicate certain kinds of information. Some people simply will not relay a problem or concern to the supervisor because it has a personal dimension that they do not wish to reveal. Some may also hesitate to point out certain problems for fear of being blamed for causing them, and for like reason they will say nothing they might consider to be self-incriminating or self-deprecating in any way.

A final but sometimes insurmountable barrier to upward communication is found in emotion and prejudice on the part of a few employees. To a limited number of nonsupervisory employees, management, even though it may be enlightened, humane, and people-centered, is to be regarded as exploitative and untrustworthy simply because it *is* management. Frequently this attitude extends so far as to regard the new supervisor moving up from the ranks as abandoning the good guys and joining the bad guys. Rarely will an employee harboring such a view of management discuss any serious concerns with the supervisor—unless the supervisor has conscientiously worked to earn the employee's trust and confidence.

## YOUR ROLE IN ORGANIZATIONAL COMMUNICATION

Have you ever found yourself, perhaps in anger or frustration, voicing the opening quotation: "The trouble with this place is there's no communication"? If the truth could be determined, we would probably discover that most supervisors have said this (or something very much like it) more than just a few times. However, the next time you feel inclined to cry "no communication," you might do well to consider that much of the supervisor's role in organizational communication depends on you and what you do and say. Before dwelling on the shortcomings that "they" exhibit—"they" being the often-blamed but never specifically identified villains of "they won't let me do it," "they didn't tell me," for example—it might prove more productive to work on your own communications practices. You cannot change someone else's habits and practices, but you can encourage them to change these for themselves and you can best do this by changing your own behavior.

Look at the simplified diagram of Figure 29–1. You, the supervisor, are in the middle. Your lines of communication run between you and other people in the organization. Your strictly formal lines of communication are those numbered 1, 2, 5, and 6; these depict the direct reporting relationships that exist between you and your employees and you and your immediate superior. Lines 3 and 4 suggest a large number of less rigid but still formal communicating relationships. These relationships are still formal because although you neither manage nor report to any of the people who work in or manage other functions and departments throughout the institution, you nevertheless require communication with many of them in the performance of your job.

First appreciate that communication along three of the six lines shown (those outgoing lines, numbered 1, 3, and 5) is completely in your hands. As the sender of a message, the originator of a communication, you have full control over all information leaving you. You control what is sent, why it is sent, how it is sent, to whom it is sent, and where it goes. And you can always send something. Even when a communication you wish to send is dependent on your first receiving something from another party, you can at least say "I don't know yet," "I'm still waiting," or "I'll call you as soon as I hear."

The point of this discussion is twofold: (1) your outgoing channels of communication are completely under your control and (2) the best way to get information moving along your incoming lines of communication is to assure that the outgoing lines are open and operating.

Of your incoming lines of communication you have the greatest degree of control over number 2, information flowing from your employees. Some of this control is due to the authority of your position; these people report to you, so most of them expect to give you certain information at certain times.

An additional measure of control will stem from your degree of success in requesting and receiving feedback from your employees. This is where assign-

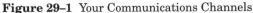

**Figure 29-1** Your Communications Channels

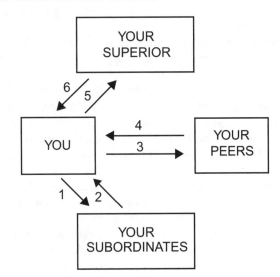

ment completion targets and deadlines and periodic reports come into the picture, along with your effective use of follow-up. In short, you can manage in a way that assures you will receive a great deal of work-related communication simply because your style tells your employees you both need it and expect it. However, there remains a sometimes considerable amount of information you would like to know as a supervisor, such as individual complaints, claims of unfair treatment, and dissension between employees, that cannot be mandated by structure or approach. You will receive this added information only by earning the trust and confidence of your employees and by showing through your actions that you are willing to communicate openly, honestly, and in confidence.

Some of the most valuable feedback you can receive from employees concerns your continuing performance and especially any mistakes you make. If an employee will tell you, willingly, honestly, and constructively, that a decision of yours appears inappropriate or that you seem to be heading in an improper direction, you will have achieved a positive communicating relationship with that employee. Many employees will say nothing if they see "the boss" getting into trouble. But if you have the employees' trust and respect, if you have proven they can be critical of you without negative repercussions, they will speak up. One of the most valuable assets you can have as a supervisor consists of employees who will prevent you from shooting yourself in the foot.

You have considerably less control over the information reaching you by way of line 4, the channel running from other organizational elements to you. You do not work for any of these people and they do not work for you. Because of your level or position you may possess some implied authority with some of these people, but you will have no authority at all with numerous others. Therefore, your communicating relationship with these people has to be based on cooperation. You must display the willingness to communicate and the ability to decide, when you are ready to send something out: who else truly needs it, who should be aware of it, and to whom it should go as a matter of information or simple courtesy.

Again, the best way to get information moving in is first to see that it is freely moving out. Do so even if you have to shake off the old "50-50 ethic," the pressure suggesting that in our communication, as well as in other endeavors, it is only "fair" for each party to go halfway. Some people will respond to your conscientious efforts in kind; others, however, will respond inadequately or not at all. Nevertheless, you should be prepared consistently to go more than halfway more than half of the time. If this sounds unfair to you, then look at it from a selfish point of view: the person who is benefiting most from your extra communications effort is you.

The one channel of communication not yet discussed, number 6, leading from your superior to you, presents more problems than the others. It is on this channel that you stand the least chance of exerting some appreciable measure of control. Obviously, you do not have positional authority to help you in this relationship; in fact, the reverse is true. Your communicating relationship with your boss, then, deserves special attention.

## Getting Your Boss to Communicate

You may be able to skim through these few paragraphs and worry not at all about what they contain if your immediate supervisor is a conscientious practitioner of the art of effective communication. On the other hand, you may have sufficient problems with this particular relationship to make these few words worth considering.

Once again, how you are communicated with is to some extent a reflection of how you communicate. The following are a few ways in which you can "tune up" your communications along line 5 in an attempt to stimulate more effective communication along line 6.

### Be Selective in What You Communicate

Do not expect your boss to do your job for you and take care of your problems. When something comes up and your initial impulse is to turn to the boss for information, advice, or assistance, before doing so make sure it is something you cannot take care of yourself. One of your legitimate functions as a supervisor is to be a "problem filter" for your boss, screening out those matters that should be resolved at a lower level.

### Do Your Homework

It has been stated several times in this book that the existence of problems is one of the major reasons for the existence of managers. No manager really needs more problems than are already present. Sufficient problems make themselves felt at all organizational levels, so what your boss needs are solutions. Even though many problems you encounter might be beyond the range of your decision-making authority, you can do more toward solving them than simply passing them one block up the organizational chart.

Remember that you are just one of several people reporting to the same superior, and what may look like a trickle of trouble to you may strike the boss as a flood of grief. Rather, when you must pass a problem up the line, you should do so having analyzed it, assessed its implications, prepared perhaps two or three alternative solutions, and possibly recommended the answer that looks best to you. In short, instead of saying, "Here's a problem. What do you want me to do?" you should be saying, "Here's a problem; here's why it's a problem; here are one or two (or however many) possible solutions; here's the answer I think is best, and here's why."

### Structure Your Communications

This is a variation of the previous point in which you were advised to do the spadework necessary to make decision making easier for your superior. When you need information, especially small bits of advice or minor decisions, put your questions in writing in such a way that they can be answered in one or two words. To cite an example, a staff education director was having difficulty obtaining a few minutes of discussion time with an extremely busy administrator on a matter of great concern to the director. Unable to get time with the administrator, the director reexamined the situation, expressing the problem in the form of three concise questions. After typing the questions on a single sheet of paper, the director left them on the administrator's telephone. The next morning the answers were on the staff education director's desk (see Exhibit 29–1).

*Make Yourself Available*

Some bosses are thoughtful enough to say something like, "The best time to get me is first thing in the morning before the telephone starts to ring," or "I'm likely to be free between 4:00 and 4:30." Even without such assistance, however, you may often find you are in a position to know your manager's comings and goings and develop a sense for the better times to try for a brief audience. Although a conscientious manager will try to be available to someone with a problem, this conscientiousness may not be particularly visible to you, because, as noted earlier, you may be but one of several supervisors reporting to this manager and the activity you see may be only the tip of the iceberg. So make yourself available to the boss, and in doing so strive to consume as little time as possible. This latter point concerning time is raised not because we are claiming the boss's time is valuable, although it certainly may be, but because your time is valuable. Most of your time belongs to your department, not to your boss.

## When the Boss Is More Than One

"Too many bosses" was cited in Chapter 10 as one of the reasons why people quit jobs. The multiple-boss situation can exist in two distinct ways: hazy lines of authority under which one is unclear as to who is actually calling the

---

**Exhibit 29–1** A Structured Commuication

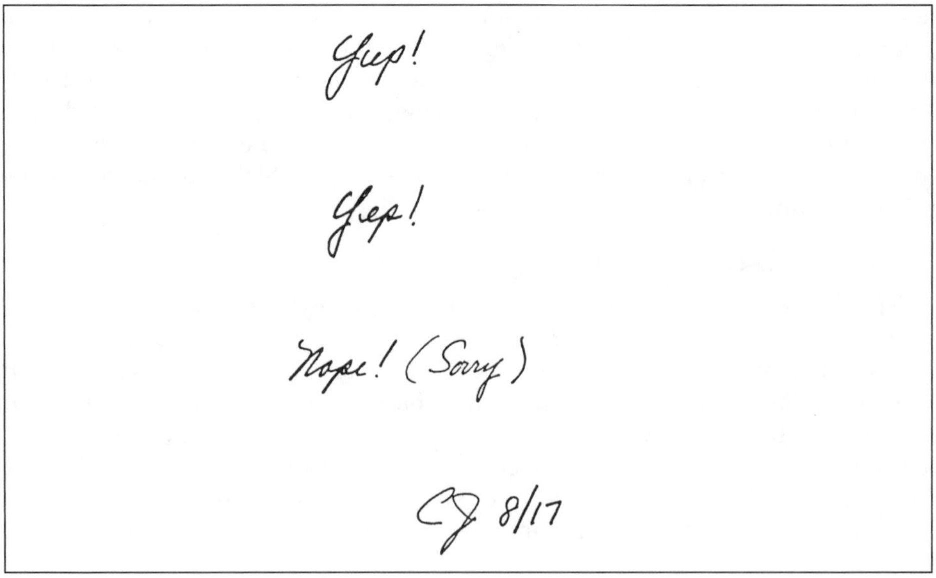

*Yup!*

*Yep!*

*Nope! (Sorry)*

*CJ 8/17*

shots much of the time and assignments that legitimately call for reporting to more than one manager. The first, the hazy lines of authority, is contrary to the basic principle of unity of command and is in fact never legitimate. The second, that of split or multiple reporting relationships, is becoming more common in health care organizations.

Multiple reporting relationships have proliferated as multidepartment, multifacility, or multilocation assignments have increased. It is becoming more and more common for an individual supervisor to have to balance reporting relationships with two and sometimes even three bosses. Consider the finance director assigned to two facilities within a large health system, reporting to each separate facility's chief executive officer as well as to the system's vice president for finance. This individual must legitimately balance the needs of three bosses.

Unfortunately, how well multiple boss arrangements work often depends more on the behavior of the bosses than on the shared supervisor. The higher manager who behaves as though his or her needs usually supersede all others' can make life miserable for the supervisor and eventually destroy the arrangement itself. Higher management has as much to learn about functioning in such arrangements as do the supervisors subject to them.

Multiple-boss arrangements work best when all parties at both levels fully understand the others' needs and understand what is expected of them individually. The supervisor who works in a successful multiple-boss assignment—without taking advantage of the freedom afforded by the usual remoteness of most or all superiors at any given time—is often rewarded with the satisfaction that comes with autonomous functioning. That is, rather than feeling like many bosses are demanding things of you, it is possible to feel more like your own boss than ever before.

## THE GRAPEVINE

What we know as "the grapevine" may be more accurately described as the communications network of the informal organization. Every organization has a formal structure, a network of reporting relationships describable by the well-known organization chart. Your formal lines of communication follow many of the relationships suggested on the organization chart. However, you also have, as everyone in the organization has, a number of informal channels of communication. Informal relationships with friends, acquaintances, relatives, and others with whom you speak in the work organization lead to the flow of communication. Furthermore, many of these relationships at least partially describe the informal organization, which is that implied structure that exists based on numerous related effects of respect, acknowledgment, deference, or prestige accorded various individuals primarily because of personality impact.

You have seen the informal organization at work when a certain two or three nonsupervisory employees happen to stand out from the group, perhaps even speaking for others, although they have no official standing, or when a single supervisor is regarded as "senior" by the work group over a number of others at the same level because of some particular trait or combination of traits. In short, interpersonal relationships and people's regard for one another describe the informal organization, at best a phantom structure that is always shifting and realigning.

People will talk. The grapevine is not required by management, and it is certainly not controlled by management. It runs merrily back and forth across departmental lines and rapidly changes its course. The grapevine is dynamic but unreliable. It carries a great deal of misinformation, but it is here to stay.

Be aware of the grapevine. Tune in; listen to what it is carrying and learn from it. As a supervisor you are likely to be isolated from some of the bits and pieces the grapevine carries, or at least you will miss a few things until they have been around awhile. How much you hear is frequently dependent on how well you relate with your employees and peers.

When you are tuned in to the grapevine you are going to hear a few things that you know are simply not correct. When you hear something that is disturbing or strikes you as inappropriate, check it out if possible. As a supervisor you are responsible for setting the facts of the story right whenever you have the opportunity to do so, but be sure you have your story straight so you do not simply heap more speculation onto a growing rumor.

The grapevine sometimes possesses the distinct advantages of speed and depth of penetration. Some bits of news can travel through the organization at an astonishing rate and often reach people who would never think to read a bulletin board or look at an employee newsletter. The grapevine can carry the good as well as the bad, and because it will always be with you, it is to your advantage to feed it some real facts whenever possible so it will have something useful to carry.

## DEALING WITH "THE UNREQUESTED INFORMATION"

Referring to the "Situation" at the beginning of the chapter, it is hoped that we all would consider the first option to be out of the question. You have been provided with a load of hearsay, and even without the admonition, "Please don't say I told you so," you would have no business taking any definitive action against anyone based on second-hand evidence (which is really no evidence at all). You certainly do not want to encourage one employee to continue being an informer.

Concerning the third choice, after hearing Mrs. Morris you will probably not be able to avoid being more than normally aware of Mrs. Greely's presence and behavior. So much for keeping an eye on Mrs. Greely; you will be fairly sensitive to everything she does for some time to come. If you thank Mrs. Morris at all you should stress the "concern for the department." However, asking her to "say nothing to anyone else" is risky in that doing so might seem to be drawing the two of you into a conspiratorial relationship.

The best option is the middle one, but it does not go far enough. You need to question her concerning what she has been telling you. If you have heard general condemnations, you should ask for specifics; for example, exactly who did precisely what and when, and how it could be proven. You need to tell her that without provable specifics you can take no action on anything she perceives as a problem.

Also, in a situation such as this you need always to watch out for factionalism—division in the ranks of your employees. Perhaps Mrs. Morris and Mrs. Greely are at the centers of opposing factions—not a far-fetched notion—and either faction would probably like to have you perceive that one as the "good" one.

You will need to keep your eyes open concerning your entire department, and step up your meetings with individual employees and small groups as possible. Undoubtedly something is going on, but based on Mrs. Morris's information you have no idea what it is. Unfortunately, all Mrs. Morris really did by coming to you was to provide you the basis for some substantial worry.

## WHICH WAY DO YOU FACE?

Your employees are likely to infer a great deal about your overall attitude as a supervisor according to how effectively you communicate. It is also likely that many such inferences will be influenced by your visibility and availability, that is, how much your employees see of you in and around the department and how readily they can get a few minutes of your time when they need it.

In our organizations there are many pressures that cause us to "face upward" and in general be most visible and available to our superiors and other members of higher management. After all, it is notice from above that leads to pay increases, promotions, and other rewards. There are some traps in this reasoning, however. Not all higher managers are necessarily impressed by your ready availability to them. In fact, some of the more effective top managers, if they see what they believe is too much of you, will begin to wonder who is running your department while you are busy looking upward.

What we are getting at, of course, is the desirability for the supervisor to spend most of the time "facing downward" toward the ranks of the employees in the department. It is there you will find the real action, the real challenges, and the true opportunities.

Supervisors must be conscious of the necessity to develop and cultivate all communicating relationships in the organization, but your most important communicating relationships will remain those that you establish with your employees. Regardless of the number and capability of the managers in any health care institution, it remains largely the nonmanagerial employees who do the hands-on work of delivering patient care. You are there to ensure that the portion of patient care for which you are responsible is accomplished in the best interest of the patients. Your primary attentions belong to the people who do the work. In the last analysis, it remains your employees who, through their job performance, can determine whether you succeed or fail as a manager.

## REVIEW QUESTIONS

1. Why is it generally more difficult for information to flow upward than downward in the work organization?
2. Why is effective communication with your fellow supervisors usually more difficult to achieve than with your employees?
3. What practice do you believe creates the greatest barrier to the upward flow of information from employees to management?
4. Is there any practical value to the "grapevine," and if so what might it be?
5. What is probably the most difficult area of communication for the supervisor to control? Why is it difficult?
6. How and why do you communicate when you believe you have nothing new of substance to communicate?

## CASE: THE CRUNCH

You and four other supervisors are at a meeting with your immediate boss, the department head to whom the five of you report. Also present are two other department heads and a member of the administrative staff. The subject of the meeting is sensitive.

Just minutes into the meeting the boss makes a statement that you know to be incorrect. You attempt to intervene, but the boss asks you to hold your comments. He seems to be focusing almost entirely on the other department heads and the visitor from administration.

Your boss proceeds to build an argument on his incorrect statement, and you can sense that he is verbally painting himself into a corner. Because you have already been silenced once you are hesitant to speak up again, and although you are sure of your information, you have no way of proving anything without making a trip to your office and rummaging through some files. Within the confines of the conference room it would simply be your word against his, and he is the boss.

What should you do? In deciding on a possible course of action, consider the implications of

- keeping quiet and allowing the boss to proceed in apparent error
- intruding, forcefully if necessary, until your information is heard by the group.

## CHAPTER 30

# Unions: Avoiding Them When Possible and Living with Them When Necessary

*If you don't have them, the best way to avoid them is to create a Theory Y environment where your people have a chance to realize their potential. If you already have unions, then deal with them openly and honestly.*
—*Robert Townsend*

## CHAPTER OBJECTIVES

☛ Explore the apparent reasons for the organizing success of many unions, with emphasis on the basic management errors often leading to unionization.

☛ Describe the circumstances that make health care a particularly fertile ground for union organizing.

☛ Describe the typical union organizing approach.

☛ Define the supervisor's active role during a union organizing campaign.

☛ Stress the importance of the supervisor's role in effective two-way communication with employees—whether or not the employees belong to a union.

## SITUATION: THE CONFRONTATION

You are head nurse of a medical-surgical unit that has been operating at full capacity for a number of months. Times have been hectic, so you have been pitching in on the floor much more than used to be necessary. On days when you have been short-staffed you have been providing lunch relief personally for one or two other nurses. This practice has caused you to change your own lunchtime to the time when the hospital cafeteria is most crowded.

Today you have just gotten your lunch and are standing in the dining room, tray in hands, looking for familiar faces and open seats, when you are approached and very nearly circled by three of your staff members. One of them says to you, "We've been meaning to talk with you, but we're all so much on the run that we haven't gotten to you. Things have got to change around here. We can't keep going the way we're going. We're thinking of asking a union to come in, and we want to talk with you about it—now."

There you stand in the middle of the noisy, crowded cafeteria dining room, tray in both hands, feeling surrounded.

*Instructions*

As you proceed through this chapter, consider the following question: How should you handle this incident?

## CAN UNIONIZATION BE AVOIDED?

A study of union organizing campaigns and their results over the recent three to four decades would likely lead to the following three conclusions, verified time and again through experience:

1. Most organizing campaigns have focused on economic issues, at least up until the 1990s when we began to see more union emphasis on job security and quality of work life. Most initial demands have been unreasonable, reflecting ignorance or indifference concerning the organizations' true financial positions. In many instances the unions won because of apparent management indifference to complaints, no response to employees' problems, and lack of credibility with employees in regard to costs and true operating circumstances.

2. In the majority of union victories, anti-management sentiment initially arises from working conditions that include poor organizational communication or arbitrary or seemingly uncaring management.

3. In many cases the anxiety produced by widespread lack of knowledge about what is truly happening provides a boost to the union cause.

In essentially all instances of elections lost to unions, it is possible to identify serious and usually long-standing morale problems among employees. Also in all such instances, management will be found to have been operating in something of a vacuum with respect to true employee feelings and opinions.

In testing the potential for unionization it is simply not enough for top management to have you talk to employees and report back on their feelings. True anti-management sentiment, potentially beneficial to a union organizer, is determined only through effective listening. Many employees—quite likely the majority—would prefer to be loyal to the organization, but the organization's seeming indifference to upward communication can discourage such loyalty. Also, the price of management indifference can be extremely high; if a union loses a bargaining election it may try again after one year has elapsed, and again and again until it succeeds, but the management need lose only once. If management does not listen to employees, the union organizers will.

There are three basic errors commonly committed by management in assessing the potential for success of union organizing efforts.

1. There is a widely prevalent management notion that most elements of worker dissatisfaction are due to wages, fringe benefits, and other economic items. However, initial organizing activity usually springs from non-economic matters involving issues that are not nearly as quantifiable as dollars. Employee dissatisfaction will ultimately be expressed in the form of financial demands. A specific financial package can be obtained by contract, but there is no contractual way to obtain less tangible items such as sympathetic listening, open communications, and humane and respectful treatment.

2. Many top managers automatically assume that all supervisors are on the side of management. However, most supervisors came up from the ranks within the functions they supervise and as such are an inte-

gral part of the work group. Also, in many institutions' first-line supervisors have been kept out of participation in real management decision-making.

3. Frequently nobody at the top of the organization has any solid idea of what is really troubling the ranks of nonmanagerial employees.

Commission of any of these basic management errors in one form or another can pave the way for a successful union organizing drive. More specifically, an institution can push its employees closer to a union by the following actions:

- introducing major changes in organization structure, job content, equipment, or operating practices without advance notice or subsequent explanation

- giving employees little or no information about the financial status of the institution or about its plans, goals, or achievements

- making key decisions in ignorance of the employees' true wants, needs, and feelings

- using pressure (authoritarian or autocratic leadership) rather than true leadership (consultative or participative leadership) to obtain employee performance

- disregarding or downplaying instances of employee dissatisfaction

In addition to the three basic management errors and the foregoing acts of managerial shortsightedness, some factors encouraging unionization are unique to health care. For a number of years, health care and industry in general have been moving in opposite directions in their appeal and suitability for union organizing. Present circumstances suggest that health care organizations will continue to be choice organizing targets for at least several years to come.

## HEALTH CARE: MORE AND MORE A SPECIAL CASE

It is no secret that the total number of jobs available in the manufacturing sector of the U.S. economy has been steadily declining for a number of years as competition and the "globalization" of business have sent an increasing number of jobs to foreign countries. Manufacturing was long the source of most union membership. However, as manufacturing jobs have been lost, the unions have shifted much of their focus to service industries. The service sector of the economy now employs more than 75 percent of the work force. Thus it comes as no surprise that many unions, having seen their membership dwindle for several years, have diversified and turned their attentions to the service industries.

Health care organizations in general, and hospitals in particular, are fertile grounds for union organizing and should continue as such for a number of years to come. From the 1970s to the present, total union membership dropped while union membership in health care continued to increase. The Department of Labor reported that during the year 2000 the percentage of American workers belonging to unions fell to 13.5 percent, the lowest in six decades.[1] As of this writing (early 2006) the percentage of the total work force that is unionized remains the smallest it has been since the late 1940s; however, the percentage of the health care work force that is unionized is presently the largest it has ever been.

Health care as an employment arena began to change dramatically during the late 1960s. Pressures intended to stem the steady increase of health care costs—which have gone up at twice or more the normal rate of inflation for years—continue to the present. Along the way, specifically in 1975, the National Labor Relations Act (NLRA) was amended to include hospitals and other health care organizations that had previously been excluded from coverage under the act. In 1975, when much of the industry was starting to see the effects of cost-containment efforts, the unions were given new opportunities in this significant segment of the service economy.

With much of health care in turmoil or near-turmoil, employees are feeling more and more uncertain about the future. In some parts of the country where hospitals are severely underutilized, many employees perceive a threat to their continued full-time employment. As health care providers attempt to meet shifting demands in the most economical fashion by adopting more staffing variations—more part-time employment, flextime and other nontraditional approaches, and job sharing and the like—employees are further threatened by the perceived uncertainty of their situation.

The survival-oriented remedies of many provider organizations have included staff cuts, mergers, downsizing, and corporate reorganizing. As a partial result, employees perceive a direct threat to the quality of the care they can provide and to their job security. The effects of health care organization restructuring—mergers, downsizing, and the rest—emerged as the number one human resources concern that hospitals faced in 1987.[2] These effects remain at the forefront of employee concern nearly two decades later; health care workers remain concerned for their jobs and their futures in health care. And while job security remains a critical issue targeted by health care union organizers, at the same time wages and benefits are becoming increasingly important to the predominantly female health care work force.

Tangibles such as pay and benefits are always prominent in the presence of labor unrest, but the turmoil in the health care industry drives far more than these economic concerns. When employees feel that their concerns are not being adequately addressed by management—and health care management is faced with some nearly overwhelming concerns, many of which seem to defy all attempts at resolution because of outside pressures and restrictions—these employees will turn to someone else who will seem to listen. Often this "someone else" is a union.

It is possible, however, for the non-unionized institution to remain that way, and the individual supervisor has an important role in keeping the institution union-free.

## THE SUPERVISOR'S POSITION

Several parts of this book have talked about the importance of the supervisor-employee relationship. As the supervisor you are the member of management whom your employees know best. You indeed may be the only member of this mysterious entity called management whom most of your employees know on a first-name basis or even know on speaking terms at all. Thus, as your employees see you, so are they likely to see all of management and the organization itself. If they see you as unconcerned, uncaring, distant, or indifferent, they are likely to view the organization as a whole that way.

It follows, then, that the supervisor is in a key position when it comes to dealing with the threat of unionization. You are the link that ties your employees to higher management and thus to the organization. Your long-term behavior will have a great deal to do with whether your department is a fertile ground for union organizing activity, and your conduct and actions during an organizing campaign will exert a significant influence on your employees' reaction to the organizing drive.

## THE ORGANIZING APPROACH

What do the first stages of a union organizing campaign look like? You might be inclined to answer this question by citing one of the first signs visible to you—"leafleting," or the distribution of union literature to employees at walkways, driveways, and parking lot entrances. However, although serious leafleting is an undeniable indication of union activity, it is ordinarily not the first step in an organizing campaign. Chances are the union has been studying the institution for weeks or even months, to judge its organizing potential, before the first literature appears.

When organizing activity actually begins, management may well know nothing about it. In fact, during the earliest stages the union may take considerable precautions to prevent management from learning about their interest. The union may send organizers into the institution simply to loiter and listen and pick up what they can from conversations in the cafeteria, snack bar, parking area, employee lounge areas, and other such places where employees congregate informally. Outsiders can move freely in many institutions, and such infiltration is especially easy in an institution that does not use employee identification badges or passes for visitors and vendors. The organizers will simply merge with the crowd and listen, picking up gripes, locating supervisory weaknesses and departments with obvious morale problems, and identifying informal leaders among the employees. They will try to learn as much as possible about the institution before revealing themselves.

The still-unannounced organizers will also attempt to pinpoint employees who have the potential to serve as internal organizers, looking especially for those employees who are popular, knowledgeable, reasonably articulate, and in some way unhappy with the organization.

Should their silent survey raise serious doubts that the institution could possibly be unionized, the organizers might simply withdraw without ever announcing their presence. However, if they believe the union stands a chance of succeeding they will likely identify themselves to a few selected employees and begin preparations to carry their message to others. Leafleting is likely to begin at about this stage.

The major exception to the usual significance of leafleting occurs in a practice sometimes referred to as a "pass-through." In a pass-through the union will devote a day or two to distributing literature at perhaps several institutions in the same general area. These are generally "cold" visits—no advance investigation has taken place. The union will simply "pass through" the area and drop off as much literature as possible with the employees of as many institutions as they can readily reach and follow up only if they receive expressions of interest from employees. (The pass-through literature usually includes a reply card to be returned for more information.)

When the organizers are out in the open and their purpose is generally known, they will step up their activities in meeting with employees and contacting them in other ways. Somewhere along the way, possibly through sympathetic employees, they will attempt to obtain a list of the names and addresses of all the institution's nonmanagerial employees. The union will most certainly be contacting many individual employees by telephone and will seek to visit the homes of others.

In talking with employees the union will attempt to uncover issues to use as rallying points for employee sympathy and support. The organizers will attempt to identify martyrs and victims of "the system" and will effectively play on emotions in spotlighting incidents of alleged unfair treatment and discrimination.

The union organizers will go to great lengths to impress on employees their right to be treated as individuals. This may seem elementary, because most of us will express strong belief in the rights of the individual. If, however, in the face of seemingly indifferent management the union organizer is the first person to tell them this, then the grounds for union credibility may exist. The organizers will make every effort to develop a communicating relationship with your employees. This should sound familiar, because the development of such a relationship is part of your role as a supervisor.

You can be sure that most issues and incidents brought to life by the union are specially selected to make management look bad. Lacking sufficient factual material, organizers frequently stage incidents intended to make the union look good and make management look foolish. The supervisor's awareness of this particular organizing tactic is critical; it is all too easy to make an inappropriate statement or incorrect decision when confronted with a trumped-up grievance or problem at an inconvenient time and under awkward circumstances (which usually includes the presence of some employee witnesses). Such matters would be rightly dealt with by administration, labor relations, or whoever else may be coordinating the institution's counterorganizing activities. However, there is a need for the supervisor to react on the spot, without making promises or commitments and without seeming to be refusing to listen to an employee. Afterward the incident can be promptly reported to the proper persons.

## UNEQUAL POSITIONS

Under the NLRA, unions and employers do not have equal clout in the organizing process. In many respects the union enjoys the upper hand. Under the act, an employer can commit an unfair labor practice and such charges can be brought against the organization by the union. If the National Labor Relations Board (NLRB), ruling on an unfair labor practice charge, upholds the union's claim, then the union may be automatically certified as a recognized bargaining agent without the necessity of a representation election. The law, however, does not work the other way around; generally, there is no such thing as an unfair labor practice committed by a union. Also, as noted earlier, if the union should lose a bargaining election it may petition for another election after one year has elapsed. The employer may well have to win year after year to remain union-free. However, the employer need lose only once and the union is in, permanently, for all practical purposes, because decertification of a union is difficult to achieve and occurs infrequently.

## YOUR ACTIVE ROLE

The guidelines pertinent to supervisory behavior during a union organizing campaign make up a sizeable collection of do's and don'ts (Exhibits 30–1 and 30–2). It is to your advantage to be sensitive to the limitations these requirements place on your actions and comments in your dealings with employees. Ideally, the supervisors in an institution undergoing organizing pressure should receive classroom training in these guidelines from a labor attorney or a labor relations expert.

---

**Exhibit 30–1** What the Supervisor *Can* Do When a Union Beckons

1. Campaign against a union seeking to represent employees, and reply to union attacks on the institution's practices or policies.
2. Give employees your opinions about unions, union policies, and union leaders.
3. Advise employees of their legal rights during and after the organizing campaign, and supply them with the institution's legal position on matters that may arise.
4. Keep outside organizers off institution premises.
5. Tell employees of the disadvantages of belonging to a union, such as strikes and picket-line duty; dues, fines, and assessments; rule by a single person or small group; and possible domination of a local by its international union.
6. Remind employees of the benefits they enjoy without a union, and tell them how their wages and benefits compare with those at other institutions (both union and nonunion).
7. Let employees know that signing a union authorization card is not a commitment to vote for the union if there is an election.
8. Tell employees that you would rather deal directly with them than attempt to settle differences through a union or any other outsiders.
9. Give employees factual information concerning the union and its officials, even if such information is uncomplimentary.
10. Remind employees that no union can obtain more for them than the institution is able to give.
11. Correct any untrue or misleading claims or statements made by the union organizers.
12. Inform employees that the institution may legally hire a new employee to replace any employee who strikes for economic reasons.
13. Declare a fixed position against compulsory union membership contracts.
14. Insist that all organizing be conducted outside of working time.
15. Question open and active union supporters about their union sentiments, as long as you do so without direct or implied threats or promises (see Shifting Ground Rules).
16. State that you do not like to deal with unions.

**Exhibit 30–2** What the Supervisor *Cannot* Do When a Union Beckons

1. Ask employees about their union sentiments in a manner that includes or implies threats, promises, or intimidation in any form. Employees may *volunteer* any such information and you may listen, but you may *ask* only with caution (see Shifting Ground Rules).
2. Attend union meetings or participate in any undercover activities to find out who is or is not participating in union activities.
3. Attempt to prevent internal organizers from soliciting memberships during nonworking time.
4. Grant pay raises or make special concessions or promises to keep the union out.
5. Discriminate against prounion employees in granting pay increases; apportioning overtime; making work assignments, promotions, layoffs, or demotions; or applying disciplinary action.
6. Intimidate, threaten, or punish employees who engage in union activity.
7. Suggest in any way that unionization will force the institution to close up, move, lay off employees, or reduce benefits.
8. Deviate from known institution policies for the primary purpose of eliminating a prounion employee.
9. Provide financial support or other assistance to employees who oppose the union, or be a party to a petition or such action encouraging employees to organize to reject the union.
10. Visit employees at home to urge them to oppose the union.
11. Question prospective employees about past union affiliation.
12. Make statements to the effect that the institution "will not deal with a union."
13. Use a third party to threaten, coerce, or attempt to influence employees in exercising their right to vote concerning union representation.
14. Question employees on whether they have or have not signed a union authorization card.
15. Use the word *never* in any statements or predictions about dealings with the union.

It is also to your advantage—at all times, but especially during a union organizing campaign—to know your employees as individuals, and know them well. Although people cannot be stereotyped, and there are few reliable generalizations concerning employees' receptiveness to a union, it is nevertheless possible for you to make some reasonable judgments as to how certain employees might react under organizing pressure. Often the employee sympathetic to the union's cause may

- feel unfairly treated by the organization and believe that reasonable work opportunities have been denied
- feel that the organization has been unsympathetic regarding personal problems and pressures
- express a lack of confidence in supervision or administration and be unwilling to talk openly with members of management
- feel unequally treated in terms of pay and other economic benefits
- take no apparent pride in affiliation with the institution
- exhibit career-path problems, having either changed jobs frequently or having reached the top in pay and classification while still having a significant number of working years remaining

- be a source of complaints or grievances more often than most other employees
- exhibit a poor overall attitude

As a supervisor it is extremely important for you to know your employees' attitudes toward the institution so you may develop a sense for how well you are communicating. Ultimately, a labor union has little to offer if employees already feel that the organization is responding to their needs.


## Shifting Ground Rules

The lists of what the supervisor can (Exhibit 30–1) and cannot do (Exhibit 30–2) in the presence of union organizing are based on interpretations of the NLRA by the NLRB. Many of these interpretations are clear-cut and have stood the test of time regardless of the composition of the NLRB. Some, however, are not clear-cut and are likely to change as the board's composition changes. The matter of management's questioning of employees about union sentiments and activities is the best illustration of this possibility.

For years it has been relatively accurate to cite the so-called "TIPS Rule" in summarizing the most important elements of what a member of management could not do during union organizing: A manager could not Threaten, Interrogate, Promise, or Spy. (You may have encountered "TIPS" as "SPIT" or "PITS," depending on the arrangement of the four prohibitions.)

In the middle 1980s the NLRB loosened its interpretation of interrogation to suggest that it is lawful for an employer to question union supporters about their union sentiments as long as the questioning carries with it no threats or promises and in no way interferes with or restrains the employees in the exercise of their rights under the NLRA.

The present posture on interrogation is hardly new; it had been an applied principle of labor relations for 30 years until 1980. In 1980, however, when the NLRB was dominated by the Democratic Party, the stricter interpretation of the interrogation prohibitions of the law was imposed. This stricter interpretation was reversed in 1984, when the NLRB composition changed again. However, even the principle as it is currently applied does not mean that most questioning of employees about union involvement is necessarily "safe." It essentially means that an unfair labor practice charge concerning interrogation will not automatically go against management but will likely be subjected to searching analysis to determine whether any aspect of the questioning may have been coercive. The "TIPS Rule" remains valid in that interrogation still carries with it a fair amount of risk.

Should you find yourself in the midst of a union organizing drive, pay strict attention to your institution's labor attorney and labor relations director (or whoever is coordinating management's counter-organizing efforts) for advice on what to do and what to avoid. Although the actions enumerated in Exhibits 30–1 and 30–2 should remain largely valid, some of them may vary in content or emphasis from one national administration to another depending on the makeup of the NLRB.

### Handling "The Confrontation"

In reference to the "Situation" presented at the beginning of the chapter, you should certainly want to hear what is on your employees' minds; however, the one clear way not to address the problem is to give in to what they want and immediately talk about their consideration of a union. You are in a sufficiently awkward position to make you suspect that this encounter was deliberately timed to catch you off guard.

However you do it, get the meeting out of the crowded cafeteria into some private space where you can all talk over lunch so that you can hold the discussion as much as possible on your own terms. Also, the slight delay involved in finding a space or setting up a time will allow the surprise effect to wear off and give you at least a few minutes in which to order your thoughts.

This encounter can be made to work to your advantage. Recall that you cannot legally ask employees about their interest or involvement in union activities (you cannot threaten, interrogate, promise, or spy). However, you can listen to what employees tell you. Just take care that the steps you take to encourage further conversation do not involve direct questioning, and avoid threatening or promising as you answer questions as best as you can.

## THE BARGAINING ELECTION

The union, working through both outside and inside organizers, will go about the business of securing sufficient employee interest to allow it to petition the NLRB for a bargaining election. Generally the indications of such support will take the form of simple cards that employees sign to indicate interest in having an election. Employees should be aware that signing a card is not an automatic "yes" vote for union representation but rather simply an expression of interest in having an election.

When sufficient signatures are gathered (usually half or more of the number of employees in the unit that the union is seeking to represent, although the union need have signatures from just 30 percent of eligible employees to legally submit its petition), the union will petition the NLRB. After what is usually a cursory investigation, the board will sanction an election and a date for voting will be set.

Election is by secret ballot, and all employees who work in the unit the union is seeking to represent are eligible to vote. If the union receives a simple majority of the vote it will then be certified by the board as the legal bargaining agent for all persons who work in the unit. Although compulsory union membership is not required by law, this usually means that all persons working in the unit must eventually join the union because this particular right of the union is usually bargained for in the initial contract.

If the union fails to achieve a simple majority and various possible legal challenges do not upset the results of the election, the union will withdraw, at least for a while if the vote was close, or perhaps for a longer period if the results were clearly one-sided.

Keep in mind, however, that some elections are little more than formalities—many elections are lost long before the organizers ever show up. If the trend in relations between employees and management is clearly in the direction of a union, this can be difficult to reverse. Reversal may, however, be accomplished through hard work and plenty of open and honest communication.

Even if a single unit of employees is lost to a union (for instance, a union representing service and maintenance employees or one representing only licensed practical nurses), then new steps aimed at creating positive communicating relationships can still pay off. A new atmosphere can make contract bargaining easier, smooth out day-to-day labor relations matters, and help keep other bargaining units out of the institution.

## IF THE UNION WINS

Shortly after the union is certified as a recognized bargaining unit, an initial contract will be negotiated. This gives supervisors a whole new set of rules and regulations to live with.

Learn the contract inside out—learn what it says, learn what it does not say, and learn why it says what it says—and comply with it faithfully. Some contracts seem top-heavy with numerous details and exacting requirements, but you may find that some parts of your job are actually easier because there are now hard and fast rules for situations that were previously subject to interpretation and judgment.

Above all, as advised by Robert Townsend in the opening quotation, be open and honest in your dealings with the union.

The presence of a union does not mean you can back off in your communications with employees and simply wave the contract at them. Complete two-way communication remains essential in establishing and maintaining your relationships with all your employees whether you do or do not have a union. After all, your employees work for the institution, not for the union. Generally the union will be the employees' voice only if the employees feel they are not recognized as individuals and are not being heard by management.

---

## REVIEW QUESTIONS

1. Why do most union demands seem to revolve around pay and benefits when we know there are a variety of reasons that can cause employees to seek representation?

2. In a union-organizing situation why might some supervisors be sympathetic toward employees as opposed to remaining solidly loyal to management?

3. Why do you believe organizing within healthcare has been expanding while union membership overall has declined?

4. Leafleting may be the first visible sign of union interest in your organization's employees. Is anything likely to have occurred before leafleting, and if so, what?

5. Why can a union legally promise unorganized employees anything its representatives wish to promise to induce people to accept the union, but the organization's management cannot legally promise anything to induce employees to reject the union?

6. How are you going to answer the long-time employee who asks you, "Should I vote for or against this union?"

---

## CASE: THE ORGANIZER

You are the central supply supervisor in a hospital presently under union organizing pressure. The union's drive has reached the stage of signature cards. You are passing through one of the nursing units when you observe an individual who you believe is a union organizer backing one of the nurse's aides into a corner and waving what appears to be a union authorization card. The aide looks worried and in considerable distress and also appears to be physically trapped in the corner by the other party. You cannot hear what the person with the card is saying, but you believe you recognize the kind of card this person is waving and you can tell this person is speaking quite forcefully.

Describe what you would do under the following sets of circumstances:

1. You recognize the probable organizer as an employee of the hospital but belonging to a department other than your own.

2. You are reasonably certain the probable organizer is not an employee of the hospital.

---

**NOTES**

1. The Associated Press, "Public Support Grows for Unions," *Democrat and Chronicle* (Rochester, NY), 30 August 2001.

2. F. Cerne, "Job Security Topped Employee Concerns in 1987," *Hospitals,* 20 December 1987, 56.

# Annotated Bibliography

**Aspen Reference Group.** *The Aspen Guide to Effective Health Care Correspondence.* Gaithersburg, MD: Aspen Publishers, Inc., 1993.
This guide provides supervisors and managers with a fairly wide range of letters that can be used as models for routine as well as specialized correspondence in most areas of health care facility operations. Rarely will one of these letters fill your specific need exactly, but if you are unsure of how to approach a certain topic in a letter, one of these may at least get you started by providing a sample you can adapt to your situation.

**Barnes, Ralph M.** *Motion and Time Study: Design and Measurement of Work.* 7th ed. New York: John Wiley & Sons, 1980.
This book is the definitive work on the analysis of work motions and the establishment of time or performance standards. It is easily the most comprehensive volume available on the tools and techniques of methods analysis. Although the book is clearly intended as a text for industrial engineers or management engineers, a number of its sections, such as those on the general problem-solving process and human engineering, are useful to anyone interested in improving work methods. This volume clearly and understandably details all the known and proven tools applied in methods improvement.

**Becker-Reems, Elizabeth D.** *Self-Managed Work Teams in Health Care Organizations.* American Hospital Association, 1984.
This book may prove helpful because of the growing interest in the use of self-managed work teams, in part a feature of many total quality management (TQM) implementations. It addresses all sides of the numerous issues surrounding the question of the feasibility of such teams while clearly advocating the benefits of self-managed teams.

**Berne, Eric.** *Games People Play.* New York: Grove Press, 1964 (original publication). Also mass-market paperbacks, 1967 and 1975 from Dell; and 1975, 1980, and 1981 from Random House Publishing Group.
Much of Berne's work presented in *Games People Play* formed the basis of the later work by Thomas Harris, *I'm O.K.—You're O.K.*, essentially making Berne, a psychiatrist, one of the founders of transactional analysis. *Games*

*People Play* is an interesting and important book in the study of the psychology of human relationships. It is not the easiest book to read, and the reading can be risky because we are likely to recognize ourselves in the deadly serious little "games" we play with each other almost every day of our lives. This book remains in print and is readily available.

**Brown, Montague**, Editor. *Health Care Financial Management*. Gaithersburg, MD: Aspen Publishers, Inc., 1992.
This work constitutes a third collection of articles from *Health Care Management Review*. This volume offers insights and techniques for more effective financial management and control of the health care organization. From this volume the supervisor can acquire guidance on financial analysis; capital purchase decisions; and cost, price, and managerial accounting.

**Brown, Montague**, Editor. *Health Care Management: Strategy, Structure, and Process*. Gaithersburg, MD: Aspen Publishers, Inc., 1992.
This work is a collection of articles from the journal *Health Care Management Review*. Although focusing on themes and topics relevant to chief executive officers, this collection is helpful to supervisors who wish to learn more about the major issues and concerns driving health care organizations. Included are articles on strategy formulation, vertical integration, hospital alliances, and total quality management.

**Brown, Montague**, Editor. *Human Resource Management in Health Care*. Gaithersburg, MD: Aspen Publishers, Inc., 1992.
This is another collection of articles from *Health Care Management Review*. Also targeted largely toward chief executive officers, this collection nevertheless provides the supervisor with insight into the broader human resource issues that concern today's health care managers. Included are useful articles on high-performance management and leadership, cultural change, performance appraisal systems, management stress, and managing the effects of mergers and downsizing.

**Cleverly, William O.** *Essentials of Health Care Finance*, 4th ed. Gaithersburg, MD: Aspen Publishers, Inc., 1997.
This is basic financial management for hospitals and other health care organizations, kept as completely up to date as possible with the ever-changing health care finance and reimbursement environment. A valuable aid in improving your understanding of the overall finances of the organization and a practical guide for making financially related decisions at the department level.

**Coile, Russell C., Jr.** *The New Medicine: Reshaping Medical Practice and Health Care Management*. Gaithersburg, MD: Aspen Publishers, Inc., 1990.
This is an extremely helpful book for the supervisor to read for a broad perspective concerning where organized health care is likely to be going beyond the 1990s. Chances are the supervisor who has remained in the system for more than just a few years has seen active involvement in one of the author's "Alternative Scenarios for the Future of Medicine in the Year 2000." In any

case, it is interesting to check out the "year 2000" predictions to see what has or has not come to pass.

**Cribbin, James J.** *Leadership: Strategies for Organizational Effectiveness.* New York: AMACOM, A Division of American Management Associations, 1981. Also a trade paperback edition in 1984, also from AMACOM.

This is a clear and readable treatment of leadership that takes a fairly down-to-earth look at the essentials of leadership from the individual supervisor's point of view. Especially helpful are the chapters concerned with organization approaches to motivation and leadership values.

**Crichton, Michael.** *Five Patients.* New York: Alfred A. Knopf. Originally published in 1970; mass-market paperback from William Morrow and Co., Inc., in 1981; mass-market paperback from Alfred A. Knopf, 1988; new hardcover edition from Sagebrush Education Resources, 1989; and new mass-market paperback edition in 1994.

Subtitled *The Hospital Explained*, this book is highly recommended to all persons interested in the management of health institutions at any level. Crichton uses five graphic illustrations—five patients and how their cases were handled—to trace the development of hospitals and their services from the days of simply custodial care to the ultimate in medical sophistication. Fully as pertinent as the day it was first published, you can read this for greater understanding of medical practice, hospital life and problems, and hospital staff and their responsibilities. *Five Patients* reads like a good novel but is medically authentic. (Best known as an author of popular suspense and science fiction, Crichton is also a physician.)

**Drucker, Peter F.** *The Practice of Management.* New York: Harper & Row, 1954; trade paperback edition, 1986, Harper Collins Publishers; paperback reissue, 1986, Harper Business; audio cassette 1990, Harper Collins Publishers; paperback reissue 1993.

Along with Drucker's *Managing for Results* (Harper & Row, 1964), *The Practice of Management* stands out as one of the highlights of this particular author's productive output. This is recommended reading for any supervisor who truly enjoys management and aspires to rise higher in the organization. One chapter of particular value is "Management by Objectives and Self-Control" (which gave us a whole "new" approach to management—management by objectives). The original hardcover is long out of print, but subsequent paperbacks are available.

**Etzioni, Amitai.** *Modern Organizations*, Prentice-Hall Foundations of Modern Sociology Series, 1964; Prentice-Hall Professional Technical Reference, 1997.

The basic premise of this rather academic work is that modern civilization depends largely on organizations as the most rational and efficient form of social grouping known. The book addresses organizational goals, organizational structure, and organizations and their social environment, providing a number of valuable insights in fewer than 120 pages.

**Fast, Julius.** *Body Language.* New York: M. Evans and Company, 1970. Mass-market paperback editions 1971, 1975, 1977, 1978, and 1980, Simon and Schuster Adult Publishing Group; new hardcover 1988, M. Evans; new hardcover 1992, Fine Communications; trade paperback, revised and updated, 2002, M. Evans.

This interesting and entertaining book deals with kinesics, the study of non-verbal human communication or "body language," which can include any reflexive or nonreflexive movement of all or a part of the body used by a person to communicate an emotional message. The implications for interpersonal communication are significant; for instance, the book cites studies that reveal the extent to which body language can actually contradict verbal communications. *Body Language* will give you some interesting and potentially helpful insights into the actions that surround or accompany a person's words.

**Goldsmith, Seth B.** *Principles of Health Care Management: Compliance, Consumerism, and Accountability in the 21st Century.* Sudbury, MA: Jones & Bartlett Publishers, 2005.

This is a textbook for students in health administration programs as well as a reference for working health care managers. The central theme of the book is accountability but its focus is effective management. It provides a foundation for the understanding of the country's health care system, reviews the essentials of health care management, looks at the critical area of corporate com-pliance, and addresses the effects of consumerism on the health care organization. Included are several useful case studies.

**Gordon, Thomas.** *Leader Effectiveness Training (L.E.T.).* New York: Wyden Books, 1977; new hardcover 2001, Penguin Group (USA) (and several updated versions between 1983 and 2001).

If you seriously delve into only one or two books described in this bibliography, *Leader Effectiveness Training* should be one of your choices. Written in a clear, easily readable style, it takes a common-sense, humanistic approach to the task of getting things done through people. This book stresses the cultivation and maintenance of open and honest interpersonal relationships. The chapter titles speak for themselves: "Doing it Yourself—Or with the Group's Help," "Making Everyday Use of Your Listening Skills," and "The No-Lose Method: Turning Conflict into Cooperation."

**Haimann, Theo.** *Supervisory Management for Hospitals and Related Health Facilities.* St. Louis: The Catholic Hospital Association, 1973. Present title is *Haimann's Supervisory Management for Healthcare Organizations.* Several revisions and new editions, involving a number of coauthors, from 1982 to the present.

This is one of the few available works specifically concerned with lower-level management in the health care setting. Although some aspects of the supervisory role are treated briefly or not at all, the book has a pair of strengths to recommend it: an extremely good grasp of management fundamentals and a full appreciation of the necessary balance between the supervisor's technical role and management role. This original edition is long out of print, but it can still be found in some hospital and university libraries.

**Harris, Thomas A.** *I'm O.K.—You're O.K.* New York: Harper & Row, 1967, and a number of subsequent printings both hardcover and mass-market paperback.

This book is most appropriately read for improved understanding of human behavior—your own as well as others'—and for deeper insight into the problems of interpersonal communication. Although much of the book consists of the definitive presentation of the field we call transactional analysis (TA), it can help you become more attuned to "where someone is coming from" in interpersonal dealings.

**Heckman, I.L., Jr., and Huneryager, S.G.** *Human Relations in Management.* Cincinnati: South-Western Publishing Co., 1960; 2nd edition 1967.

This is a collection of readings, questions, and bibliographies originally intended as a college text. Although difficult to read in places and with the bibliographies somewhat out of date, this book is nevertheless a gold-mine of information. Included in their original form, for example, are **A.H. Maslow's** "A Theory of Human Motivation," **Douglas McGregor's** "The Human Side of Enterprise," and **Gordon Allport's** "The Psychology of Participation." Although this book is out of print, it remains available in many college and university libraries and is well worth searching for.

**Jay, Antony.** *Management and Machiavelli.* New York: Holt, Reinhart & Winston, 1967; revised and updated, trade paperback 1994, Pfeiffer and Company.

Subtitled *An Inquiry into the Politics of Corporate Life*, this book is decidedly slanted toward the overall management of entire organizations. It has its basis in Jay's interpretation of the psychology and conduct of modern corporations paralleling the principles of management employed in the medieval political state. If you have an interest in the rights and wrongs of corporate management, you will get something from *Management and Machiavelli* that applies to all types of organizations, especially those of the bureaucratic and institutional form we may work for (large hospitals, various associations, state and federal agencies, etc.). The original is out of print, but the revised edition can be found.

**Liebler, Joan Gratto, McConnell, Charles R.** *Management Principles for Health Professionals*, 4th ed. Sudbury, MA: Jones & Bartlett Publishers, 2004.

This book is intended for health care personnel who have been called on to manage the work of others without having had extensive education in management. It provides basic management theory to individuals whose education has been largely or completely clinical or technical, and it serves as a health care management textbook for students of the health professions. It is a helpful volume overall, and its organization makes it useful as a reference for looking up specific management topics.

**Likert, Rensis.** *New Patterns of Management.* New York: McGraw-Hill, 1961.

This is a most valuable work in promoting understanding of the "systems of management" that exist in our work organizations. The basic organizational differences attributable to health institutions are not the differences of "hospital" versus "industry" but rather the differences between organizations doing repetitive work and those doing varied work. *New Patterns of Management* sheds considerable light on understanding the varying styles of supervision related to the different kinds of work the organizations do. Although out of print, this book continues to be quoted and excerpted in various publications, and it remains available in numerous college and university libraries.

**Lombardi, Donald N.** *Handbook for the New Health Care Manager,* 2nd ed. San Francisco, CA: Jossey-Bass, Inc., 2001.

This book is described in its preface as "a practical guidebook for anyone who enjoys passionately the responsibilities and satisfaction of health care leadership and management." It covers a broad range of pertinent topics, including an interesting chapter titled "Managing the Nonplayers," which provides advice for dealing with those employees whose behavior is a continuing challenge for the manager. This book is probably most appropriate to "new" managers who enter with some management knowledge and a reasonable familiarity with the health care environment.

**Manion, Jo.** *Create a Positive Health Care Workplace!* 2005, Health Forum, Inc., American Hospital Association.

This book addresses such issues as how to find good employees and how to keep them, and considers how to keep present employees fully engaged and committed to their work. In a fairly readable manner it suggests how to create a strong positive work environment and develop a competitive edge in attracting and retaining high quality employees.

**Maynard, H.B.,** Editor-in-Chief, *Industrial Engineering Handbook*, 3rd ed. New York: McGraw-Hill, 1971; 4th ed., as *Maynard's Industrial Engineering Handbook*, **William K. Hodson** and **H.B. Maynard,** 1992 and 5th ed. by **Kjell B. Zandin** and **H.B. Maynard.**

This weighty volume, consisting of more than 1,500 pages containing the contributions of more than 100 authors, is primarily a reference book for practicing industrial engineers. However, it is also especially useful to supervisors and managers whose work is affected by that of industrial or management engineers or who become actively involved in methods improvement projects. It makes an especially handy reference for a methods improvement project team involved in the analysis of work. This book is out of print but remains available on a limited basis and is usually found in university libraries or, specifically, engineering school libraries.

**McCay, James T.** *The Management of Time.* Originally published 1959, Prentice-Hall, Inc., and reprinted literally dozens of times. Trade paperback in 1973, new hardcover in 1984, and trade paperback reprint in 1995, all Prentice-Hall Professional Technical Reference.

This book addresses practical means of addressing present-day time pressures and preparing to meet greater time demands in the future. It takes a considerably longer-range view of time management than we usually associate with seminars and workshops and such on the topic of time management. It is well organized, with each of its four parts summarized in turn, and loaded with useful advice.

**McConnell, Charles R.** *The Health Care Manager's Guide to Performance Appraisal.* Gaithersburg, MD: Aspen Publishers, Inc., 1993.

This book is suggested as an adjunct to Chapter 12, "Performance Appraisal: Cornerstone of Employee Development," for those who wish to further pursue the topic of performance appraisal. Appraisal is briefly examined in philosophy and principle. Guidance is provided for handling the individual elements of appraisal and for designing and developing an appraisal system. Appraisal's relationship to job descriptions and other source documents is established, and basic variations in appraisal practices are examined. Presently out of print.

**McConnell, Charles R.,** Editor. *The Health Care Supervisor Series.* Sudbury, MA: Jones & Bartlett Publishers, 1993.

This is a six-volume series of collected articles that appeared initially in the journal, *The Health Care Supervisor.* The volumes deal with *Career Development, Effective Communication, Effective Employee Relations, Law, Productivity,* and *Professional Nursing Management.* On each topic the series presents a wide range of information in the perspective of the first-line supervisor or middle manager.

**McConnell, Charles R.** *Umiker's Management Skills for the New Health Care Supervisor.* 4th ed. Sudbury, MA: Jones & Bartlett Publishers.

An updating and expansion of William Umiker's original work, this book provides basic grounding in the supervisory skills required in the health care setting. It is an especially helpful introduction for the individual who is new to both health care and supervision. Its straightforward language and list-and-bullet-point style make it useful as a handy reference for individual topics.

**Metzger, Norman,** Editor. *Handbook of Health Care Human Resources Management.* 2d ed. Gaithersburg, MD: Aspen Publishers, Inc., 1990.

This is a collection of more than 70 helpful articles on a variety of aspects of "people management." Although oriented primarily to the needs of human resource personnel, this book has much to offer anyone who supervises the work of others. Overall it provides a great deal of help in determining how to get the maximum possible benefit from your organization's human resource function.

**Metzger, Norman.** *The Health Care Supervisor's Handbook.* 3d ed. Gaithersburg, MD: Aspen Publishers, Inc., 1988.

This is a helpful book for supervisors in health care organizations, especially in matters of personnel relations such as evaluating performance, disciplining, handling grievances, and relating to a labor organization. Its detailed table of contents and its checklist approach to presenting much information make it a handy "look-it-up" reference for specific problems or topics.

**Monagle, John F., and Thomasma, David C.** *Health Care Ethics: Critical Issues*. Gaithersburg, MD: Aspen Publishers, Inc., 1994.

This is a contributed volume involving nearly 60 authors addressing essentially all aspects of medical ethics in some 46 chapters. Chances are this book has something to say about any medical ethical issue you care to inquire about, from those most frequently encountered (abortion, end-of-life, etc.) to those more recently entering the spotlight (e.g., genetic manipulation, for example), plus issues of medical entrepreneurship and the ethics of health care as a business.

**Nierenberg, Gerard, and Calero, Henry.** *Meta-Talk*. New York: Simon & Schuster, 1973; paperback edition 1975, Pocket Books.

If you are seriously interested in learning more about oral communication, this is a book to be reread and studied. Subtitled *Guide to Hidden Meanings in Conversations*, the book deals with the kinds of things we say and why we probably say them—and not with the exact words we happen to be using but rather with the messages and meanings "between the words." One reading of Meta-Talk—or two or three readings, for that matter—will not make you an expert on hidden meanings. However, the book should provide insights that cannot help but enhance your ability to understand others better. The book's message is essentially that no "meaning" is ever absolute, and that true meaning lies in the combination of speaker, listener, and circumstances. This book remains out of print, but it is occasionally available used.

**Odiorne, George S.** *How Managers Make Things Happen*. 2nd ed. Englewood Cliffs, NJ: Prentice Hall Professional Technical Reference, 1987; issued on (4) audio cassettes, 1995.

An excellent, easily readable rendering of the basics of management in modern work organizations, this work covers how to change poor work habits into good ones, how to know when to criticize and when to praise, and how to combat carelessness and indifference. Odiorne's chapter on decision-making is especially well done. This book is out of print, but it remains available on a limited basis.

**Osborn, Alex F.** *Applied Imagination: Principles and Procedures of Creative Thinking*. New York: Charles Scribner's Sons, 1953. Revised and reissued 1993, 3rd edition, Creative Education Foundation, Inc.

This is one of the best books you could delve into for help in "getting your mind in gear." It may well stand as the definitive work on creativity, at least as presented for a general audience; certainly it is among the most entertaining and readable works on the subject. Much of what the book contains might strike you as old, familiar stuff, but it is presented appealingly and most of it still holds true. The original hardcover is out of print, but it can still be found in larger libraries and is occasionally available used.

**Parkinson, C. Northcote.** *Parkinson's Law*. Boston: Houghton-Mifflin Company, 1957. Mass-market paperback 1957, Ballantine Books, Inc.; Mass-market paperbacks 1975 and 1977, Random House Publishing Group; in hardcover as *Parkinson: The Law*, 1980, Houghton Mifflin Company; hardcover edition 1993, Buccaneer Books, Inc.; trade paperback 1996, Global Publications Association.

This book is essentially the forerunner of the many volumes that take a humor-in-the-bitter-truth approach to the problems of management and administration. Parkinson's elaborate and pompous style is exactly suited to the sometimes outlandish ideas he presents. Although you may be inclined to believe the author rarely entertained a serious thought—for instance, he concedes that serious books on public or business administration have their place "provided only that these works are classified as fiction"—you may also find that a single reading provides a great deal of insight into organizational behavior. The best chapter is the opening one, "Parkinson's Law or the Rising Pyramid." The "law" itself is stated in the book's opening sentence: *Work expands so as to fill the time available for its completion.*

**Peter, Laurence J., and Hull, Raymond.** *The Peter Principle*. New York: William Morrow and Company, 1969, an early mass-market paperback, an edition in library binding in 1996 (also Morrow), and a new hardcover edition in 2001.

This highly successful book presents some deadly serious messages in a wholly entertaining manner. The "Principle" states simply: *In a hierarchy every employee tends to rise to his level of incompetence.* The author is suggesting that we rise just so high, and no higher, in any organization, and that the level at which we stop is just a bit over our heads. It follows, Peter suggests, that eventually every position tends to be occupied by someone who is incompetent to carry out its duties, and that the real work is accomplished by people who are still on the way up to their levels. (This book was followed by *The Peter Prescription* in 1972 and *The Peter Plan* in 1973, both by Laurence J. Peter alone. *The Peter Principle* remains far superior to these latter two books.)

**Smalley, Harold E.** *Hospital Management Engineering: A Guide to Improvement of Hospital Management Systems*. Englewood Cliffs, NJ: Prentice-Hall, 1982.

This book represents another step in the abandonment of the term industrial engineering in favor of management engineering in health care (an earlier version by **Harold E. Smalley** and **John R. Freeman,** 1966, used *Industrial* instead of *Management* in its title). It is somewhat specialized in that its target audience consists of persons working in management engineering in the hospital setting. Nevertheless, this book is a primary reference for managers looking for information about methods improvement. For instance, a supervisor with a physical space problem might find help in the chapter on "Facilities Design and Space Utilization," and one attempting to restructure jobs in the department might turn to "Job Analysis and Evaluation." This book is out of print.

**Snook, I. Donald, Jr.** *Hospitals: What They Are and How They Work*. 2d ed. Gaithersburg, MD: Aspen Publishers, Inc., 1992.

By some standards a relatively basic book for people who know their way around a hospital, this book is an excellent primer for a newly appointed supervisor in health care or potential supervisor who is new to the hospital setting. Especially helpful to the latter are the author's straightforward descriptions of each traditional hospital department and the functions it performs.

**Strunk, William, Jr., and White, E.B.** *The Elements of Style,* 3rd ed. Englewood Cliffs, NJ: Prentice Hall, 1994.

According to E.B. White, who in 1957 was commissioned to revise Strunk's original 1919 publication for the college market and the general trade, this book was Strunk's attempt to "cut the vast tangle of English rhetoric down to size and write its rules on the head of a pin." The attempt was successful; the book is a tight summation of the case for cleanliness, accuracy, and brevity in the use of written language. Even at considerably fewer than 100 pages, it is arguably the most valuable book about writing available. Should you limit yourself to only a single book about writing, *The Elements of Style* should be your choice. It has been constantly in print for many years.

**Toffler, Alvin.** *Future Shock.* New York: Random House, 1970; mass-market paperbacks 1971, 1984, and 1991, Bantam Doubleday Dell Publishing Group, numerous printings of each edition; and an edition in library binding.

An immensely popular book, *Future Shock* is most valuable in creating a full appreciation of the rate at which all aspects of life and living are changing around us. Also of note are the author's observations concerning the ways people cope—or fail to cope—with accelerating change. Anyone seeking insight into the impact of change and the origins of resistance to change would do well to examine the lengthy table of contents and read a few selected sections, especially those relating to health and work and work organizations.

**Townsend, Robert.** *Up the Organization.* New York: Alfred A. Knopf, 1970; mass-market paperback, 1970, Fawcett World Library. Revised and expanded as *Further Up the Organization,* 1984, Alfred A. Knopf.

This is an entertaining book. It is arranged in alphabetical order by topic, and since no topic requires more than a few minutes reading time, it is a book that can be read in bits and pieces with no loss of impact. Townsend's approach is energetic and people centered; his is a management style that depends heavily on a basic belief in the willingness of most people to produce, given the proper environment. Although aimed largely at top management, there is much in the book's pages for the first-line supervisor. Sections on "Delegation of Authority" and "People" are recommended. Read this book with some caution, however; much of its gutsy leadership style is personality based, and not everyone is a Robert Townsend. Although based largely on humanity and common sense, in practical terms the Townsend style will reform an organization only when applied from the top down.

**van Servellen, Gwen.** *Communication Skills for the Health Professional.* Gaithersburg, MD: Aspen Publishers, Inc., 1997.

The primary emphasis of this volume is communication between clinicians and patients. As such it is a comprehensive rendering of the issues encountered in health professionals' communication with patients or clients and families, including plenty of good advice for addressing certain sensitive situations (e.g., terminal illness). Also, the book's initial three chapters, comprising Part I: Theoretical Foundations for Understanding Communications, provide some helpful generic information on communications theory applicable in all human communication.

**Zinsser, William.** *On Writing Well: An Informal Guide to Writing Nonfiction.* 5th ed., revised. New York: Harper, 1994.
Lively and readable in its own right, this is also a helpful reference for people who are seriously interested in learning how to improve their writing in general. It is not a textbook, and certainly not an English grammar lesson. This book will give you valuable guidelines for writing with simplicity and clarity in today's world. The book's main theme is that there is no subject that cannot be made accessible if the writer writes with humanity and cares enough to write well.

# List of Quotations

Chapter 1     "Nothing in progression can . . ."
Source: Jacob M. Braude, *Lifetime Speaker's Encyclopedia*
(Englewood Cliffs, NJ: Prentice Hall, 1962), Vol. 1, 94.

Chapter 2     "The end product . . ."
Source: Rensis Likert, *New Patterns of Management* (New
York: McGraw-Hill, 1961).

Chapter 3     "As we are born . . ."
Source: Oliver Goldsmith

Chapter 4     "Good leadership is . . ."
Source: A.M. Sullivan

"Wishing . . ."
Source: Anonymous

Chapter 5     "One of modern management's . . ."
Source: Earle Brooks

Chapter 6     "Time is . . ."
Source: Jacob M. Braude, *Lifetime Speaker's Encyclopedia*
(Englewood Cliffs, NJ: Prentice Hall, 1962), Vol. 2, 815.

Chapter 7     "Technical training . . ."
Source: Jacob M. Braude, *Lifetime Speaker's Encyclopedia*
(Englewood Cliffs, NJ: Prentice Hall, 1962), Vol. 1, 393.

Chapter 8     "The best man . . ."
Source: Anonymous

Chapter 9     "I know . . ."
              Source: Anonymous

Chapter 10    "Real leaders . . ."
              Source: Jacob M. Braude, *Lifetime Speaker's Encyclopedia*
              (Englewood Cliffs, NJ: Prentice Hall, 1962), Vol. 1, 423.

Chapter 11     "The only way . . ."
              Source: Frederick R. Herzberg, "Does Money Really Moti-
              vate?" Copyright 1970 by Frederick R. Herzberg, Case West-
              ern University.

Chapter 12    "The privilege . . ."
              Source: Anonymous

Chapter 13    "Indifference is . . ."
              Source: Jacob M. Braude, Lifetime Speaker's Encyclopedia
              (Englewood Cliffs, NJ: Prentice Hall, 1962), Vol. 1, 152.

Chapter 14    "In so complex a thing . . ."
              Source: George Eliot

Chapter 15    "I use not only . . ."
              Source: Anonymous

Chapter 16    "I look upon the simple . . ."
              Source: Ralph Waldo Emerson

Chapter 17    "All decisions . . ."
              Source: Robert Townsend, *Up the Organization* (New York:
              Alfred A. Knopf, 1970), 27.

Chapter 18    "Have no fear . . ."
              Source: Robert Moses

Chapter 19    "I have made . . ."
              Source: Blaise Pascal

Chapter 20    "Meetings . . ."
              Source: Anonymous

Chapter 21    "A budget . . ."
              Source: Anonymous

Chapter 22     "Quality never costs . . ."
Source: Anonymous

"We are not at our best . . ."
Source: John W. Gardner, "Thoughts on the Business Life,"
*Forbes,* January 17, 1983, p. 126.

Chapter 23     "Man's greatest discovery is not fire, nor . . ."
Source: B. Brewster Jennings

Chapter 24     "There's a way . . ."
Source: Thomas A. Edison

Chapter 25     "The future never . . ."
Source: V. Clayton Sherman, *Creating the New American Hospital: A Time for Greatness* (San Francisco: Jossey-Bass, 1993).

Chapter 26     "Your education . . ."
Source: Oliver Wendell Holmes

Chapter 27     "Laws should be . . ."
Source: Clarence Darrow

Chapter 28     "The purpose of . . ."
Source: Dwight D. Eisenhower

"It is difficult to make . . ."
Source: Theodore Roosevelt

Chapter 29     "The trouble . . ."
Source: Anonymous

Chapter 30     "If you don't . . ."
Source: Robert Townsend, *Up the Organization* (New York: Alfred A. Knopf, 1970), 77.

# Index

# About the Author

Charles R. McConnell retired following 18 years in health care human resource management with the affiliated organizations of ViaHealth, Rochester, New York; 11 years as a senior consultant with the Management and Planning Services (MAPS) division of the Hospital Association of New York State (HANYS), and a prior career in industrial engineering. He presently works as an independent human resource management consultant and freelance writer and editor. He is the author or editor of 17 previous books and approximately 340 published articles, and he is the editor of the professional journal, *The Health Care Manager*. Mr. McConnell holds a BS degree in engineering, as well as an MBA from the State University of New York at Buffalo.